Pharmacy Simplified: A Glossary of Terms

F. James Grogan, Pharm.D.
President
Grogan Communications, Inc.

DELMAR
✳ ™
THOMSON LEARNING

Australia Canada Mexico Singapore Spain United Kingdom United States

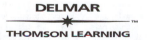

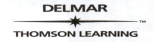

DELMAR

™

THOMSON LEARNING

Pharmacy Simplified: A Glossary of Terms
by F. James Grogan, Pharm.D.

Health Care Publishing Director:
William Brottmiller

Product Developmental Manager:
Marion Waldman

Product Development Editor:
Jill Rembetski

PTR Editorial Assistant:
Robin Irons

Executive Marketing Manager:
Dawn F. Gerrain

PTR Channel Manager:
Gretta Oliver

Technology Project Manager:
Laurie Davis

Production Editor:
Mary Colleen Liburdi

Cover Design:
Mary Colleen Liburdi

Library of Congress Cataloging-in-Publication Data has been applied for

ISBN 0-7668-2858-1

NOTICE TO THE READER

Contents

Dedication

This book is dedicated to my wife Donna, our children Jennifer, Dan, and Claire, and our grandchildren, present and future.

Acknowledgments

As solitary as a writer may feel at the keyboard, no book is written in a vacuum. A completed book represents a community of effort, a collaboration of intellectual, emotional, and professional support.

Such is the case with this book. The original idea grew from discussions with friend and former co-worker, Michael Austrin. *Pharmacy Simplified* is, in fact, a companion to Michael's ground-breaking book, *Managed Health Care Simplified: A Glossary of Terms*. Besides handing me the idea for this book and nudging me to pursue it, Michael also provided a wide range of advice while I developed my editorial plan. His valuable counsel continued throughout the writing phase.

Three of my colleagues, pharmacists Robin Hemby, David Flowers, and Rachel Palos, have contributed in ways they probably cannot imagine. Through sometimes bleary eyes and at times when they had other things that needed their attention, they diligently reviewed the original manuscript and provided valuable suggestions.

And then there are the professionals at Delmar Thomson Learning who shepherded this project to completion. Without the efforts and talents of Marion Waldman, Penny Cartwright, Robin Irons, Jill Rembetski, and their co-workers, this book would still be just a pile of papers on my desk.

And most of all I want to acknowledge the help of my wife, Donna. Without her support I could not have done this or a lot of other things.

Preface

Every industry has its own jargon. Executives, sales representatives, and other employees in diverse industries—insurance companies, corporate benefit managers, government agencies, and even pharmaceutical companies themselves—find that they have to deal with mysterious and confusing aspects of pharmacy, including pharmacy's peculiar language. Most of these professionals, while highly proficient at their chosen specialties, lack the health care background to deal with this "language barrier." Consequently, they find themselves in the uncomfortable position of administering programs that they cannot fully understand. This book serves as a tool to help them with their jobs.

Over the course of hundreds of meetings, I often found myself acting as a "translator" for health insurance executives, self-insured corporate clients, and even with pharmacy benefit management company executives and pharmaceutical company sales representatives. In addition to presenting and discussing my own analyses of costs, trends, clinical impact of management decisions, and potential interventions during these meetings, I also needed to explain pharmacy-related terms and concepts such as open and closed formularies, neurotransmitters, AWP, MAC, WAC, and antibiotic resistance. On several occasions I was asked to give extemporaneous mini-lectures to provide background on pharmacy-related issues.

Pharmacy Simplified: A Glossary of Terms is the solution to that problem. It captures 4,288 terms commonly used in pharmacy and pharmacy-related businesses and defines them in plain, **user-friendly** English. It is the first book that helps readers without health profession backgrounds to understand the pharmacy-related terms they must use in their businesses.

Audience

Pharmacy Simplified: A Glossary of Terms is intended for these specific groups:

- Health insurance companies

  In order to preserve their financial viability, heath insurers (indemnity plans, HMOs, PPOs, etc.) must manage the costs of their programs. The pharmacy benefit is the fastest growing expenditure in health care. Insurance executives desperately seek tools to help them manage these costs. Understanding pharmacy terminology is essential to managing the pharmacy benefit.

- Pharmaceutical companies

  Many sales representatives for pharmaceutical companies have no health care background. Without a thorough knowledge of pharmacy-related terminology, they have great difficulty promoting their products to health care professionals.

- Employer groups

  Almost all corporations with 1,000 or more employees are self-insured. This means that they assume all costs and pay all legitimate claims for their employee health insurance plans. Typically, these programs are administered through the corporate human resources department. Human resource (HR) managers typically have a good understanding of the administrative aspects of employee benefit programs, but usually do not have a technical background in health care.

- Pharmacy benefit management companies

  Only a small percentage of people who work for pharmacy benefit management companies (PBMs) have a technical knowledge of pharmacy. These companies administer pharmacy claims, sell their services to health insurers and employer groups, and try to control pharmacy program costs.

- Government

  The United States. government is the largest single insurer in the country and Medicaid is the largest single pharmacy insurance plan. Each state and many counties have their own public aid departments that pay claims for prescription drugs.

- Consumers

  Consumers who are interested in health topics in general and pharmacy in particular will find this book to be a valuable reference tool.

How Terms Were Selected

Entries in *Pharmacy Simplified* were chosen because they fit one or more of the following criteria:

Common abbreviations used in relation to pharmaceuticals or the conditions they treat—ACE, HIV, BPH, b.i.d., p.r.n.

Common medical conditions that may be treated with pharmaceuticals or may be side effects of drug therapy—benign prostatic hyperplasia, depression, anxiety, insomnia, leukemia

Common diagnostic or treatment procedures—angioplasty, electroconvulsive therapy, electrocardiogram

Common laboratory tests—culture and sensitivity, liver function test, white blood cell count

Drug class name—penicillins, barbiturates, benzodiazepines, antidepressants

Health insurance terms and abbreviations related to pharmacy—carve out, PMPM, copayment

Health systems—accreditation, hospital, hospice, ambulatory care

Medical specialties—oncology, pediatrics, bariatrics

Pharmacologic properties—absorption, distribution, metabolism, elimination

Physiologic terms—adrenergic, cholinergic, digestion

Regulatory terms frequently used by FDA, DEA, or other agencies—Controlled substance, orphan drug, schedule II

I excluded specific drug names and common English terms that do not have a special meaning in this context.

Please email me through my web site www.grogancommunications.com if you have terms to suggest for future editions.

—F. James Grogan, Pharm.D.

About the Author

F. James Grogan is an independent consultant, writer, and editor. He has more than twenty years' experience in virtually all aspects of pharmacy, including retail and hospital pharmacy, hospital-based clinical practice, home health care, pharmacy benefit management, and academics.

A winner of the American Health Book Award for his consumer-oriented book *The Pharmacist's Prescription: Your Complete Guide to the Over-the-Counter Drugs That Work Best*, Dr. Grogan has written and edited for both the professional and lay press. As a speaker, he has delivered research findings at national meetings, presented continuing education seminars to professional groups, spoken to consumer groups on a wide variety of pharmacy-related topics, and made numerous television and radio appearances.

Dr. Grogan has advised some of the country's largest insurance plans and employer groups. Clients have included Blue Cross Blue Shield of Missouri, Blue Cross Blue Shield of Iowa, Blue Cross Blue Shield of Arizona, Blue Cross Blue Shield of Kansas, Wausau Insurance Companies, HealthPlus of Michigan, Borg-Warner Automotive, UniGroup (United and Mayflower Van Lines), Cracker Barrel, Drummond Coal, Amway, Illinois Business Coalition, Wisconsin Electric, Mead Paper, and others.

Most recently, Dr. Grogan has published patient education brochures and written and edited for internet-based Channel-Health.com. He has worked extensively on aspects of *Mosby's GenRx* and *Mosby's Patient GenRx*. He has also consulted on electronic versions of the following Mosby publications: J. H. Stein, *Internal Medicine*; P. Rosen et al., *Emergency Medicine*; D. E. Longnecker et al., *Principles and Practice of Anesthesiology*; and D. R. Mishell et al., *Comprehensive Gynecology*.

Dr. Grogan earned a bachelor of science degree in pharmacy from St. Louis College of Pharmacy and a doctor of pharmacy degree from the University of Tennessee. He has been on the faculties of Northwestern University, Washington University, the University of New Mexico, and St. Louis College of Pharmacy.

A

a. – Abbreviation commonly used on prescriptions for the Latin term *ante*, meaning before.

a- – Prefix meaning without. For example, *afebrile* means without fever.

aa – Abbreviation commonly used on prescriptions for the Latin term *ana*, meaning of each.

AAC – *See actual acquisition cost.*

abbreviated new drug application (ANDA) – A shortened form of the application a drug company makes to the United States Food and Drug Administration (FDA) for approval to market a product. This abbreviated process is primarily used in the case of generic drugs.

The main difference between a new drug application (NDA) and an abbreviated new drug application (ANDA) is that the filer of the ANDA does not have to repeat the full range of animal and human clinical trials the NDA filer had to perform and report. The ANDA filer, however, must still submit data relating to the new drug's manufacturing processes and proof that the new product's bioavailability characteristics meet standards. In other words, the manufacturer of the generic product must prove to the FDA that patients will experience no significant clinical differences between the original brand name product and the new generic. *See also new drug application.*

abdomen – The part of the body between the diaphragm at the bottom of the ribcage and the pelvis. Also colloquially called the stomach.

abdominal – Pertaining to the abdomen.

abortion – The expulsion of a fetus before it is able to live separately from its mother. In the medical sense, the term abortion includes surgical abortions as well as spontaneous miscarriage. Some drugs in their package inserts are described as being capable of producing abortion because they may cause miscarriage as a side effect if taken during pregnancy. *See also therapeutic abortion, and threatened abortion.*

abrasion – A scraping. On the skin, an abrasion is a scraping away of some of the top layer of skin.

abscess – A localized infection that causes a pocket of pus. In most cases antibiotics have little effect on abscesses because the drug cannot reach the bacteria inside the pocket. The usual treatment is to physically drain the abscess, then administer antibiotics if they are still necessary.

absolute neutrophil count (ANC) – Number of neutrophilic white blood cells (neutrophils) in a cubic millimeter of blood. Neutrophils are the white blood cells that are most important in fighting infection.

absorption – The ability of a drug to pass through a barrier. In order to be absorbed, drugs taken by mouth typically pass from the intestinal fluids through the intestinal wall (the barrier) and into the bloodstream. A drug given by intramuscular injection passes from the muscle (the barrier) into the bloodstream.

Some drugs are not intended to be absorbed. For example, a laxative suppository is expected to exert its effect in the rectum and never pass from there. Other drugs that are not intended to be absorbed, nevertheless are. When the antibiotic neomycin is used as a bowel or bladder irrigant, small amounts are absorbed and can cause side effects for susceptible people.

abstinence syndrome – Characteristic symptoms that appear when an addicting drug is withdrawn from a user. Addictive drugs cause their own distinctive pattern of symptoms. Stimulant drugs like amphetamine cause users to experience excessive drowsiness and lethargy. Depressant drugs like narcotics and alcohol tend to stimulate users during withdrawal, causing tremors and insomnia.

abuse – Improper or excessive use that may be intentional or unintended. In the case of drugs, the abused drug may be legal or illegal and available with a prescription or not.

Abuse of a health insurance plan is the excessive use of benefits. In this context the abuse is unintended. Intentional misuse of insurance benefits is considered fraud and may be a crime.

A

abuse liability – *See abuse potential.*

abuse potential – The propensity for a drug to be misused. Most drugs with high abuse potential either stimulate (e.g., amphetamines) or depress (e.g., alcohol) the functions of the central nervous system. However, the misuse of androgenic steroids, male sex hormones, by athletes has led to their classification as controlled substances. *See controlled substance.*

a.c. – Abbreviation commonly used on prescriptions for the Latin term *ante cibos*, meaning before meals.

academic detailing – The process of presenting alternative prescribing information to physicians. The term is derived from the so-called detailing activities drug companies orient toward physicians. Generally, a drug company sales representative makes a sales call to a physician to give the doctor the "details" about the company's drugs in order to convince the doctor to prescribe those products.

To counter this, some hospitals and managed care organizations have developed academic or counter detailing programs. In these programs the organizations present physicians with alternative information in an attempt to blunt the drug companies' sales efforts.

Academy of Managed Care Pharmacists (AMCP) – The professional organization of pharmacists who work in or are otherwise affiliated with the managed health care industry. Located in Alexandria, Virginia.

accelerated approval – An expedited process for passing a new drug application through the United States Food and Drug Administration (FDA). Accelerated approval is usually reserved for drugs intended to treat fatal (e.g., AIDS, cancer) or otherwise devastating diseases. In this case the FDA does not require the same amount of detail from drug sponsors as it ordinarily would. *See also new drug application.*

access – The ability to obtain health care within a health insurance plan. In this sense, access includes the availability of contracted hospitals, clinics, doctors, dentists, pharmacies, etc.

A

account representative – An individual at a health insurance company who works with corporate clients. An employer's benefits administrator is usually assigned to a specific contact person at the insurance company to coordinate health benefits, register new employees, solve problems, etc.

accreditation – Process of certifying that an organization has met industry standards. Accreditation is usually voluntary on the part of the organization being surveyed and is not performed by any government agency. Accreditation bodies are nonprofit companies, usually founded by the industry itself.

For hospitals, clinics, and home care companies, the largest accrediting organization is the Joint Commission on Accreditation of Health Care Organizations (JCAHO). For managed care organizations, the largest accrediting body is the National Committee for Quality Assurance (NCQA).

ACE – *See angiotensin-converting enzyme.*

ACE inhibitor – *See angiotensin-converting enzyme inhibitor.*

acetylcholine – A chemical released from the ends of certain nerve fibers. Acetylcholine stimulates other nerves or muscle fibers to act.

achlorhydria – Absence of hydrochloric acid in the stomach and intestinal tract. Achlorhydria may occur with advancing age, pernicious anemia, or as a side effect of some drugs.

acid neutralizing capacity – The amount of acid an antacid can deactivate.

acidosis – A clinical state where the pH of the blood drops significantly below 7.35.

acne – A skin condition characterized by inflammation of the oil-producing glands and ducts. Acne can occur on any skin surface and present itself at any age. As many as 20% of adults may have one or more patches of acne at any time.

acneform – Any skin eruption that looks similar to acne.

acne vulgaris – Acne of the face, upper back, and chest that primarily affects adolescents during puberty.

A

acquired – A disease or condition that was not present at birth but has developed during life.

acquired immune deficiency syndrome (AIDS) – A disorder of the immune system attributed to a specific virus. People with this immune disorder are at risk of fungal and protozoal infections and skin cancers that are not usually seen in people with intact immune systems. Although there is no known cure, the progression of AIDS can often be slowed or controlled by use of antiviral drugs.

acquired immunity – Resistance to a communicable disease either by being exposed to the infectious agent or by having been vaccinated against it.

actinic keratosis – A thickening of a patch of skin caused by long-term sun exposure. Actinic keratosis is often a precursor to skin cancer.

action letter – A communication from the United States Food and Drug Administration informing a drug sponsor of an official decision. These letters normally inform a sponsor that its drug has been approved, is approvable with further action on the part of the sponsor, or is not approved for release.

activator – An agent that makes another molecule, enzyme, or drug functional. For example, tissue plasminogen activator is a drug that splits plasminogen into its component parts, one of which dissolves blood clots.

active immunity – *See acquired immunity.*

active ingredient – The portion of a pharmaceutical preparation that contains the actual medicine. For example, a cough syrup may contain a cough suppressant as the active ingredient but it also contains water, sugar, dye, and flavorings as inactive ingredients.

actual acquisition cost (AAC) – The net price a pharmacy pays for a medication after considering all discounts and rebates.

actuarial table – A table or graph that illustrates insurance rates, eligibility, or risks for any specific group. Actuarial tables are developed by actuaries.

actuary – A person in the insurance industry who calculates the costs of coverage and determines premiums for any specific group. An actuary considers both the extent of coverage desired and the degree of risk within the group.

acute – Of short and intense duration.

acute care – Treatment of short duration. This term is usually used in the context of treatment of a medical emergency or the initial phase of treatment for a long-term illness.

Hospitals may be referred to as acute care (e.g., general hospitals) or chronic care (e.g., long-term mental health facilities).

acute disease – A medical condition characterized by an abrupt onset and short duration. Acute diseases may be potentially fatal and difficult to treat (e.g., acute leukemia) or self-limited, usually requiring no specific treatment (e.g., acute pharyngitis).

a.d. – Abbreviation commonly used on prescriptions for the Latin term *aurio dextra*, meaning right ear.

ad – Latin term commonly used on prescriptions meaning *to* or *up to*.

adaptation – Some cellular receptors react to drugs by changing or adapting themselves to the presence of a drug. When they do this the receptors become less responsive or even totally unresponsive to the effects of the drug.

ADD – *See attention deficit disorder.*

addiction – Originally, physiologic dependence on a chemical substance such as alcohol, heroin, cocaine, etc. Currently the term is applied more broadly to include psychological dependence upon a substance or activity over which an individual has no control. Addicting activities include gambling and sex.

adherence – Often used synonymously with compliance. *See compliance.*

adipose – Pertaining to fats or lipids.

adipose tissue – The type of cells that store body fat. Aside from the obvious health implications of too much or too little fat, adipose tissue is significant in pharmacy because it stores certain drugs.

A

In some cases, these drugs continue to be released into the bloodstream long after the last dose.

adjudication – The processing of an insurance claim. During adjudication, the claim passes through a number of edits and approvals before the claim is paid.

adjuvant – An ingredient added to a pharmaceutical preparation that changes the effect of the active ingredient. For example, an adjuvant might slow the absorption of the active ingredient, making it work longer.

ad lib. – Abbreviation commonly used on prescriptions for the Latin term *ad libitum*, meaning at pleasure.

ADME – Abbreviation for absorption, distribution, metabolism, and elimination. These are the basic components of the science of pharmacokinetics.

administer – The act of giving a dose of medication. For example, certain medicines may be administered by mouth, under the tongue, by injection, directly to the skin, and by many other means. Each dosage form of a medicine is intended to be administered in a specific way.

administration route – *See route of administration.*

administrative services only (ASO) – An arrangement between an insurance company and a large client where the client agrees to assume all risk for claims and the insurance company agrees to provide the necessary resources (administrative services) to run the program.

admitting physician – A physician who arranges for a patient to be let into a hospital, skilled nursing facility, or other inpatient care setting. The admitting physician may be the patient's personal physician or may be someone else, for example a consulting physician or emergency room physician.

adolescent medicine – A subspecialty of pediatrics that deals with the diagnosis and treatment of illnesses in the adolescent population.

adren- – Prefix that relates to the adrenal gland.

adrenal- – Prefix that relates to the adrenal gland.

adrenal gland – Glands located next to the kidneys. The adrenal glands secrete a wide variety of essential hormones that include aldosterone, cortisol, and epinephrine. Epinephrine is sometimes called adrenaline.

adrenergic – Pertaining to the sympathetic nervous system. The term adrenergic is derived from the fact that many of the functions of the sympathetic nervous system are controlled by epinephrine, sometimes called adrenaline.

adreno- – Prefix that relates to the adrenal gland.

adrenocortical – Pertaining to the outer portion (cortex) of the adrenal gland.

adsorption – The property some solids have of attaching other solids, liquids, or gases to their surfaces. The best example of an adsorbant is activated charcoal. Because of its porous surface, activated charcoal can cause other materials to attach to it. This property makes it valuable in treating poisonings in children and filtering air and water.

adult – A fully grown and mature person or animal.

adulterant – An impurity.

adulteration – The addition of one or more impurities.

adult medicine – That branch of medicine that deals exclusively with adult patients.

adult-onset diabetes – *See diabetes mellitus.*

advance directives – Legal documents that specify actions to be taken in the event the signatory becomes incapacitated. Advance directives include living wills and powers of attorney.

adverse drug reaction (ADR) – An unwanted side effect of a medication.

A

aerobe – An organism that can live in ordinary air. This term is often applied to bacteria and other microorganisms that need a supply of oxygen to live. Opposite of anaerobe.

aerobic – Pertaining to an aerobe.

aerosol – A liquid or fine powder that is sprayed in a fine mist. In pharmacy, aerosols are frequently used as medication delivery systems. In these cases, a medication is packaged inside a canister and a propellant is added before the canister is sealed. The patient positions the spray outlet in or over the area to be medicated and then releases the spray.

The most commonly used aerosols are the respiratory treatments for asthma and the skin sprays. While most aerosolized medicines are liquids, some are powders whose particles are small enough to pass through the spray apparatus.

See also metered dose inhaler.

aerospace medicine – The specialty of medicine that deals with diagnosis and treatment of conditions related to aviation and space travel.

affect – In psychology and psychiatry, affect is the mood or feelings a patient expresses.

affective disorder – A condition characterized by inappropriate moods. Examples include depression and manic-depressive illness, also called bipolar affective disorder.

aftereffect – The properties that persist after a treatment or procedure is finished. In pharmacy, an aftereffect is the change induced by a drug after treatment has been completed. Depending upon the treatment, aftereffects may either be beneficial or detrimental.

afterload – The pressure the heart must push against when it ejects blood into the circulation system. In congestive heart failure, reducing afterload becomes critically important because it decreases the amount of work the heart has to do. This, in turn, reduces symptoms of the condition and may lengthen the patient's life.

A

agent – A drug or other substance that produces an effect. For example, a suspending agent is used in some products to help hold up an insoluble medicine in a liquid long enough for a dose to be poured. A beta-blocking agent is a drug that blocks beta receptors.

aggregation – A coming together or a clumping. The term is commonly applied to the process where platelets clump together (aggregate) to form a blood clot. While platelet aggregation is important to control bleeding, inappropriate aggregation can lead to heart attacks and strokes. Aspirin and other drugs are used to inhibit inappropriate platelet aggregation.

agonist – A drug or other agent that mimics the effects of another substance or function. It may do this by interacting at a cellular receptor. The opposite of antagonist.

agranulocytosis – A condition characterized by a deficiency of the white blood cells known as granulocytes. The most important of these are the neutrophils, which are needed to fight infections.

AHF – *See antihemophilic factor.*

AIDS – *See acquired immune deficiency syndrome.*

AIDS-related complex – Infection with the human immunodeficiency virus (HIV) and early symptoms of illness (e.g., enlarged lymph nodes) but absent any signs of immune deficiency, opportunistic infection, or skin lesions.

airway – The passageway for air in the respiratory tract. The airway begins at the mouth and nose and extends to the alveoli in the lungs.

akathisia – Inability to sit still. Akathisia is a common side effect of antipsychotic medications.

akinesia – Difficulty in initiating muscle movement. Akinesia is a common symptom of Parkinson's disease. It is also a common side effect of antipsychotic medications.

a.l. – Abbreviation commonly used on prescriptions for the Latin term *aurio laeva*, meaning left ear.

A

albumin – The major protein in the blood plasma. Some drugs bind themselves to albumin. The drug molecules that are bound to albumin or other plasma proteins are pharmacologically inactive and do not become active again until they detach themselves from the protein.

albuminuria – Presence of albumin in the urine. May be a sign of kidney disease.

alcohol – While most people think only of ethanol, also called grain alcohol, as alcohol, there are many other alcohols. Any organic chemical that has a hydroxyl group (-OH) attached to a carbon atom is an alcohol.

alcohol abuse – Misuse of the drug alcohol. While most often used in the context of addiction to alcohol (alcoholism), alcohol abuse relates to any misuse of the drug.

alcohol dependence – The physical or psychological need to use the drug alcohol in order to function. *See also alcoholism.*

alcoholic – A person who has the disease of alcoholism. Also, the adjective form of alcohol.

alcoholism – A disease characterized by the chronic abuse of alcohol. Alcoholism is a lifelong disease that, unless controlled, leads to physical illness and social dysfunction. Long-term alcohol abuse can lead to disease of the central nervous system and gastrointestinal system. Abrupt cessation of drinking in the absence of medical supervision can lead to a rigorous, potentially fatal, withdrawal syndrome.

aldosterone – A hormone produced in the adrenal glands, aldosterone regulates the balance of sodium, potassium, and water in the body.

alkaloid – Alkaline, nitrogen-containing, naturally occurring chemicals found almost exclusively in plants. Over 2,000 alkaloids have been identified in nature, many of which are used or have the potential to be used as drugs or poisons. Examples include morphine (used for pain), pilocarpine (glaucoma), and theophylline (asthma). Also caffeine, nicotine, and cocaine.

A

alkalosis – A state where the pH of the blood rises significantly above the normal of 7.4. Alkalosis may be due to drug side effects or disease states.

alkylating agent – One of the oldest classes of cancer chemotherapy drugs. Alkylating agents bind to DNA molecules, not allowing DNA to replicate during cell division. Alkylating agents are effective in treating a wide variety of cancers. Cyclophosphamide (Cytoxan) is one example of this class.

allergen – A substance capable of initiating an allergic reaction. Most commonly, allergens are proteins that are foreign to the body. Examples include animal dander and pollen. *See also allergic reaction.*

allergic reaction – The interaction between the immune system and an allergen. Upon recognizing the presence of an allergen, the immune system attempts to destroy it. This works well when the allergen is part of a virus, bacterium, or other potentially harmful invader. However, what we normally think of as an allergic reaction is an overreaction to the situation.

Mild allergic reactions may be manifested by skin rash, itching, or sneezing. More serious reactions may cause wheezing, shock, and even death.

allergic rhinitis – Inflammation of the nose that narrows breathing passages and produces excess mucus. Allergic rhinitis may be seasonal (occurring at specific times of the year) or perennial (present throughout the year).

allergist – A physician who specializes in the diagnosis and treatment of conditions caused by allergies.

allergy – A reaction to a food, drug, or environmental condition or substance triggered by the body's immune system. While all allergies to drugs are considered side effects, not all side effects are allergies. The immune system must be involved in order for a drug reaction to be considered an allergy.

allogenic – Pertaining to differing gene patterns within the same species. For example, differing blood types between two people are the result of differences in the genes that determine blood type.

allogenic transplant – Transplantation of tissues or organs that are not an exact genetic match. Since only identical twins have identical gene patterns, transplant teams try to find the best match possible. Minimizing genetic differences reduces the chances that the immune system will recognize the transplanted material as foreign and reject it.

allopathic – Pertaining to allopathy.

allopathic physician – A medical pratctitioner of allopathy. Normally used to describe a practitioner of traditional Western medicine, as opposed to an osteopath, chiropractor, etc.

allopathy – A type of treatment that uses a therapeutic intervention to oppose the effects of a disease or condition; for example, using antihypertensive medications to reduce high blood pressure or surgery to remove or repair a diseased organ.

alopecia – Loss of hair from anywhere on the body or the condition of baldness.

alpha-adrenergic blocker – A drug that blocks receptors for norepinephrine and other substances that stimulate receptors in the alpha portion of the sympathetic nervous system. Stimulating alpha-adrenergic receptors usually increases blood pressure. Therefore, drugs that are alpha-adrenergic blockers may be useful for treating hypertension.

alpha-blocker – *See alpha-adrenergic blocker.*

ALS – *See amylotrophic lateral sclerosis.*

alternative medicine – Any health practice that does not follow mainstream or allopathic medicine. Examples include massage therapy, aromatherapy, herbalism, osteopathy, homeopathy, nutritional therapy, meditation, chiropractic, and yoga.

Practices such as physical therapy, dentistry, occupational therapy, and psychotherapy are all well accepted by traditional medicine and are not considered alternative.

alveoli – Plural form of alveolus.

A

alveolus – A small cavity at the end of the airway. The alveolus is the place where the lungs remove carbon dioxide from the blood and exchange it for oxygen.

Alzheimer's disease – A chronic, progressive form of dementia causing loss of memory, confusion, and disorientation. Pathologically, the brain atrophies and exhibits neurofibrillary tangles and senile plaques.

AMA – *See American Medical Association.*

ambulatory – Able to walk. The term is usually applied to someone who is not required to stay in bed due to disease.

ambulatory care – Medical care that is given on an outpatient basis. Patients are able to come and go to an office or clinic for diagnostic tests or treatments.

ambulatory surgery – A procedure where a nonhospitalized patient comes into a facility for an operation and leaves the same day. Also called outpatient surgery.

AMCP – *See Academy of Managed Care Pharmacists.*

amebiasis – A condition caused by infection with ameba (*see also ameba*). Amebiasis often produces severe diarrhea and may invade the liver or skin.

amendment to a new drug application – Additional information that is filed with a new drug application (NDA).

amenorrhea – Absence of menstrual periods. Amenorrhea may be caused by a hormonal imbalance or as a side effect of a drug.

American Medical Association (AMA) – The professional organization representing the interests of physicians. Located in Chicago, Illinois.

American Pharmaceutical Association (APhA) – The professional organization of pharmacists who work in any setting. Located in Washington, D.C.

American Red Cross (ARC) – American branch of the international organization. Services include disaster relief, blood collection, and blood and blood product distribution.

A

American Society of Health-system Pharmacists (ASHP) – Originally called the American Society of Hospital Pharmacists, this organization represented the interests of pharmacists who worked in hospitals, now, a professional organization representing the interests of pharmacists who work in practically any health care setting. Located in Bethesda, Maryland.

amino acid – An organic acid that contains at least one -NH_2 group. Amino acids are the building blocks for all proteins.

aminobisphosphonate – A class of drugs that inhibits bone resorption, the process where minerals leach out of bone tissue. Bone resorption leads to loss of bone mass and increased risk of fractures. Aminobisphosphonates are used primarily to treat osteoporosis.

aminoglycoside – A class of antibiotics that are most commonly used against Gram-negative bacteria. Aminoglycosides are most commonly used intravenously or topically. Systemic use of aminoglycosides is limited by their potential for causing damage to the kidneys and inner ear.

amnesia – Loss of memory, usually memory of a specific period of time. *See also anterograde amnesia.*

amoeba – A single-celled organism found in soil and water. *See also amebiasis.*

amphetamine – A class of drugs that chemically resemble ephedrine. Amphetamines are central nervous stimulants whose uses include treatment of attention deficit disorder, narcolepsy, and obesity. Amphetamines have potential for abuse.

ampul – *See ampule.*

ampule – A sealed glass container that usually contains a single dose of medicine. The top of the ampule must be broken off in order to open the container.

amylotrophic lateral sclerosis (ALS) – A devastating disease of the central nervous system causing profound wasting and weakness of the muscles. Eventually the muscles responsible for breathing become too weak to function. The condition is always fatal. Also known as Lou Gehrig's disease.

A

anabolic – Pertaining to anabolism.

anabolic steroid – A derivative of the alcohol sterol that increases anabolism. All anabolic steroids have properties similar to the male hormone testosterone. Although many of them are used legitimately for men and women with testosterone deficiencies, the anabolic steroids are often misused by individuals who seek enhanced athletic performance. Both men and women use these drugs primarily to stimulate protein formation, which leads to greater strength and endurance.

anabolism – The process of building complex molecules in the body from simpler materials. In a state of good health and proper nutrition, the body uses simple nutrients (amino acids, fats, glucose, vitamins, etc.) to build the basic chemicals that support cellular function and sustain life. Opposite of catabolism.

anacidity – Deficiency or absence of hydrochloric acid in the stomach and digestive tract. Synonymous with achlorhydria.

anaerobe – A bacterium or other microorganism that can live without oxygen. In many cases, oxygen introduced into their environment can kill these organisms. During specimen collection, special handling techniques are required to prevent anaerobic bacteria from dying before a patient's specimen can be tested in a laboratory.

anaerobic – Pertaining to an anaerobe.

anaerobic infection – An invasion of one or more body tissues by anaerobic bacteria. The most common sites for anaerobic infection include the abdomen, intestinal tract, and gynecologic tissue.

analeptic – A stimulant drug that may be used to reverse the effects of anesthetics or other sedatives. These drugs are seldom used except in emergency situations because of the possibility of causing seizures.

analgesia – The relief of pain.

analgesic – A drug that relieves pain. Analgesics may or may not be narcotics.

analog – Something that is similar or comparable to something else. As applied to pharmacy, an analog is usually a drug that is chemically similar to another drug. For example, all of the barbiturate sedatives are analogs of each other.

anaphylactic shock – A life-threatening allergic reaction. Anaphylactic shock is characterized by a drop in blood pressure and is often associated with difficulty breathing. Anaphylactic shock is usually fatal unless appropriate emergency treatment is given.

anaphylaxis – An immediate and serious allergic reaction following exposure to a drug or other chemical. *See also anaphylactic shock.*

anatomy – The study of the physical structure of living organisms.

ANC – *See absolute neutrophil count.*

ANDA – *See abbreviated new drug application.*

androgen – A male sex hormone. Testosterone is the most common naturally occurring androgen. Medicines have been developed that mimic the effects of testosterone. These are also called androgens or androgenic steroids.

androgenic – Pertaining to androgen.

androgynous – Pertaining to androgyny.

androgyny – Having both male and female features and characteristics.

anemia – Deficiency of red blood cells. There are many causes and forms of anemia. The most common type, iron deficiency anemia, is due to either insufficient dietary iron or to the inability to absorb and utilize iron properly. Other forms of anemia may be genetic in nature (e.g., sickle cell anemia) or may be caused by toxic drugs or chemicals (e.g., benzene, cancer chemotherapy).

anergy – Lack of allergic reaction to a substance (e.g, poison ivy) that most people adversely react to.

anesthesia – Loss of sensation. Anesthesia can be limited to a small area (local anesthesia) or can cause loss of sensation and consciousness through the whole body (general anesthesia).

A

anesthesiologist – A physician who specializes in administering anesthetics and treating pain.

anesthesiology – The medical specialty that deals with administration of anesthetics and treatment of pain.

anesthetic – A drug that causes anesthesia. Anesthetics are available in many different forms and serve different purposes. General anesthetics may be given by inhalation or by injection prior to surgery. Local anesthetics may be injected into specific areas (as in dentistry), applied directly to intact skin or an abrasion, or may be used in special dosage forms such as gargles (for sore throats) or suppositories (for hemorrhoids).

anesthetist – A nurse who has been trained to administer anesthetics. In most cases anesthetists have a master's degree in nursing and pass a certification examination.

aneurysm – Abnormal dilation of a blood vessel within a distinctly limited area. *See also dissecting aneurysm and intracranial aneurysm.*

angiitis – Inflammation of a blood vessel.

angina – Originally, any sharp, constricting pain could have been called angina. Now, angina is usually synonymous with angina pectoris. *See angina pectoris.*

angina pectoris – Sharp pain usually felt in the chest or arm. The pain occurs when the heart does not receive a sufficient amount of oxygen to support its workload. Anginal pain most commonly follows exertion. Angina may also be produced by a temporary spasm of one or more of the coronary arteries.
See also Prinzmetal's angina.

anginal – Pertaining to angina pectoris.

angio- – Prefix referring to blood vessels.

angiocardiogram – An x-ray of the blood vessels supplying the heart muscle. *See angiography.*

angiogram – An x-ray of a blood vessel. *See angiography.*

angiography – X-ray visualization of blood vessels. In most cases a radiopaque dye is injected into blood vessels that supply the

A

area to be studied. X-ray photographs are taken as the dye passes through the subject area. The dye will fill the blood vessel and indicate if there are obstructions or aneurysms present in any of the blood vessels under examination.

angioplasty – Surgical reconstruction of one or more blood vessels. Often this is done by passing a balloon-tipped catheter into a vascular area that has been occluded by plaque or blood clots. The balloon is inflated, opening the narrowed space. In some cases a stent, basically a small metal retaining cylinder, is left in place to keep the vessel open.

angiotensin – A family of naturally occurring chemicals that constrict blood vessels and raise blood pressure.

angiotensin I – A precursor to angiotensin II. Angiotensin I does not by itself affect blood pressure. However, angiotensin-converting enzyme (ACE) chemically alters angiotensin I to form angiotensin II.

angiotensin II – The most potent known vascular constricting agent. Angiotensin II also causes release of aldosterone, another agent that increases blood pressure.

angiotensin-converting enzyme (ACE) – The substance that causes the formation of angiotensin II from angiotensin I. Usually abbreviated ACE.

angiotensin-converting enzyme (ACE) inhibitor – A drug that prevents angiotensin-converting enzyme (ACE) from producing angiotensin II. ACE inhibitors are used to treat hypertension and congestive heart failure. See also angiotensin II.

angiotensinogen – A substance produced in the liver that, in the presence of renin, forms angiotensin I.

angiotensin receptor blocker – A drug that prevents angiotensin from interacting with its receptor in vascular smooth muscle. By blocking these receptors, angiotensin II cannot raise blood pressure. Angiotensin receptor blockers are used to treat hypertension. They are being studied for potential use in congestive heart failure.

A

anhedonia – The inability to experience pleasure. Anhedonia may be caused by a medical or mental illness such as depression or by a drug that affects hormones or mental status.

animal – Any living organism that is not a plant or bacterium. Animals range in complexity from single-celled creatures to humans.

animal experiment – A scientific study using animals as subjects. In this context, animals are considered to be any nonhuman animal.

animal testing – *See animal experiment.*

ankylosing spondylitis – An arthritic condition of the spine that may lead to fusion of two or more vertebra.

anorectal – Pertaining to both the anus and the rectum.

anorectic – Pertaining to a state of anorexia. Also, a person who has the condition of anorexia nervosa.

anorexia – Loss of appetite.

anorexia nervosa – A complex psychological state characterized by the fear of being fat. Often, patients' perceptions are distorted to the extent that they believe they are overweight despite appearing to others to be emaciated. Without proper treatment, anorexia nervosa may be fatal.

anorexiant – A drug that decreases appetite.

anorexic – Pertaining to a state of anorexia. Also, a person who has the condition of anorexia nervosa.

anovulation – The inability to produce ova or to release them from the ovaries.

antacid – A drug that chemically neutralizes acid in the digestive tract. Antacids interact with hydrochloric acid in the stomach and small intestine to relieve the pain of hyperacidity or even peptic ulcer. The combination of an antacid with digestive acid produces water and carbon dioxide gas.

antagonist – A drug or other agent that blocks or antagonizes the effects of another substance or function. The opposite of agonist.

A

antalgesia – A drug or other agent that increases pain perception. Opposite of analgesic.

ante- – Prefix meaning before.

anterior – Referring to the front of something. Opposite of posterior.

anterograde – Adjective indicating something that extends forward from some point in time. See *anterograde amnesia*.

anterograde amnesia – Loss of memory of events during a specific period of time after the occurrence of a precipitating event. Some drugs (e.g., alcohol, sleeping pills, tranquilizers) cause loss of memory of the events that occur in the hours following a dose, even though the person with the condition acted normally. When caused by an episode of heavy alcohol consumption, this is often call a blackout period.

anthracycline – A class of cancer chemotherapy drugs.

anti- – Prefix meaning against.

antiarrhythmic – A drug used to treat abnormal heart rhythms. These drugs work by either changing the pattern of electrical impulses in the heart or by changing the way the heart muscle reacts to these impulses. A disturbing side effect of antiarrhythmic drugs is their ability to cause new, sometimes more dangerous, abnormal heart rhythms.

antiarthritic – A drug or other treatment intended to control symptoms of arthritis.

antibacterial – A drug or chemical used to kill or inhibit the growth and reproduction of bacteria.

antibiotic – Technically, an antibiotic is an antibacterial drug that is derived from a natural source rather than a synthetic source. The most common sources of antibiotics are molds and other bacteria. Sulfa drugs, though they are effective for treating many bacterial infections, are not truly antibiotics because they are derived from synthetic sources. In common usage, however, this distinction is rarely made.

antibody – A substance developed within the immune system and designed to identify and destroy foreign substances. For example, antibodies formed during a viral infection attack and attempt to destroy those viruses. In some cases antibodies may continue to be produced for years, thus preventing future infections from that specific strain of virus.

anticholinergic – Pertaining to an agent that blocks the effects of acetylcholine in the nervous system. Anticholinergic drugs may be used to treat spasms in the digestive and urinary tracts. Many drugs produce anticholinergic side effects.

anticholinergic side effect – Unintended drug effects that result from blocking the function of acetylcholine. Anticholinergic side effects include dry mouth, dry eyes, inhibition of sweating, constipation, and urinary retention.

anticoagulant – A drug that reduces the ability of blood to clot. Anticoagulants are often mistakenly called blood thinners. These drugs do not make blood thinner. Anticoagulants are used to treat or prevent cardiovascular disease including heart attacks and strokes.

anticonvulsant – A drug used to treat or prevent epileptic seizures.

antidepressant – A drug used to treat or prevent depression. Some antidepressants are effective for treating specific forms of anxiety and other mental illnesses.

antidiarrheal – A drug used to treat diarrhea.

antiemetic – A drug used to treat vomiting.

antiepileptic – A drug used to treat or prevent epileptic seizures. *See anticonvulsant.*

antiestrogen – A drug that either prevents the formation of estrogen, blocks estrogen receptors, or produces an effect opposite that of estrogen. Some forms of breast cancer grow faster in the presence of estrogen. Antiestrogens are commonly used to treat these types of cancer.

antiflatulent – A drug intended to reduce intestinal gas. Most antiflatulents, however, only make it easier to expel gas that has already formed.

A

antifungal – A drug that kills or inhibits reproduction of fungi. These drugs may be applied directly to the skin, given by mouth, or by intravenous injection. The route of administration depends upon the site of infection.

antigen – A substance that stimulates formation of antibodies. *See also antibody.*

antihemophilic factor – A blood component that is missing in people with hemophilia. Blood factors are necessary for normal blood clotting to take place. People with hemophilia are not able to produce a sufficient amount of at least one of these factors. In these cases, the missing factor, the antihemophilic factor, may be given by intravenous infusion to treat bleeding episodes. Antihemophilic factor, often referred to as AHF, is either extracted from donated blood or produced by genetic engineering. *See also genetic engineering.*

antihistamine – A drug that prevents histamine from interacting with its receptors. Antihistamines are typically used to treat allergic conditions. Those that cause drowsiness as a side effect are sometimes used to treat insomnia.

antihypertensive – An agent that reduces high blood pressure.

anti-infective – An agent that may be used to treat an infection due to a microorganism. This term encompasses antibacterial, antiviral, and antifungal agents.

ant-iinflammatory – Any of several drug groups that reduce inflammation. Anti-inflammatory drugs include corticosteroids like prednisone and the so-called nonsteroidal anti-inflammatory drugs (NSAIDs) like aspirin and ibuprofen.

antimalarial – A drug that kills or inhibits the reproduction of malaria parasites.

antimetabolite – A drug that prevents normal metabolic function inside a target cell. The cancer drugs fluorouracil and methotrexate are antimetabolites.

antimicrobial – A drug that can kill or inhibit the reproduction of a microorganism. This is a very general term that can be applied to antibiotics, antifungals, and antivirals.

A

antimitotic – A drug, usually an antineoplastic drug, that arrests cell division.

antimycotic – A drug that kills or inhibits reproduction of fungi.

antinauseant – A drug that relieves nausea and prevents vomiting.

antineoplastic – A drug that kills or inhibits reproduction of cancer cells.

antioxidant – A chemical that prevents oxidative reactions. Antioxidants may be effective for preventing heart disease. Commonly used antioxidants include vitamins A and E.

antiparasitic – A drug or chemical that kills or inhibits reproduction of parasites.

antiparkinsonian – A drug that helps to control symptoms of Parkinson's disease.

antiplatelet – A drug that inhibits normal platelet function, usually by reducing their ability to aggregate and inappropriately form blood clots.

antipruritic – A drug or other material that reduces itching.

antipsychotic – A drug that relieves symptoms of psychosis. Antipsychotics are most commonly used to treat condtions such as schizophrenia.

antipyretic – A drug that reduces fever.

antirheumatic – Most commonly, a drug that reduces the symptoms of rheumatic conditions such as rheumatoid arthritis.

antiseptic – A chemical that kills or inhibits microorganisms upon making physical contact. The term antiseptic is used to describe agents that are used on intact skin. Disinfectants are used on inanimate objects (e.g., countertops, floors).

antispasmodic – A drug that relieves involuntary smooth muscle contractions (spasms). Antispasmodics are most commonly used to treat spasms in the digestive or urinary tracts.

antitoxin – An antibody that forms in response to a toxin produced by an infecting microorganism. The most commonly administered antitoxins are active against diphtheria and tetanus toxins.

antitubercular – An agent that kills or inhibits the growth of the microorganism that causes tuberculosis.

antitussive – A drug that reduces coughing. Also called a cough suppressant.

antivenin – An antibody specific for an animal poison. Examples are rattlesnake antivenin and black widow spider antivenin.

antiviral – A drug that kills or inhibits reproduction of a virus.

anuria – Inability to produce urine.

anuric – Pertaining to anuria.

anus – The last part of the digestive tract. The anus is the opening through which feces pass.

anxiety – A clinical state characterized by apprehension and dread. Forms of anxiety include generalized anxiety disorder, obsessive-compulsive disorder, and post-traumatic stress disorder. Drugs used to treat anxiety are called anxiolytics.

anxiolytic – A drug intended to treat anxiety.

any willing provider – A requirement that any provider (pharmacy, physician, etc.) willing to accept an insurer's terms and conditions of participation be allowed to participate in a health plan. In most cases, the key issue on the part of the provider is accepting the insurer's level of payment. The requirement is usually mandated by a government agency.

aorta – The largest blood vessel in the body, the aorta is the artery that receives blood directly from the left ventricle of the heart. The aorta branches into smaller arteries and supplies blood to the arterial side of the circulatory system.

aortic – Pertaining to the aorta.

aortic stenosis – A narrowing of the passageway from the heart into the aorta. This condition places extra stress on the heart because it must work harder to eject blood into circulation.

aortic valve – The flap at the opening to the aorta that prevents blood from coming back into the heart.

APhA – *See American Pharmaceutical Association.*

aphasia – Inability to speak due to a brain disorder. Some people with aphasia are unable to communicate in writing, by signing, or in other ways.

aplastic anemia – A devastating, often fatal, form of anemia in which bone marrow fails to produce adequate amounts of blood cells. Aplastic anemia causes a profound drop in the levels of red blood cells, white blood cells, and platelets. Drugs, radiation, or environmental toxins may cause aplastic anemia.

apnea – Absence or severe reduction in breathing.

apoplexy – An obsolete term for stroke. *See stroke.*

apothecary – A pharmacist or a pharmacy.

appendectomy – The surgical removal of the appendix.

appendicitis – An inflammation of the appendix. Acute appendicitis usually causes intense pain in the abdomen, fever, and vomiting.

appendix – An attachment to the end of the large intestine. The appendix has no known purpose.

applied research – The use of research in practical situations.

approval letter – Official notification from the United States Food and Drug Administration (FDA) that a drug sponsor has been granted permission to release an investigational drug to the market. In some cases, the approval allows a drug already on the market to be sold for an additional purpose. For example, the manufacturer of an antidepressant may receive an approval letter from the FDA allowing it to be promoted for treating anxiety.

Approved Drug Products with Therapeutic Equivalence Evaluations – Better known as the Orange Book. The Orange Book registers the official position of the United States Food and Drug Administration on the bioequivalence of generic drug products. Many states use the Orange Book as a guide to help them deter-

A

mine which generic drugs may be substituted at the pharmacy for brand name products.

aq – Abbreviation commonly used on prescriptions for the Latin term *aqua*, meaning water.

aqueous – Pertaining to water.

ARC – *See* AIDS-*related complex or American Red Cross.*

area under the curve (AUC) – A concept that indicates how much of a drug is absorbed. The term derives from a chart that indicates blood levels of a drug over a specific period of time. The area under the curve of that chart is a measure of the total amount of drug in the body at any time point on that chart.

armamentarium – All of the tools available to treat disease. Often called a therapeutic armamentarium.

arrhythmia – An irregular heartbeat or a heart that beats with an irregular rhythm. Some arrhythmias are harmless while others are immediately fatal. Another term for arrhythmia is dysrhythmia.

arrhythmogenic – Pertaining to a factor that causes heart arrhythmias. These factors can include drugs or concurrent disease.

arsenical – An obsolete type of medicine previously used to treat infections, particularly syphilis.

arteri- – Prefix that relates to arteries.

arterial – Pertaining to an artery or arteries.

arterio- – Prefix that relates to arteries.

arteriogram – An x-ray image of an artery. The procedure is done by injecting a radiopaque dye into the artery to be examined and then using x-rays to photograph the dye as it passes through the area in question.

arteriography – The process of doing an arteriogram.

arteriole – A small blood vessel on the arterial side of the circulatory system. Arterioles are the small blood vessels that make the transition from the arteries to the capillaries.

A

arteriosclerosis – Hardening of the arteries. The most common form of this is atherosclerosis. *See also atherosclerosis.*

arteriosclerotic – Pertaining to arteriosclerosis.

arteritis – Inflammation of one or more arteries.

artery – Specialized blood vessel that carries blood away from the heart and distributes it to the rest of the body. Arterial walls have smooth muscle that contracts in order to keep blood flowing. The main function of the arteries is to distribute blood to all parts of the body.

arthralgia – Pain in a joint. Arthralgia is the term normally used to describe pain in a joint that is not due to arthritis.

arthritis – Inflammation in a joint. Among the many forms of arthritis, the two most common are rheumatoid arthritis, which involves the immune system, and osteoarthritis, which does not. *See also juvenile rheumatoid arthritis, osteoarthritis, psoriatic arthritis, ankylosing spondylitis, and rheumatoid arthritis.*

arthro- – Prefix that relates to joints.

arthrography – X-ray of a joint. In some cases a radiopaque dye is injected into the joint before the x-ray photograph is taken.

arthroscope – An instrument designed to look inside a joint. Arthroscopes are designed so that surgical instruments can be inserted through them. This way a surgeon who finds minor damage to a joint can perform the surgery without a large incision.

arthroscopic – Pertaining to an arthroscope.

arthroscopic surgery – An operation done on a joint through an arthroscope. Arthroscopic surgery avoids making large incisions into joints and reduces the pain and time required for postsurgical rehabilitation and recovery.

arthrosis – Any disease of a joint. Usually some degree of degeneration of the joint is present.

articulate – The ability of a joint to bend and flex.

A

artifact – An unwanted and unintended substance in a specimen or piece of data in a laboratory test. For example, a urine specimen may contain not only samples of bacteria causing an infection, but also other bacterial artifacts that contaminate the specimen and must be ignored.

artificial saliva – A solution that mimics the composition of saliva. Artificial saliva is used to relieve the discomfort of dry mouth in people who take drugs that cause dry mouth or have had surgical or radiation treatment that affect the salivary glands.

artificial tears – A solution that mimics the composition of tears. Artificial tears relieve discomfort from contact lenses or conditions that cause reduced tear production.

ascites – Abnormal accumulation of large amounts of fluid in the abdomen. Ascites is usually caused by severe liver disease.

asepsis – Condition of being free of bacterial contamination.

aseptic technique – A procedure where bacterial contamination is avoided. For example, pharmacists practice aseptic technique when preparing intravenous solutions. They take elaborate precautions to assure that bacteria do not enter IV bags or bottles during manipulations of the solutions.

ASHP – See *American Society of Health-system Pharmacists.*

ASO – See *administrative services only.*

assay – Test of purity. This term is commonly applied to analysis of purity of drug products or for tests of drug concentrations in blood or other body tissues.

assignment – Permission from a patient for a health provider to directly bill the patient's insurer. A health provider who accepts assignment agrees to accept payment from the insurer without further charge to the patient.

asthenia – Weakness, debility, or loss of strength.

asthma – Originally, this term was applied to any condition where breathing was difficult or labored. Now, it is used almost exclusively to mean bronchial asthma. *See bronchial asthma.*

A

asthma attack – An acute episode of bronchial asthma.

astringent – An agent that contracts tissue, usually the skin. An astringent causes drying and wrinkling of tissue. Astringents (e.g., calamine lotion) are used to relieve itching and burning.

asymptomatic – Having no symptoms. Lack of symptoms may be a desired goal of treatment. In other circumstances, having no symptoms may cause a physician to miss a diagnosis.

ataxia – Muscle incoordination. Ataxia is often a sign of toxicity of a drug that affects the central nervous system.

ataxic – Pertaining to ataxia.

atherosclerosis – A form of arteriosclerosis characterized by deposits of cholesterol and other fats on the sides of blood arteries. These deposits narrow the effective diameters of the affected arteries, thus diminishing the amount of blood that can flow through. Atherosclerosis is a common cause of coronary artery disease.

atherosclerotic – Pertaining to atherosclerosis.

atherosclerotic plaque – A well defined patch of cholesterol or other lipid material attached to the inner wall of a blood vessel. These plaques are usually the result of lipids precipitating out of blood. Atherosclerotic plaques can develop into thrombi. Also called atheromatous plaque.

athetosis – A neuromuscular disorder characterized by slow, writhing movements of the head, arms, legs, and even the trunk. Athetosis can be a side effect of antipsychotic drugs and drugs for Parkinson's disease.

athlete's foot – A fungal infection of the foot. Athlete's foot usually starts between two toes and can spread to other toes, the bottom of the foot, the toenails, or any other surface on the foot. More properly called tinea pedis.

atopic – Pertaining to atopy.

atopic dermatitis – A chronic or recurring skin lesion characteristic of an allergic reaction. Atopic dermatitis lesions usually itch intensely and are treated with a topical corticosteroid.

A

atopy – A tendency toward allergic reactions, usually in a person with a strong family history of allergies.

atria – Plural form of atrium.

atrial arrhythmia – *See supraventricular arrhythmia.*

atrioventricular (AV) – Pertaining to both the atria and ventricles of the heart.

atrioventricular (AV) node – A small knot of cardiac muscle fibers located at the juncture of the right atrium and right ventricle. The primary role of the atrioventricular node, also called the AV node, is to receive electrical impulses from the right atrium and spread those impulses through the ventricles. These impulses cause the ventricles to contract, and consist of the major portion of a heart contraction.

atrioventricular valve – The flap of tissue that prevents blood from moving backward into the atria of the heart when the ventricles contract. Without valves sealing off the various chambers of the heart, blood would flow both backward and forward with each heartbeat.

at risk – Responsible for costs. In a typical health plan, the insurance company is at risk for claims expenses. However, in a capitated plan, the health care provider (e.g., pharmacy, physician, dentist) accepts responsibility for providing care in exchange for a guaranteed monthly payment from an insurance company. The term derives from the fact that the health care provider is at risk of loss if the cost of care exceeds insurance payments.

atrium – One of the two small chambers that sit at the top of the heart. The roles of the right atrium are to receive blood as it returns from the circulation into the heart, to initiate the heartbeat, and to pump blood into the right ventricle that sits directly below it. The roles of the left atrium are to receive blood from the lungs, and then to pump that blood into the left ventricle. Formerly called auricle.

atrophic – Pertaining to atrophy.

atrophy – Wasting. This term is most commonly applied to wasting

A

away of muscle tissue due to disease, disuse, or poor nutrition. The term can also be applied to wasting of any other organ or tissue.

attending physician – A physician who has full privileges at a hospital, clinic, or other medical facility. An attending physician is not a medical student, intern, or resident.

attention deficit disorder (ADD) – A disorder primarily affecting children and adolescents characterized by the inability to focus attention, leading to behavior problems and learning disabilities. The condition is more common in boys than in girls and is usually treated with psychotherapy and stimulant drugs.

attenuated – Pertaining to attenuation.

attenuation – The process of reducing disease-producing potential. This procedure is most commonly applied in the development and production of live vaccines. Through laboratory manipulations, successive generations of bacteria or viruses are developed lacking a toxin, enzyme, or some other normal constituent that causes symptoms of disease. Without attenuation, vaccination with live organisms would likely cause the disease it was trying to prevent.

a.u. – Abbreviation commonly used on prescriptions for the Latin term *aures utrae*, meaning each ear.

AUC – *See area under the curve.*

audiogram – The written record of a hearing test.

audiologist – A person who conducts and evaluates hearing tests.

aura – A sensation a person feels before the onset of other symptoms. People with epilepsy or migraine headaches may experience aurae before the onset of a seizure or headache. Aurae manifest themselves as haloes around objects, unusual colors, odors, or sounds.

aurae – Plural form of aura.

auricle – *See atrium.*

A

authorization – The approval for medical care. Such approvals are usually given by insurance companies. *See also prior authorization.*

autoantibody – An antibody is a substance developed within the immune system and designed to identify and destroy foreign substances. An autoantibody mistakes the body's own tissue as abnormal and attempts to destroy it. *See also autoimmune disease.*

autoclave – A sterilizing machine. An autoclave uses a combination of heat, steam, and pressure to sterilize equipment.

autoimmune disease – A medical condition caused by an autoanti-body response. These conditions are the result of the interaction between autoantibodies and normal tissue. Examples include rheumatoid arthritis, lupus, and multiple sclerosis.

autologous transplantation – A form of tissue replacement where the donor and recipient are the same person. Examples include blood or bone marrow collection and skin grafting. For example, individuals who are scheduled for surgery may bank some of their own blood in the weeks prior to surgery. If the blood is needed, the patient is sure of the source and avoids the risk of contracting a blood-borne communicable disease from an unknown donor. Skin grafts are autologous transplants since they are taken from one part of the body and transplanted to another site on the same person's body.

autonomic nervous system (ANS) – The portion of the nervous system that controls vital functions such as heart rate, blood pressure, and hormone release. The autonomic nervous system is responsible for balancing most of the important functions within the body. For example, the autonomic nervous system raises blood pressure and heart rate during an emergency and lowers them during rest periods.

AV – Abbreviation for atrioventricular.

average wholesale price (AWP) – The published wholesale price of a drug. In the past this was the price pharmacies paid for a drug purchased through a wholesaler. Because of changes in purchasing and contracting practices, the average wholesale price, or AWP, only roughly reflects the actual cost of a medicine. Most insurance reimbursements to pharmacies, however, are still based on AWP.

avirulent – Not toxic or capable of causing disease.

AV node – *See atrioventricular node.*

AWP – *See average wholesale price.*

B

β-lactam – *See beta-lactam.*

β-lactamase – *See beta-lactamase.*

bacilli – Plural of bacillus.

bacillus – A general term used to describe any rod-shaped bacterium. Bacilli are widely distributed in nature. Most are harmless but some are extremely toxic and are associated with infections as varied as diarrhea, pneumonia, and plague. Also refers to a member of the genus *Bacillus*.

backache – Pain that may occur anywhere from the base of the neck to the lower spine. Backache may be due to injury, muscle strain, or problems with the structure of the spine itself. Some infections (e.g., urinary tract infections) may also cause backache.

bacteremia – A general term that indicates the presence of bacteria in the blood. While the blood is normally sterile, it is not unusual for bacteria to be present without presenting any symptoms or problems. Bacteria may enter the blood following an infection anywhere in the body, a dental procedure, surgery, cut, or any other injury that breaks the skin. Unless symptoms of infection are present (e.g., fever, chills, lack of energy, etc.) most cases of bacteremia go unnoticed and do not need treatment.

bacteri- – Prefix meaning bacteria.

bacteria – Plural form of bacterium.

bacterial endocarditis – An infection of the heart caused by bacteria. Bacterial endocarditis is a life-threatening infection that requires immediate treatment with high doses of antibiotics. Bacterial endocarditis may damage heart valves, requiring surgery after recovery from the infection. Formerly called subacute bacterial endocarditis.

bacterial resistance – The ability of bacteria to adapt themselves to survive an exposure to antibiotics. Bacteria are capable of adapting themselves in many ways. For example, some bacteria form special enzymes that destroy antibiotics. In other cases, bacteria may adapt their cell walls so that antibiotics cannot penetrate them.

B

bactericidal – Capable of killing bacteria. Typically used in reference to antiseptics, disinfectants, or antibiotics. Contrary to common belief, many antibiotics do not kill bacteria. Whether they kill bacteria or not, all antibiotics rely on the immune system to cure infections. *Also see bacteriostatic.*

bacterio- – Prefix meaning bacteria.

bacteriologic – Pertaining to bacteria or the study of bacteria.

bacteriological – Pertaining to bacteria or the study of bacteria.

bacteriology – The study of bacteria. Bacteriology is a division of the science of microbiology, the study of microorganisms. *Also see microbiology.*

bacteriophage – A type of virus that uses bacteria for part of its life cycle. Typically, bacteriophages enter bacteria, use bacterial enzymes and proteins to reproduce themselves, and then escape the bacteria. Depending upon the specific type of bacteriophage, the host bacteria may or may not be harmed.

bacteriostatic – Capable of stopping the growth and reproduction of bacteria. Typically used to describe antibiotics that inhibit bacterial growth without killing the bacteria. Bacteriostatic antibiotics suppress reproduction and growth of bacteria until the body's immune system can kill the bacteria. *Also see bactericidal.*

bacterium – A single-celled organism capable of sustaining life by itself and of multiplying by cell division. Bacteria may be innocuous, helpful, or harmful. Some bacteria live freely by themselves while others are parasites.

A bacterium is sometime colloquially referred to as a bug or germ.

bacteriuria – The presence of bacteria in urine. Since urine in the bladder is normally sterile, bacteriuria may indicate the presence of a urinary tract infection. In some cases, however, bacteria found in a urine specimen may simply be contamination that occurred during the urine collection process.

bad cholesterol – A colloquial term for low-density lipoprotein (LDL). *See low-density lipoprotein.*

B

balance – An instrument used in a pharmacy to weigh ingredients for a pharmaceutical preparation. Often mistakenly called a scale, a balance measures the weight of a substance by counterbalancing it against a known weight.

Also, the state of equilibrium in the body. For example, acid-base balance is the relationship between acidic and alkaline substances in a tissue or organ.

balance billing – The fee that remains after a patient makes a copayment. The balance due is billed to the insurance carrier.

Balance billing may also refer to the practice of some providers of billing patients for charges not fully covered by insurance. This type of balance billing is illegal for Medicare and Medicaid recipients and may be a violation of a managed care contract.

balloon angioplasty – A procedure where a special catheter is passed into an obstructed blood vessel, usually in the heart. Once the catheter is in place, its balloon tip is inflated. The inflated balloon pushes against the obstruction, often a cholesterol plaque, and if all works well, reopens the blood vessel so that blood may flow through unobstructed. *Also see angioplasty.*

balloon catheter – A thin, flexible tube that has an inflatable collar. Once the catheter is in place, the balloon portion is inflated to hold the catheter in proper position.

balm – A scented ointment.

barbiturate – A class of drugs derived from barbituric acid. Barbiturates may be used to produce sedation, sleep, anesthesia, or treat seizure problems. All barbiturates have potential for abuse and dependence. Phenobarbital is the most commonly prescribed barbiturate.

bariatric – Pertaining to obesity.

bariatric medicine – A medical specialty that deals with the treatment of obesity and its complications.

bariatric physician – A medical doctor who specializes in the treatment of obesity and its complications. Bariatric physicians employ a wide variety of treatments that may include diet, exercise, medication, hypnosis, and/or acupuncture. They may also make referrals for surgery.

bariatrics – See *bariatric medicine.*

barium sulfate – A chalky chemical used to facilitate x-ray evaluation of the gastrointestinal tract. Barium sulfate is dense enough to stop x-rays from passing through and appears white on x-ray film. Because it fills in craters and crevices and forms around obstructions, it can be used to help diagnose peptic ulcer, diverticulosis, and other gastrointestinal problems.

Barium sulfate may be swallowed for x-rays of the upper gastrointestinal tract or may be inserted rectally as an enema for viewing the lower gastrointestinal tract.

baro- – Prefix meaning weight or pressure.

baroreceptors – Nerve endings that act as blood pressure monitors within the body. Baroreceptors are found in the walls of the heart and major blood vessels. Baroreceptors transmit messages to the brain when they sense the blood pressure is too high or too low.

Barrett esophagus – An ulceration of the lowest portion of the passageway between the mouth and the stomach. The syndrome may follow long-standing gastroesophageal reflux (*see gastroesophageal reflux disease*) where the corrosive effects of stomach acid on the esophagus causes changes in the cells lining the lower part of the esophagus. About 10% of people with Barrett esophagus, also known as Barrett syndrome, develop esophageal cancer.

barrier – An obstruction. In relation to drug therapy, a barrier obstructs the passage of a drug through a tissue. Most barriers probably developed as a protective mechanism against poisons in the primitive diet. *Also see blood-brain barrier.*

barrier contraceptive – An agent that prevents the union of a sperm cell with an egg by obstructing sperm flow within the female reproductive system. A diaphragm is an example of a barrier contraceptive.

B

base – The vehicle for preparing a medication dosage form. For example, a topical antibiotic might be dispensed in an ointment base. In this case a pharmacist or pharmaceutical company physically mixes a precise amount of antibiotic into a measured amount of petrolatum. The preparation may then be applied to the skin.

Also an alkaline substance such as sodium hydroxide.

basic benefits – The specific insurance coverages listed in a certificate of insurance plus any unlisted items that are required by state law.

basic coverage – The standard benefits provided by an insurance company.

basophil – A white blood cell that displays blue granules when dyed with a basic stain. The granules contain heparin and histamine. Basophils normally comprise less than 1% of the total number of white blood cells, but this percentage can rise during allergic reactions. The functions of basophils are not clearly understood.

BBB – See *blood-brain barrier.*

beaker – A glass container with a spout on its lip and usually with volumes marked or etched on the outside. In pharmacy, beakers may be used to mix liquids during prescription compounding.

bedsore – See *decubitus ulcer.*

behavioral health care – Diagnosis and treatment of mental illness and substance abuse. Behavioral health care may be delivered in either inpatient or outpatient settings. Insurance for behavioral health care may have different limits than other health care.

belly – Colloquial term for the abdomen, stomach, or uterus.

bellyache – Colloquial term for a pain in the abdomen or stomach.

benchmarking – The practice of comparing one's products, standards, practices, or outcomes against those of either another similar organization or an industry standard. A hospital, for example, might compare its rate of medication errors against the error rate of a similar hospital. Accrediting agencies such as the Joint Commission on Accreditation of Healthcare Organizations (JCAHO) require health facilities to perform benchmarking.

B

beneficiary – A person who is eligible to receive insurance benefits. In the case of health insurance, beneficiaries are typically the spouse of the insurance subscriber and the subscriber's children under 19 years of age. Most health insurance policies allow coverage to children up to 24 years of age as long as they are enrolled full-time in a college or university.

benefit – The services or expenses an insurance company will pay for. Also, the actual amount of money an insurer will pay for a service.

benefit limit – Any constraint that restricts coverage, other than an outright policy exclusion, without regard to the medical necessity of a product or service. Some pharmacy plans, for example, limit the dollar amount of coverage over the course of a quarter or a year. Prescription drug purchases beyond that limit are not covered by the policy.

benefit package – Services or perquisites an employer offers to employees in addition to salary. The benefit package may include health insurance, life insurance, 401k plans, sick leave, vacation time, tuition reimbursement, parking, and others.

benefit period – The length of time covered by an insurance policy. Most employer-sponsored health insurance policies cover a 12-month period. An individual plan may only provide coverage from month to month.

benefit-to-risk – An estimate of the probability of a desirable outcome with a treatment versus the likelihood of side effects or other adverse event. For example, the benefit-to-risk of treating pneumonia with an antibiotic is high. The benefit of treatment is potential cure of the infection (highly probable). The main risk is an allergic reaction to the antibiotic (low probability, especially if the patient has not had an allergy to this medicine in the past). A further risk is potential death if no treatment is given.

benign – Capable of doing little or no harm. Often used to describe a nonmalignant tumor.

benign prostatic hyperplasia (BPH) – A noncancerous enlargement of the prostate gland. An age-related condition common in men

B

over 60 years old, BPH can cause urine retention and difficulty passing urine. Drug therapy is usually tried first but men who do not respond adequately may need surgery. Also called benign prostatic hypertrophy.

benzodiazepine – A large class of medications most commonly used to treat anxiety and insomnia.

best price – The lowest fee a health care provider offers to its most valued customers. Some insurance companies and government contracts require providers to bill them the lower of either the provider's best price or the published price the payer is willing to pay. For example, if a pharmacy offers to the public or to a select group a deep discount on a specific prescription drug, it must offer that same price to any payer that includes a best price clause in its contract.

beta-adrenergic agonist – A drug or hormone that acts through the sympathetic nervous system and whose effects include increasing heart rate, dilating bronchial tubes in the lungs, and reducing the force and rate of uterine contractions during labor. Beta-adrenergic agonists are commonly referred to simply as beta-agonists.

Drugs with primarily $beta_1$–agonist activity act mainly on the heart, increasing heart rate and raising blood pressure. These medicines are sometimes used to treat shock and cardiac arrest. Drugs with primarily $beta_2$-agonist activity act mainly on the lungs and uterus. They are used to treat asthma and premature labor.

beta-adrenergic blocker – A drug that inhibits the effects of endogenous beta-adrenergic agonists. Commonly referred to simply as beta-blockers, these drugs are used to treat hypertension and a wide variety of disorders. They may also cause recurrence or worsening of asthma or other breathing problems in susceptible persons.

beta-agonist – *See beta-adrenergic agonist.*

beta-blocker – *See beta-adrenergic blocker.*

B

beta-lactam – A chemical structure found in all penicillin and cephalosporin antibiotics. The beta-lactam ring is essential for their activity as antibiotics. These drugs are sometimes referred to as beta-lactam antibiotics.

beta-lactamase – An enzyme secreted by some bacteria that destroys the beta-lactam ring of some penicillins and related antibiotics. Destroying this ring destroys the antibiotic effectiveness of the drug. Once highly sensitive to penicillin, over 95% of *Staphylococcus aureus* bacteria are now resistant to penicillin because they produce this enzyme. Beta-lactamase is sometimes called penicillinase.

bi- – Prefix meaning two or double.

biceps – A muscle in the upper arm. Each of the muscles has two attachments to bone.

b.i.d. – Abbreviation for the Latin *bis in die*, meaning twice in a day. A common abbreviation on written prescriptions indicating that the medicine is to be taken twice a day.

bilateral – Pertaining to two sides. For example, a bilateral tremor is one that affects both sides of the body.

bile – A yellowish brown or greenish fluid that aids in digestion. Bile is formed in the liver and stored in the gallbladder. Bile's main functions are to facilitate absorption of fat from food and to assist in the elimination of waste.

bile acid – A group of chemicals formed in the liver from cholesterol and other biochemicals. Bile acids assist with dietary fat and fat-soluble vitamin absorption.

bile acid sequestrant – A group of drugs that chemically combine with bile acids in the intestine, causing these bile acids to be eliminated from the body. Bile acid sequestrants are prescribed to lower blood cholesterol and other blood lipid levels. Bile acids are made from cholesterol. By chemically bonding with bile acids and forcing their elimination from the body, bile acid sequestrants force the liver to use additional blood cholesterol to replace the missing bile acids. Thus, blood cholesterol is depleted.

B

biliary – Pertaining to bile.

bilirubin – A pigment released into blood after the destruction of old or damaged red blood cells. The liver recycles bilirubin into new hemoglobin.

bilirubinemia – Excessive levels of bilirubin in the blood. Bilirubinemia is usually an indication of liver disease.

bio- – Prefix meaning life.

bioassay – Measurement of the potency of a drug or other agent by administering the drug to an animal or live tissue culture and evaluating response. Bioassay is used when chemical analysis does not adequately indicate a drug's potency.

Potencies of drugs that are standardized by means of bioassay are usually indicated as units or international units. Insulin and vitamin E are examples.

bioavailability – The degree to which a drug releases itself from its dosage form (e.g., tablet, capsule, suspension) to become accessible for its intended effect.

biochemical – Pertaining to biochemistry.

A substance produced as the result of a chemical reaction within a living organism.

biochemistry – The study of the chemical reactions that occur within a living organism. The chemistry of life.

bioengineering – See *biomedical engineering*.

bioequivalence – The determination of whether two or more drug products release their contents in equal amounts over the same amount of time. Drug products that have similar dissolution and absorption characteristics are said to be bioequivalent.

biologic response modulator – A drug or other agent that either increases or decreases the activity of the immune system.

biomedical – Relating to the sciences that underlie medicine. These include pharmacology, anatomy, physiology, microbiology, pathology, and biochemistry.

B

biomedical engineering – The application of physical, mechanical, and mathematical theories and practices to medical needs. Biomedical engineering is used to develop pumps, respirators, monitors, telemetry, and other medical equipment.

biopharmaceutics – The study of the chemical properties of drug dosage forms (e.g., tablets, capsules, suspensions, injections).

biopsy – A surgical procedure where a piece of tissue is removed for further diagnostic study. Some biopsies require general anesthesia while others are minor procedures done with local anesthesia or even no anesthesia at all.

In most cases, a pathologist examines biopsied tissue samples under a microscope. Changes in cell types or cell structures often allow for diagnosis of a clinical problem.

biosynthesis – Formation of chemical substances within a living organism.

biotechnology – The process of using live organisms to produce drugs or hormones for human use.

Insulin was the first commercial product produced by biotechnology. In this case, human genes responsible for producing insulin were spliced into E. *coli* bacteria. As these bacteria reproduced and grew, they secreted insulin chemically identical to that made by humans. The human insulin produced in this fashion is easier to harvest and causes fewer side effects than the beef and pork insulin previously used.

bipolar affective disorder – A mental illness characterized by periods of extreme excitation (mania) and deep depression. Contrary to the popular notion, it usually takes months to move from one of these extremes to the other. Some patients have predominantly manic episodes or depressive episodes. Few patients experience the classic swing from mania to depression and back. Also called manic-depressive illness.

birth control pill – An oral tablet (not a pill) intended for contraception. Birth control pills contain either a progesterone-like hormone called a progestin alone or in combination with an estrogen. Birth control pills work by inhibiting ovulation, inhibiting

B

implantation of fertilized eggs, thickening cervical mucus to make it more difficult for sperm to enter the uterus, or by a combination of these effects.

bisphosphonate – A class of drugs that prevent calcium loss from bone. Bisphosphonates are most often used to treat osteoporosis. In some cases, bisphosphonates actually increase bone calcium content and replenish some lost bone tissue.

blackout – A temporary loss of consciousness or memory due to trauma to the head or an adverse drug reaction. Blackouts may occur following episodes of heavy drinking. Tranquilizers and sleeping medicines may cause a type of blackout called anterograde amnesia.

-blast – Suffix indicating an immature cell form. For example, an erythroblast is an immature erythrocyte (red blood cell).

bleed – To lose blood.

bleeder – A blood vessel that is losing blood.

Also, a colloquial term for someone who has a disorder that makes blood clotting difficult (e.g., hemophilia).

blemish – An abnormal and cosmetically unappealing patch of skin. Blemishes are not necessarily indicative of a skin disease.

blepharitis – Inflammation of one or both eyes.

blepharo- – Prefix meaning eyelid.

blepharoptosis – A drooping eyelid caused by either a weakness of the muscle in the eyelid or by inadequate nerve stimulation to the muscle.

blepharospasm – Involuntary contraction of the muscles in the eyelids. Blepharospasm may cause uncontrollable blinking or even complete eye closure.

blinded – Pertaining to a research study in which the subjects and/or the investigators do not know which treatment is the investigational treatment and which is the reference standard. Blinding is one technique to try to minimize the effects of subject or investigator bias.

B

block – A stoppage or obstruction to flow or passage. For example, a regional block is a technique for administering local anesthesia where pain impulses from an entire area of the body are blocked from reaching the brain. Atrioventricular block is an obstruction to the flow of electrical current from the right atrium to the right ventricle of the heart.

blockade – The temporary obstruction of function. Blockade typically involves altered nerve function, usually because of a desired or undesired drug effect.

blocker – An agent that produces a blockade, for example, a beta-adrenergic blocker.

blocking agent – See *blocker*.

blood – The fluid pumped through the circulatory system. The blood consists of water, cells (e.g., red blood cells, white blood cells), proteins, carbohydrates, fats, hormones, and electrolytes. Blood is the tissue that delivers oxygen and nutrients to all the cells of the body and picks up cellular waste material for detoxification and elimination.

blood bank – A facility, most commonly in a hospital, where blood is collected, stored, tested for blood type, and prepared for administration to patients.

blood-brain barrier (BBB) – A selective impediment to the passage of ions and large molecules from the blood into the brain. This function protects the brain from poisons and even some of the body's own chemicals that might otherwise interfere with nerve functions.

The blood-brain barrier can also hinder some types of drug therapy. For example, most antibiotics have great difficulty reaching the brain in high enough concentrations to treat infections there.

blood cholesterol – See *cholesterol*.

blood clot – See *clot*.

blood count – The number of blood cells per cubic millimeter of blood. Normal blood counts are usually considered to be in the following ranges:

Red blood cells: 4.6–6.2 million/mm³ (adult males) and 4.2–5.4 million/mm³ (adult females)

Total white blood cells: 4,500–11,000/mm³

Platelets: 150,000–350,000/mm³

blood level – The concentration of a substance in the blood. In pharmacy, blood level relates to the concentration of a drug in blood. Blood levels are often used to adjust doses to maximize clinical benefit while minimizing side effects.

blood pressure – The force blood exerts against the walls of the blood vessels. Blood pressure is influenced by the amount of blood the heart pumps, the volume of blood in the circulatory system, and the squeezing force of the smooth muscle in blood vessel walls. Normal blood pressure is usually said to be 120/80 millimeters of mercury.

blood thinner – Colloquial term for an anticoagulant. Anticoagulants do not affect the viscosity or thickness of blood. Instead, they reduce the amounts of the blood protein factors that are responsible for clotting blood.

blood type – A system of classification of blood that reflects the presence or absence of specific antigens on the surface of red blood cells. The most commonly used classification system is the ABO system, which detects the presence of A antigens (type A blood), B antigens (type B blood), both A and B antigens (type AB blood), or neither antigen (type O blood). Transfusion of antigenically incompatible blood (e.g., giving type A blood to a type B patient) can result in serious, even fatal, reactions.

board certified – A health care professional, usually a physician, who has completed the training requirements and passed a rigorous examination for official recognition in a given specialty. For example, a physician who successfully completes a residency in internal medicine and passes the internal medicine certification examination is recognized as board certified in internal medicine.

Board certification is a step beyond licensure.

B

board eligible – A health care professional, usually a physician, who has completed the training requirements for examination in a given specialty. For example, a physician who successfully completes a residency in internal medicine and a fellowship in cardiology is eligible to take the cardiology specialty board examination.

board of pharmacy – An administrative body that regulates the practice of pharmacy in each state. Although laws vary from state to state, members of a state board of pharmacy are usually appointed by the governor for a specific term. Board members normally include pharmacists and consumers. Functions of the board of pharmacy include licensing pharmacists, disciplining pharmacists, and promulgating regulations to protect the public health.

boil – A painful, localized skin infection, usually caused by staphylococcus, characterized by a raised pustule surrounded by inflammation. Boils most often start in hair shafts, oil glands, or in an underlying layer of skin. Boils usually affect underlying blood vessels, forming a core of clotted material. In time, boils dissolve, but more commonly they are surgically lanced and drained.

bolus – A single, large dose or application of an agent. For example, an intravenous bolus is a large dose of medication injected rapidly into a vein to produce an immediate effect.

bone – The hardened connective tissue that comprises the skeleton. Bones consist of a matrix of connective tissue, blood vessels, and minerals, particularly calcium phosphate. The human skeleton is composed of 206 bones.

bone marrow – The soft tissue that fills the inside of bones. Bone marrow is the site of production of red blood cells, platelets, and most white blood cells.

bone marrow depression – A condition where the cell production of bone marrow is reduced. Bone marrow depression may be the result of disease or drug toxicity.

bowel – *See intestine.*

B

bowel movement – Defecation. The passage of solid waste from the gastrointestinal system.

BPH – *See benign prostatic hyperplasia.*

brady- – Prefix meaning slow.

bradyarrhythmia – Any irregular heart rhythm accompanied by a slower than normal heart rate.

bradycardia – A slower than normal heart rate. A rate of less than 60 beats per minute is normally considered to be bradycardia.

bradykinesia – Extremely slow movement. Bradykinesia may be a sign of neurological disease (e.g., Parkinson's disease) or drug toxicity.

brain – The mass of nerve tissue located inside the skull. The brain is the highest functioning level of the central nervous system and the organ that commands the activities of most of the organs and tissues of the body.

bran – The portion of grains such as wheat and oats that is not digestible. Bran passes through the digestive tract intact and provides bulk for bowel movements. Adequate amounts of dietary bran help to prevent constipation.

brand-brand interchange – The act of dispensing of one brand prescription drug product in place of another when the two drugs are chemically equivalent. Brand-brand interchange may only be performed when allowed by state law.

brand name – A specific, trademarked designation given to one company's product. For example, Kodacolor is the registered trademark of a specific type of film produced by the Eastman Kodak Company of Rochester, New York.

brand name drug – A specific, trademarked designation given to one company's version of a generic drug. For example, Tylenol is the registered trademark of the drug acetaminophen. Tylenol is sold exclusively by McNeil Consumer Products. Other companies that make and sell acetaminophen products may not use the Tylenol name without the permission of the trademark holder (McNeil).

B

broad spectrum antibiotic – An antibiotic that is effective against a wide range of bacterial species.

bronchi – Plural form of bronchus.

bronchi- – Prefix meaning bronchi.

bronchial – Pertaining to the bronchi.

bronchial asthma – A respiratory condition characterized by difficulty exhaling and by wheezing. Bronchial asthma, normally simply called asthma, is caused by smooth muscle spasms in the airways, especially the bronchi, that reduce airflow, and cause inflammation and accumulation of mucus in the air passages. Asthma is more common in children.

In susceptible individuals, causes of asthma attacks include allergic reactions, exercise, changes in weather or altitude, and upper respiratory infections.

bronchiectasis – A chronic dilation of the bronchi. Bronchiectasis is usually caused by long-term inflammation or obstruction in the lungs. It is commonly seen in chronic obstructive pulmonary disease.

bronchiole – The respiratory passageway between a bronchus and the alveoli. Bronchioles are less than one millimeter in diameter and contain no cartilage. The diameter of bronchioles is controlled by smooth muscle in their walls.

bronchiolitis – An inflammation in the bronchioles that commonly occurs with bronchopneumonia.

bronchitis – An inflammation, usually due to infection, of the mucous membranes lining the bronchi.

broncho- – Prefix meaning bronchi.

bronchoconstriction – A sudden reduction of the diameter of the bronchial tubes. Bronchoconstriction may occur during an asthma attack or as a side effect of drug therapy.

bronchoconstrictor – An agent that causes bronchoconstriction.

bronchodilator – An agent that widens the diameter of the bronchial tubes. Bronchodilators, including beta-adrenergic agonists and

B

xanthines, are commonly used to treat and prevent asthma attacks.

bronchopneumonia – An acute inflammation of the bronchial passages, most often due to infection. Bronchopneumonia may spread to the alveoli or be the result of infection that has spread from the alveoli.

bronchoscope – A specially designed endoscope that is intended for examination of the internal passages of the lungs.

bronchospasm – A sudden contraction of the smooth muscles within the bronchi and bronchioles. Bronchospasm reduces the lumen of these structures, making air passage more difficult.

bronchus – One of the large air passages that branch off from the trachea and conduct air to the bronchioles. The bronchi are supported and protected by cartilage. Smooth muscle within the bronchi regulates the degree of dilation of the structures.

buccal – Pertaining to the inside of the cheek. Some drugs are administered buccally, placed between the gum and cheek and allowed to dissolve there. Once dissolved, the drug is absorbed through the mucous membranes in the mouth.

bug – Colloquial term for a microorganism.

bulk-forming laxative – An agent that produces bowel movements by increasing the volume of the intestinal contents. Doing so causes the bowels to try to eliminate their contents.

burn – Disruption or destruction of a tissue that has been exposed to excessive energy or a toxin. Burns may be minor and quick to heal (e.g., sunburn) or may be extensive and fatal (e.g., chemical burns, thermal burns).

bursa – A pad-like sac of fluid located near joints. Bursae reduce the friction caused as tendons move over bone structures during muscle movement.

bursae – Plural of bursa.

bursitis – An inflammation of one or more bursae. Bursitis most often occurs in the shoulders, hips, or knees. Bursitis causes intense pain with movement.

B

business coalition – A group of companies that have formed themselves into an association for the purpose of negotiating better terms for health coverage. Business coalitions usually involve companies in a specific geographic area (e.g., Memphis, St. Louis, Birmingham, Central Illinois). By placing all of their collective employees into a large insurance pool, these companies are able to exert pressure on insurance companies for the purpose of negotiating better insurance premiums.

bypass – A physical shunt around an obstruction or nonfunctioning structure. For example, a coronary bypass involves transplanting a small length of vein to form a bridge to convey blood around an obstructed coronary artery. A cardiopulmonary bypass temporarily shunts blood through an external pump (heart-lung machine) during heart surgery.

C

c – Abbreviation commonly used on prescriptions for the Latin term *cum*, meaning with.

Ca – Abbreviation for cancer or carcinoma, or calcium.

cachectic – Pertaining to cachexia.

cachexia – Severe weight loss and wasting. Usually associated with malnutrition or prolonged illness. Cachexia is particularly common in the late stages of cancer although it may appear with many noncancerous conditions.

CAD – *See coronary artery disease.*

cadaver – A dead body. Often used in the context of the specimen students examine and dissect in a medical school anatomy laboratory.

cadaverous – Having the appearance of a cadaver (pale, waxy skin color), even if still alive.

cafeteria plan – A benefit plan where an employer allows employees to choose their own combination of benefits. In most cases, the employer offers some standard, basic benefits (e.g., sick leave, vacation time) and allows employees to choose which type of health plan (indemnity, health maintenance organization, preferred provider organization) and other benefit options suit them best.

Cal – Abbreviation for a kilocalorie.

cal – Abbreviation for a calorie.

calcification – Deposition of calcium salts. Usually applies to the process where calcium deposits itself in newly forming tissue during bone and tooth development. Calcification can also occur in muscles and joints as a complication of injury.

calcium channel antagonist – *See calcium channel blocker.*

calcium channel blocker (CCB) – A class of drugs that restricts the movement of calcium through its normal passageways in vascular smooth muscle. Blocking calcium movement inhibits smooth muscle contraction. Calcium channel blockers are used to treat angina pectoris, hypertension, and some irregular heart rhythms.

C

calculi – Plural form of calculus.

calculus – A stone. Calculi most commonly form in the kidneys or gallbladder. Stones may be formed from uric acid, cholesterol, amino acids, or a wide variety of inorganic compounds.

caloric – Pertaining to a calorie.

calorie (cal, Cal) – The amount of heat needed to raise the temperature of one gram of water by one degree Celsius at sea level. The term calorie is often misused. The calories listed on food labels actually refer to kilocalories, the amount of heat needed to raise the temperature of 1,000 grams of water by one degree Celsius at sea level.

cancer (Ca) – A general term that applies to a wide variety of illnesses characterized by uncontrolled accumulation of abnormal cells, the ability to spread to other parts of the body, and the tendency to recur if not completely eradicated by treatment.

Depending upon the type and location of the cancer, it may be treated with drugs (chemotherapy), radiation, surgery, or any combination of these. Some cancers are relatively easily treated while others show little response to aggressive treatment.

Virtually any normal tissue can generate a cancerous growth.

cancer chemotherapy – The drug therapy used to treat cancer. In most cases, combinations of drugs with complimentary actions are used. Depending upon the properties of the individual drugs, they may be given by mouth or by injection. In some cases, they are continuously infused intravenously over a period of several days.

Although there are exceptions, chemotherapy is generally extremely toxic. Chemotherapy may cause severe vomiting, hair loss, and low blood counts that lead to fatigue and increased risk of infection. Fortunately, treatments have been developed to reduce the severity of many of these side effects.

candidiasis – An infection caused by the candida yeast. Candidiasis most often affects warm, moist areas such as skin folds, the mouth, diaper areas, and the labia and vagina. Candidiasis sometimes follows treatment with a broad spectrum antibiotic

C

such as tetracycline. Candidiasis is a common complication of diaper rash.

cap. – Abbreviation for capsule, commonly used on prescriptions.

capillary – The smallest blood vessel in the cardiovascular system. Capillaries are the vessels that actually allow the blood to distribute oxygen and nutrients to individual cells and pick up carbon dioxide and waste products. Blood is fed to the capillaries by the arterioles and passes through to the venules.

capitation – A predetermined fee paid by a health insurance plan to a health care provider (e.g., physician, pharmacy, dentist, clinic) per health plan member assigned to that provider. Providers and health plans usually commit to the capitation rate for one calendar year and the insurance plan makes prorated payments monthly.

The term is derived from the Latin word for head, thus capitation is a payment per head. In a capitation plan, the provider receives a set payment every month regardless of how many patients use the service. Consequently, the provider makes money on patients who need little or no service and loses money on patients who need more care.

capsule – A medication dosage form where the drug is contained in an external shell. Capsule shells are usually made of hard gelatin and enclose or encapsulate powder or medication beads. However, soft gelatin capsules are used for drugs that only appear in the liquid form. Vitamin E capsules are an example of soft gelatin capsules.

carbapenem – A class of antibiotics usually given intravenously and reserved for Gram-negative infections.

carbohydrate (CHO) – A chemical compound composed of one or more simple sugars. Carbohydrates are composed of carbon, hydrogen, and oxygen in a ring structure or a linked series of ring structures.

A carbohydrate may be as simple as one (e.g., dextrose, fructose) or two (e.g., sucrose, lactose) sugar molecules or may be composed of long chains of molecules (e.g., starches). These are often called simple or complex carbohydrates, respectively.

carbuncle – A deep-seated abscess that forms in a hair follicle. Carbuncles may grow, connecting to and involving many other follicles. Carbuncles most commonly appear after an illness.

carcino- – Prefix relating to cancer.

carcinogen – An agent that can cause cancer. Carcinogens may include drugs, chemicals, environmental toxins, radiation, or viruses.

carcinogenesis – The process of causing cancer to begin.

carcinoma (Ca) – A malignancy that starts in epithelial cells. Epithelial cells and epithelial tissue generally form the lining of organs such as the skin, stomach, intestines, and many glands.

card program – An arrangement where a health insurance program participant is issued an identification card to use in conjunction with the pharmacy benefit. The card, either in plain language or through coding, indicates which individuals are eligible for prescription drug benefits, which drugs are allowed and disallowed, and the level of copayment.

Besides the direct interaction of the participant with the pharmacy, a card program also directs reimbursements to pharmacies and initiates cost management activities on the part of the payer.

cardiac – Pertaining to the heart.

cardiac arrest – The absence of a productive heartbeat. Cardiac arrest may occur spontaneously or following trauma or drowning. In most cases, however, cardiac arrest occurs in people who have a serious, preexisting heart condition.

Cardiopulmonary resuscitation, the treatment for cardiac arrest, must be started immediately to prevent death. Even if the heart recovers, there is risk of damage to other organs due to interruption of blood supply to the body.

cardiac arrhythmia – *See arrhythmia.*

cardiac catheterization – A surgical procedure in which a thin, narrow, sterile tube (catheter) is inserted into a vein and threaded up to the heart. When the catheterization is intended for diag-

C

nosis or evaluation of the state of coronary blood vessels, a radiopaque dye is injected through the catheter allowing for x-ray visualization.

If the coronary blood vessels are found to be diseased, the physician may decide to proceed with coronary angioplasty. *See angioplasty.*

cardiac enzymes – Organic catalysts found in heart tissue. These enzymes are necessary to perform metabolic functions within the heart cells. When the heart muscle is injured, as in a myocardial infarction (heart attack), heart cells die and release their contents, including these enzymes, into the blood. In the blood, these enzymes are harmless but measuring their concentration in blood is a valuable part of the diagnostic work-up for myocardial infarction.

cardiac glycoside – A class of drugs that increases the force of heart contractions. Cardiac glycosides are found in the foxglove plant. First discovered by William Withering in the 18th century, one of these drugs (digoxin) is still commonly used to treat congestive heart failure and some abnormal heart rhythms.

cardiac output – The amount of blood the heart pumps with each contraction. The primary function of the heart is to provide enough blood supply to support the metabolic needs of the rest of the body. Conditions such as congestive heart failure and cardiac arrhythmias progressively decrease cardiac output.

cardiac workload – The amount of work the heart must perform in order to pump blood. Reducing preload and afterload helps to reduce the heart's workload in conditions such as heart failure. *See preload and afterload.*

cardio- – Prefix relating to the heart.

cardiogenic shock – Dangerous decrease in blood pressure due to a rapid decrease in cardiac output. Cardiogenic shock is a serious complication of myocardial infarction.

cardiologist – A physician who specializes in diagnosis and treatment of diseases of the cardiovascular system.

cardiology – The medical specialty that deals with the cardiovascular system. Cardiology encompasses the functions and malfunctions of the heart and blood vessels. It includes all the metabolic and hormonal factors that influence the health of the heart and blood vessels.

cardiomegaly – Enlargement of the heart. Cardiomegaly often occurs during the course of congestive heart failure as the heart is stretched by the volume and pressure of blood returning through the venous circulation. Cardiomegaly is usually a sign of a weakened heart.

cardiomyopathy – Disease of the heart muscle. Usually involves deterioration of function of cardiac muscle fibers.

cardiopulmonary resuscitation (CPR) – An emergency procedure that attempts to revive a person in cardiac arrest. CPR involves establishing an airway, assisted breathing, and chest compression to provide a semblance of circulation. Drug therapy administered during CPR may include cardiac stimulants and antiarrhythmics. *See cardiac arrest.*

cardioselective – Specific for the heart. This term is commonly applied to beta-adrenergic blockers that exert their effects on the heart with minimal effects on the lungs. *See beta-adrenergic blocker.*

cardioselectivity – The property of a drug or chemical agent to exert a greater effect on the heart or cardiac tissue than on other tissues or organs.

cardiotonic – Of benefit to the heart. For example, digoxin is sometimes described as a cardiotonic glycoside because it exerts a beneficial effect for people with heart failure.

cardiotoxic – Pertaining to a noxious effect on the heart or cardiac tissue. For example, the antineoplastic drug doxorubicin is said to be cardiotoxic because it often causes heart failure when used for long periods.

cardiotoxicity – Adverse effects on the heart. This term is applied to drugs and chemicals that impair the functions of the heart.

C

cardiovascular (CV) – Pertaining to the heart and blood vessels.

cardiovascular disorder – A medical condition or disease of the heart and/or blood vessels.

cardiovascular surgeon – A physician who specializes in surgical treatments of the heart and blood vessels.

cardiovascular system – The part of the body involved with the blood circulation. Includes the heart and blood vessels.

carditis – An inflammation of heart tissue. Carditis may be due to infection or an immune system problem.

caregiver – A person responsible for the medical care of another person. Examples of caregivers include a parent taking care of a child or a paid aide taking care of an adult.

caries – A specific site of tooth decay. Most commonly called a tooth cavity.

cariogenic – An agent that causes dental caries. Sugar is the most common cariogenic material.

carrier – A person who is capable of spreading an infection to others. Carriers do not have symptoms of the disease they carry. In some cases they may have been ill with the disease and appear to be cured, yet they still carry and are capable of spreading virulent microorganisms.

In insurance terms, a carrier is an insurer, government agency, or other organization that administers insurance programs.

carryover – A provision where deductible medical expenses from one year may be applied or carried over to the next year. This is most commonly done when a deductible is met near the end of a calendar year but the illness or injury extends into the next year.

cartilage – Connective tissue that provides form or support for an anatomical feature. Cartilage is more pliable than bone. Cartilage gives form to the nose and supports the functions of joints.

carve-out benefit – A health benefit that is removed from an insurance plan. Employer groups often carve out pharmacy, vision,

C

mental health, or dental benefits from their standard insurance policies and then bid them out to companies that specialize in those benefits. For example, a company may choose to carve out the pharmacy benefit from its health insurance plan, then arrange for a pharmacy benefit management company to administer the company's drug benefit. Sometimes employer groups carve out certain benefits because they do not wish to pay for those services.

case management – A process where a health insurer assigns a health care professional, (e.g., registered nurse, physician, social worker) to monitor the progress of patients with specific health care needs. Case managers may intervene with the insurance company, health care facility, or the patients' physicians to coordinate care. In some cases the patients themselves may be active participants in the process.

case manager – A person who practices case management.

catabolic – Pertaining to catabolism.

catabolism – The metabolic breakdown of stored proteins, carbohydrates, or fats to provide energy. While catabolism occurs continuously to some degree in every living being, excessive catabolism leads to wasting of tissues. Opposite of anabolism.

catalyst – A chemical that facilitates the reaction of two or more other chemicals without itself being permanently changed. Catalysts that are composed of organic material are called enzymes.

cataract – An opacity of the lens of the eye. As the lens becomes more opaque, less light passes and visual acuity is reduced. Cataracts occur commonly with advancing age. Cataracts may also be a side effect of prolonged use of anti-inflammatory eye drops.

catecholamine – One of a group of chemicals produced in nervous tissue. Catecholamines regulate a wide range of functions, including thought processes, hormone secretions, heart rate, and blood pressure. The most common catecholamines are epinephrine, norepinephrine, dopa, and serotonin.

cathartic – An agent that produces a bowel movement. A laxative.

C

catheter – A hollow tube intended to either administer fluids or drain fluids. For example, urinary catheters are passed into the bladder to remove urine. Intravenous catheters are inserted into veins to administer intravenous fluids.

cavity – A hollow area (e.g., abdominal cavity). Also a colloquial term for dental caries.

c.c. – Abbreviation for cubic centimeter. The preferred term for this unit of measurement is milliliter (ml), one thousandth of a liter. A cubic centimeter and a milliliter are virtually identical in size.

CCB – *See calcium channel blocker.*

CCU – *See coronary care unit.*

CDC – *See Centers for Disease Control and Prevention.*

cell – The smallest unit of life that can live independent of a larger creature. Even simple cells are highly organized, consisting of a cell wall or membrane, cytoplasm, and usually a nucleus. Some creatures, for example a bacterium, exist as a single-celled life form. Most life, however, exists as structures of multiple cells.

Cells may be highly specialized. For example, adipose cells store fat in the body while muscle cells contract to allow movements.

cellulitis – An infection of the subcutaneous tissue. Cellulitis is usually caused by an injury that pierces the outermost layer of skin and allows bacteria to reach the lower layers. Cellulitis is usually painful and is capable of spreading rapidly over a large area. Cellulitis is often treated with intravenous antibiotics.

census – The number of patients occupying a hospital or other residential health care facility.

Centers for Disease Control and Prevention (CDC) – A division of the United States Public Health Service. The Centers for Disease Control and Prevention analyze data on infectious diseases and track epidemics worldwide. The CDC makes recommendations on immunization programs in the United States and determines immunization needs of Americans traveling abroad. CDC also provides consultative services to physicians and public health departments. Located in Atlanta, Georgia.

central nervous system (CNS) – The primary communication and control system in the body. The central nervous system consists of the brain, spinal cord, and the nerves that branch out from those structures. The central nervous system controls nerve functions as varied as abstract thought to involuntary smooth muscle movement.

cephalosporin – A class of antibiotics effective against both Gram-positive and Gram-negative organisms. The cephalosporins share many properties with penicillins, including allergic reactions. Cephalosporins affect a wider range of bacteria than do the penicillins.

cerebral – Pertaining to the cerebrum of the brain and its functions.

cerebral embolism – A blood clot that breaks away from the wall of a blood vessel and then lodges in a blood vessel in the cerebrum portion of the brain. Cerebral embolism is the leading cause of stroke.

cerebral hemorrhage – Bleeding from a blood vessel in the cerebrum. Cerebral hemorrhage may result from an aneurysm or head trauma.

cerebral thrombosis – A blood clot that forms in a blood vessel in the cerebrum portion of the brain.

cerebro- – Prefix relating to the cerebrum.

cerebrospinal fluid – The protective and cushioning fluid that forms around the brain and the spinal cord. Small amounts of cerebrospinal fluid can be tapped and examined for diagnosis of some diseases and infections of the central nervous system.

cerebrovascular – Pertaining to the blood vessels or blood circulation in the cerebrum.

cerebrovascular accident – *See stroke.*

cerebrum – The largest portion of the brain. Functions include cognition, memory, movement, emotions, and sensory perception.

cerumen – Earwax.

C

cervical – Pertaining to a cervix. The term may apply to either the uterine cervix (the narrow opening to the uterus) or the neck of the body (the structure that supports the head).

cervical mucus – The clear, viscous fluid secreted from the uterine cervix. The cervical mucus changes viscosity during the menstrual cycle and is sometimes used as a rough indicator of fertility.

cervicitis – Inflammation of the uterine cervix.

cervix – A general term meaning neck. Most commonly, the term is applied to the uterine cervix, the neck-like structure at the lower end of the uterus.

CFC – *See chlorofluorocarbon*.

chain pharmacy – One of a group of four or more pharmacies owned by an individual or a corporation.

channeling – The process of using either incentives or rigid plan requirements to persuade insurance plan members to use designated care providers.

chargeback – A system where a pharmaceutical manufacturer repays a drug wholesaler for drugs sold to a pharmacy at a contracted price. Chargebacks are most commonly applied in situations where a high volume purchaser (e.g., a hospital group, a group purchasing organization, a mail order pharmacy) contracts with a drug manufacturer for a volume discount. When a qualified pharmacy buys contracted drugs through its wholesaler, the wholesaler charges the pharmacy the contract price for the drug. This price is usually lower than the price the wholesaler itself pays for the drug. The wholesaler then charges back to the drug manufacturer the difference in costs plus a handling charge.

chart – The clinical record relating to a patient's care. A chart may be written on paper or stored in an electronic medium. Typically, a chart contains demographic information, insurance information, laboratory test values, and health care workers' notations regarding the patient's specific problems, diagnosis, treatments given, and changes in status.

CHD – *See coronary heart disease*.

chelation – The chemical combination of a metal with a water-soluble molecule. Originally, one or more chelating agents were given to patients with symptoms of heavy metal (e.g., arsenic, mercury, lead, iron) poisoning. The water-soluble compound formed by the combination of a chelating agent with the metal is easier for the body to eliminate than is the metal itself. Now, a more common application of chelation is to combine a chelating agent with a nutritionally valuable (e.g., manganese, potassium, chromium) mineral. The resulting complex is claimed to be better absorbed than the more traditional metal salts.

chemical conjunctivitis – Inflammation, due to direct contact with a substance, of the mucous membrane that covers the exterior of the eye and the inside of the eyelid.

chemical peel – A dermatologic procedure where irritating agents are applied to the skin. The outer layer of skin sloughs off and leaves behind more attractive and more elastic skin.

chemical synthesis – The process of combining two or more compounds to form a new entity. This term is most commonly applied to organic chemical reactions.

chemist – A person trained in the science of chemistry. Pharmacists are called chemists in much of the English-speaking world.

chemoreceptor trigger zone (CTZ) – The portion of the brain that initiates feelings of nausea. If stimulated strongly enough, the chemoreceptor trigger zone sends a message to the brain's true vomiting center and vomiting ensues. The physiologic purpose of the chemoreceptor trigger zone is to detect poisons in the blood and produce vomiting to clear them from the digestive tract. Most antinauseant drugs suppress the function of the chemoreceptor trigger zone.

chemotaxis – A process where chemicals attract or repel cells or organisms. For example, a torn blood vessel releases chemicals that attract platelets. These platelets clump together at the site of the injury to form a clot.

chemotherapeutic agent – A drug used in chemotherapy.

C

chemotherapy – In the broadest sense, chemotherapy is treatment of a medical condition with a chemical agent. Most often, the term is applied to drug treatments of cancer. Sometimes the term is also used in the context of antibiotic treatment of infections or antipsychotic drug treatment of mental illness.

CHF – *See heart failure.*

child-resistant packaging – Product packaging intended to make it more difficult for children to open a container. Child-resistant packaging has proven itself effective in saving thousands of children's lives. In most cases, the packaging causes children under five years old to lose interest in the contents of the container and move on to some other activity. Unfortunately, some adults also have difficulty opening these containers.

chill – A feeling of cold, often accompanied by shivering. Chills may be caused by hypothermia but more often they are part of the body's response to fever.

chiropractic – An alternative medical practice that relies on compression or manipulation of the spinal column to treat illnesses or relieve symptoms.

chiropractor – A practitioner of chiropractic. In addition to spinal treatments, chiropractors may also choose to use other alternative treatments such as acupuncture, aromatherapy, massage, and herbal therapy.

Chiropractors hold doctor of chiropractic (D.C.) degrees and must pass state licensing examinations.

chlamydia – A microorganism capable of causing urinary tract infections and infections of the cervix, endometrium, and fallopian tubes in women and the urethra, epididymis, and prostate in men. Chlamydia infections are usually passed through sexual contact.

chlorofluorocarbon (CFC) – An organic chemical that contains chlorine and fluorine. Chlorofluorocarbons have been used as propellants in aerosols. These chemicals have been associated with depletion of the earth's ozone layer.

C

CHO – *See carbohydrate.*

cholecystectomy – The surgical removal of the gallbladder.

cholecystitis – Inflammation of the gallbladder. May be caused by infection or the presence of stones.

cholesterol – A fatty alcohol with a steroid nucleus. Cholesterol is found in highest concentration in animal muscles and organs. Cholesterol does not exist in plants.

Cholesterol is essential for certain cell structures; however, excess cholesterol can deposit in blood vessels and lead to cardiovascular disease.

cholinergic – Relating to nerve functions that are regulated by acetylcholine. The effects of acetylcholine and cholinergic drugs include skeletal muscle contraction, slowing heart rate, increasing gastric acid secretion, intestinal stimulation.

chorea – Spasmodic muscle movements, usually abrupt in nature. Chorea may be the result of a neurologic disorder (e.g., Huntington's chorea) or may be drug-induced. Chorea is a common side effect of antiparkinson drugs.

choreoathetoid – Pertaining to choreoathetosis.

choreoathetosis – Abnormal movements that consist of components of both chorea and athetosis. Typically, these movements start as an abrupt motion (chorea), then end with a writhing action (athetosis). Choreoathetosis is one manifestation of tardive dyskinesia, a complication of treatment with antipsychotic drugs.

chromosome – The structure that holds an organism's genes. Chromosomes are usually located in the cellular nucleus. Humans have 46 chromosomes arranged in 23 pairs.

chronic – Of long duration. There is no specific delineation between the point where acute ends and chronic begins.

chronic bronchitis – A long-term condition of inflammation of the bronchioles in the lungs. Chronic bronchitis is one manifestation of chronic obstructive pulmonary disease, the other being emphysema.

C

Chronic bronchitis usually results from many years of physical or chemical insult to the lungs. The most common cause is long-term smoking. People with chronic bronchitis typically have a chronic cough that produces large amounts of mucus. Infections are common.

chronic disease – A medical condition of long duration. Chronic disease is typically of years' duration and follows a slowly progressive course.

chronic obstruction lung disease (COLD) – Abbreviation for chronic obstructive lung disease. *See chronic obstructive pulmonary disease.*

chronic obstructive pulmonary disease (COPD) – A long-term, slowly progressive lung disease characterized by a decreased ability to exhale due to decreased elasticity of lung tissue. Patients with COPD typically have elements of both chronic bronchitis and emphysema and experience frequent lung infections. Lung infections are common in people with COPD. The condition is most commonly caused by long-term smoking or exposure to dust particles. Black lung disease is a form of COPD associated with coal mining.

chronic pain – Discomfort of long duration. Unlike acute pain, which is short-term and typically caused by an injury (e.g., scraped knee, fractured bone, etc.) or short-term illness (e.g., tension headache), chronic pain may last for years, despite treatment. Chronic pain may be due to psychological or neurological conditions or may be the result of a chronic disease such as cancer. Although narcotics may be effective in controlling chronic pain, the benefit of pain relief must be weighed against the risk of addiction. Depending upon the cause of the pain, other treatments include nonnarcotic drugs, surgery, physical therapy, psychotherapy, acupuncture, massage therapy, and chiropractic.

chronopharmacology – The study of the effects of time of day on drug effects. In some cases, drug effects and side effects change slightly at different times of the day because the body releases some hormones and other chemicals at different rates as the day goes by.

churning – The practice of performing a service more often than necessary in order to collect additional reimbursement. For example, a physician may churn patients by having them come back to the office more often than necessary or a pharmacist may churn by dispensing small amounts of medicine in order to collect more dispensing fees on the refills.

chylomicron – A small fat globule that travels through the blood. Chylomicra (or chylomicrons) are formed in the digestive tract and are released from there into the blood and collected by the liver. The primary purpose of chylomicra is to transport fat from the intestines to the liver, where they are metabolized. Fat-soluble vitamins may also be carried in chylomicra.

chyme – The partially digested contents of the stomach and upper intestinal tract. Chyme is composed of food, hydrochloric acid from the stomach, and digestive enzymes.

-cide – Suffix meaning to kill. For example, a fungicide is an agent that kills fungus.

ciliary – Pertaining to hair or hair-like structures.

circulation – The route of blood through the heart and blood vessels.

circulatory system – The anatomic structures that support blood flow. Circulation is initiated by the pumping function of the heart. The heart starts the process by pushing blood into the aorta. From there, blood flows into the arteries and then to the arterioles. Arterioles distribute blood to the capillaries, which provide oxygen and nutrients to individual cells in the body and pick up their waste. From the capillaries, blood flows into the venous side of the circulation to begin its return to the heart. Venules are the smallest vessels in the venous circulation. Venules receive blood from the capillaries and direct it into the veins. The veins empty into the vena cava and the vena cava returns blood to the heart.

cirrhosis – A collective term for diseases that cause slowly progressive deterioration of liver function. Cirrhosis is characterized by damage to the functional cells of the liver and by scarring. The liver forms nodules as it tries to regenerate itself. Eventually, blood flow through the liver is impaired and the ability of the liver to

C

function diminishes and the liver fails.

Cirrhosis may result from long-term alcohol abuse, heart failure, environmental toxins, or hepatitis.

cirrhotic – Pertaining to cirrhosis.

Cl – Chemical symbol for chlorine or chloride.

claim – A request to an insurance company for payment for a covered benefit. A claim may be filed by a covered person or by a service provider (e.g., hospital, physician, pharmacy).

claim denial – A decision on the part of an insurance company that a claim is not to be paid. The denial may be generated because:

- the service provided did not meet the criteria for coverage (e.g., a drug that the plan does not cover),

- the claim was not submitted properly (e.g., a form was not completed correctly), or

- required procedures were not followed (e.g., absence of a second opinion before elective surgery).

Insurance companies typically provide a mechanism for appealing claim denials.

claim form – The document used to file an insurance claim. Claim forms may be paper or electronic and may be completed by either the insured person or by the service provider. In pharmacy, most claims for prescription drugs are filed electronically at the time the prescription is filled. In most cases, the patient only needs to sign a log to indicate that service was provided.

claims processor – A company that administers payments on behalf of an insurance company. In pharmacy, these companies are usually referred to as pharmacy benefit management companies or PBMs.

The most basic role of the PBM is to receive a claim either directly from the pharmacy at the time a prescription is filled or from the patient via a mail-in form. The PBM uses information provided by the insurance company to verify that the patient is eligible for the service being billed. If everything is correct, the PBM mails out a check to the pharmacy or patient and then bills the

C

insurance company for the payment plus a handling fee. *See also pharmacy benefit management company.*

claims review – A part of the approval process an insurance company uses to assure the legitimacy of claims filed before authorizing payment.

claudication – Limping. In general usage, claudication has come to be synonymous with intermittent claudication. *See intermittent claudication.*

clearance – Removal of a substance from the blood. In pharmacy, clearance is usually expressed in the context of the rate of removal of a drug by the kidneys. Measurement of clearance can determine whether or not a drug is being eliminated from the body at a proper rate. Excessive clearance may make the drug less effective while slow clearance may cause drug accumulation and toxicity.

clinic – A medical facility where ambulatory patients receive evaluation, diagnosis, and treatment. A clinic may be either a single office or a building. In common usage, a clinic is usually part of a hospital or governmental agency. In some cases (e.g., Mayo Clinic, Menninger Clinic, Cleveland Clinic), the term clinic applies to a whole complex of hospitals and other treatment facilities.

clinical – Pertaining to a clinic or treatment of a patient. The term may also be applied to the actual characteristics of a patient's disease (e.g., the clinical course of an illness) rather than to the theoretical or expected course.

clinical pathologist – A physician who specializes in the diagnosis of disease through examination of body tissues. Clinical pathologists may make these diagnoses by examination of cadavers at autopsy or by microscopic examination of tissues removed through biopsy or surgery.

clinical pathway – A detailed plan for diagnosis and treatment of a specific disease. Clinical pathways, sometimes called treatment algorithms or critical pathways, are usually drawn out as diagrams.

C

Clinical pathways may be developed by a single expert or more commonly by a multidisciplinary team of specialists within a professional organization, university, or hospital. The purpose of a clinical pathway is to assure proper and uniform treatment of a disease. Clinical pathways provide enough detail to offer guidance for nearly every eventuality.

clinical pharmacist – A pharmacist whose practice is oriented toward patient care. Although there are many exceptions, clinical pharmacists most commonly work in an institutional setting such as a hospital or clinic.

Clinical pharmacists may act as drug therapy advisors to physicians, nurses, and other health professionals. In some cases, they have patients assigned to them for medication monitoring. They may also participate in educational programs for patients or health care professionals.

Most clinical pharmacists have a doctor of pharmacy (Pharm.D.) degree, but that degree is not a requirement.

clinical pharmacologist – A physician who has had special training in drug therapy.

clinical practice guideline – See *clinical pathway*.

clinical privileges – Permission for a nonemployee health care professional to practice at a specific institution, usually a hospital. Clinical privileges may be limited (e.g., admitting privileges but not surgical privileges) according to the qualifications of the applicant. Among the professionals who need clinical privileges are physicians, dentists, and psychologists.

Clinical privileges often correspond to an applicant's specialty. For example, a pediatrician may be granted full privileges in the children's section but not elsewhere. A radiologist may be granted certain privileges but not be allowed to do thoracic surgery.

clinical protocol – A guideline for diagnosis or treatment of a specific condition. Clinical protocols are usually less detailed than clinical pathways.

clinical psychologist – A person who diagnoses and treats mental illnesses. Clinical psychologists must possess a master's degree or

C

a doctorate in clinical psychology. They must also complete a supervised training period prior to licensing by the state.

Clinical psychologists evaluate patients by testing, interviewing, and observing. They employ a wide variety of therapies, depending upon the needs of the patient and their own training. In most states, clinical psychologists cannot prescribe medications.

clinical response – The reaction of a patient to a treatment or other stimulus. For example, the desired clinical response to a dose of aspirin for a person with a headache is relief of pain. Clinical responses may be beneficial or harmful. A treatment may totally correct a medical condition (beneficial) or may cause a side effect (harmful).

clinical study – See *clinical trial.*

clinical trial – An evaluation of a treatment or diagnostic procedure using human subjects. Well-organized clinical trials provide for the safety of the subjects and include techniques to minimize any bias on the part of the investigators.

clinician – A health professional who works directly with patients.

clone – A cell, group of cells, or even an entire plant or animal that was developed from a single cell without the normal process of reproduction. A cloned cell has exactly the same genetic make-up as the cell it was developed from.

cloning – The process of making a clone.

closed access – A type of health insurance plan that requires patients to select a primary care physician from the plan's list of contracted doctors. The patient must see that physician for all care. Only that physician is permitted to make referrals for specialized care. Also called a gatekeeper model.

Despite the closed access provision, a plan may make exceptions to the gatekeeper feature. For example, a woman may be allowed an annual visit with a gynecologist without going through her primary care physician. Emergency services are also exceptions, although specific procedures may apply.

closed formulary – A list of drugs the plan covers. In the case of a closed formulary, only those specific drugs are covered and no others. If a physician prescribes a drug other than one on the closed formulary, either the prescription must be changed to a covered drug or the patient must pay the full price for the medicine. In special cases, the physician may appeal to the health plan to request an exception. In these cases the physician must usually provide the plan with documentation or other evidence that the patient cannot use a formulary drug. The insurance company may approve or deny such requests. *See also formulary.*

closed panel – An exclusive list of health care providers approved to participate in an insurance plan. Providers (e.g., pharmacies, physicians, dentists) who are not on this panel will not be reimbursed by the plan, even if they provide service to a plan member. Special provisions are usually made for emergency care.

clot – A soft mass intended to stop bleeding. Clots are comprised of platelets and fibrin and form at the point where a blood vessel is cut or broken. Unfortunately, clots sometimes form spontaneously inside blood vessels and obstruct blood flow. These clots can break away and cause heart attacks or strokes.

clotting factor – One of a group of blood chemicals that interact with each other to form blood clots. In order for a clot to form, each clotting factor must be present in sufficient concentration. Lack of a single clotting factor causes clotting to fail. In hemophilia, patients are unable to produce at least one clotting factor.

cluster headache – An intense pain in the head, similar to migraine headache. The pain of a cluster headache is severe and is usually localized to a specific area. They are called cluster headaches because they usually occur in bunches. A patient may have several of these each day for several days. Weeks or months may intervene before another cluster occurs.

cm – Abbreviation for centimeter.

CMV – *See cytomegalovirus.*

CNS – *See central nervous system.*

co- – Prefix meaning with or along with.

coagulant – An agent or substance that facilitates blood clotting.

C

coagulation – The process of blood clotting.

coalition – An alliance of large employers who pool their resources and buying power to negotiate more favorable insurance rates. The businesses in these coalitions are usually located in a single metropolitan area or state.

COB – *See coordination of benefits.*

COBRA – *See Consolidated Omnibus Budget Reconciliation Act.*

cochlea – A portion of the inner ear essential for hearing and balance.

cochlear – Pertaining to the cochlea.

cocktail – A liquid that contains a mixture of drugs. For example, the Brompton's cocktail, a mixture that was used for decades as a treatment for cancer pain, contained a narcotic, a stimulant, and an antiemetic.

The advantage of a cocktail is that it reduces the number of doses of medicine a patient must take. The disadvantage is that the proportions of ingredients are fixed and the dose of one medicine cannot be changed without changing the dose of all of them.

coenzyme – An organic chemical that must combine with an enzyme in order for the enzyme to function. Unless they combine with an enzyme, coenzymes usually have no function of their own. Most vitamins are coenzymes.

cofactor – A molecule that is necessary for another molecule to function. Coenzymes are one type of cofactor.

cognition – The process of knowing. Cognition includes thinking, perception, recognition, judgment, memory, and imagination.

cognitive – Pertaining to thought processes.

cognitive disturbance – A mental or emotional disorder that impairs or hinders thought processes.

cognitive services – In pharmacy, cognitive services are the consultative services some pharmacists provide aside from drug dispensing. These services may include patient interviewing, evaluation, teaching, or counseling. Pharmacists may charge for these services or bill insurance companies for compensation.

cohort – A group of people or a population selected for a study.

coinsurance – The portion of health care costs paid for by a patient. In many cases, insurance plans do not require coinsurance beyond a copayment. Many indemnity plans and preferred provider organizations (PPOs) require 20% coinsurance, often after meeting an annual deductible.

COLD – Abbreviation for chronic obstructive lung disease. *See chronic obstructive pulmonary disease.*

cold – *See common cold.*

cold sore – A blister or lesion in or around the mouth. Also called herpes labialis. Cold sores are caused by the herpes simplex virus. These sores most commonly occur during times of physical stress.

colic – Painful spasms in the colon. The term is most commonly applied to a condition in infants characterized by crying, swallowing air, cramps, and increased gas.

colicky – Pertaining to the symptoms of colic.

coliform – Pertaining to the bacteria that are normally found in the large intestine.

colitis – Inflammation of the large intestine.

collagen – The primary protein found in bone, cartilage, and connective tissue. Collagen provides strength and support for these structures.

collagen disease – A group of disorders characterized by an attack of the immune system upon the host's own connective tissue. Rheumatoid arthritis is an example of a collagen disease.

collateral circulation – A network of small blood vessels that serves as a back-up for normal circulation. For example, people who slowly develop a coronary artery obstruction utilize collateral blood vessels to carry blood around the obstruction.

C

Collateral circulation needs time to develop itself. While collateral circulation helps to supply the metabolic needs of the heart in the above example, it is not adequate if the blockage is sudden.

colon – The large intestine. Also called the large bowel.

colonic – Pertaining to the colon. In some cases an enema is referred to as a colonic.

colony – A growth of cells, usually cells grown in a laboratory environment. When studying bacteria, a colony typically develops from the isolation of a single organism.

colony stimulating factor (CSF) – A naturally occurring protein that stimulates the bone marrow to produce white blood cells. Colony stimulating factor can now be produced commercially and administered to patients with low white blood cell counts. CSF is commonly used to treat people who have low blood counts due to cancer or cancer treatment.

colorectal – Pertaining to both the colon and rectum.

colostomy – A surgically produced opening that links the large intestine to the outside of the body. Colostomies become necessary when a medical condition prevents the colon from functioning normally.

coma – A deep state of unconsciousness from which the individual cannot be aroused.

comarket – An agreement between two pharmaceutical manufacturers in which both companies promote the same drug. In a typical case, a company with a small sales force contracts with a larger company to help sell one of the smaller company's products. The combined sales force is able to increase market awareness of the product. The larger company is compensated for its efforts.

comatose – The state of being in a coma.

combination drug – A medication that contains more than one active ingredient. The ingredients may be combined in order to treat a wider spectrum of symptoms, to decrease side effects, or to increase the effectiveness of one of the ingredients.

combination therapy – A treatment that has more than one component. Examples of combination therapies include using two or more drugs at the same time, drug therapy plus psychotherapy, or surgery plus physical therapy.

comedo – The basic lesion of acne. Comedos are caused when the flow of oil from a pore is obstructed and inflammation results. Comedos are often referred to as pimples, whiteheads, blackheads, or zits.

comedone – *See comedo.*

commercial carrier – A private company that provides insurance coverage to a group.

common cold – An upper respiratory infection caused by a virus. Symptoms include sneezing, runny nose, and nasal congestion and usually last from three to five days. Common cold is usually not associated with fever. Fever or illness lasting more than a week may be indications of a different problem.

communicable – Capable of being spread from one place to another. Most commonly used in the context of communicable disease, an infection that is spread from one person to another.

community-acquired infection – An infectious disorder contracted outside of a hospital. Community-acquired infections often have different characteristics (e.g., virulence, antibiotic sensitivities) than hospital-acquired infections.

community hospital – A health care facility established to serve the medical needs of its specific geographic area. Formerly, community hospitals were established as not-for-profit facilities. Community hospitals were often founded by religious groups or other civic minded organizations.

comorbidity – The presence of at least two unrelated disorders. For example, a person may have both hypertension and diabetes. Comorbidity increases medical costs, plus the presence of one condition may complicate treatment of the other.

compatible – In pharmacy, the ability of two medications to be physically mixed together without either drug altering the chemical properties of the other.

C

compensation – A process where a diseased organ, organ system, or other organ system alters its normal functions in order to continue to survive. For example, in response to poor circulation due to heart failure, the heart tries to beat faster and the kidneys retain water. Unfortunately, some compensatory mechanisms are counterproductive.

Also, payment for a service.

competence – The ability to perform necessary functions. For example, abnormal rhythms decrease the heart's competence.

complement – A group of proteins in the blood that assist (complement) the function of antibodies in the immune system. Complements attack some bacteria and are involved in inflammation.

complete remission – The total disappearance of symptoms of a disease. The term is most commonly applied to cancer. Remission, however, is not necessarily a cure. Cancers and chronic diseases may recur after a quiet period.

complex carbohydrate – A long chain of sugar molecules. Starches derived from grains and vegetables are common examples of complex carbohydrates.

complex partial seizure – A form of epilepsy caused by abnormal electrical discharges in the temporal lobe of the brain. The disorder commonly manifests itself very differently from one person to another. Symptoms may include loss of consciousness, loss of memory of events during the seizure, emotional outbursts, physical or verbal violence, or uncontrolled physical shaking.

compliance – The process of following medical instructions. Compliance relates to correctly taking medication, keeping appointments, and following instructions of clinicians regarding diet, exercise, or other treatments.

complication – An unwanted and undesirable event that occurs in relation to a medical condition. A complication may range in severity from benign to fatal.

compounded prescription – A preparation of medicine that has more than one component. Most commonly, compounded prescriptions are medicines that must be put together by a pharmacist. Compounded prescriptions may be prepared as lotions, ointments, suppositories, capsules, solutions, or other forms.

compress – A bandage.

compulsion – An overwhelming urge to perform some physical act. Commonly encountered as part of obsessive-compulsive disorder, a type of anxiety where an individual has repetitive thoughts (obsession) that lead to repetitive or ritualistic actions (compulsion).

con- – Prefix meaning with or along with.

concentration – The amount of a chemical in another substance. Concentrations are usually measured in terms of parts per million or percentage strength.

Also, a mental process that allows a person to focus thoughts on a single topic.

concomitant – Accompanying or going along with.

concomitant therapy – The simultaneous use of two or more treatments or types of treatment. For example, a person receiving physical therapy for arthritis might also be taking concomitant drug therapy.

concurrent drug evaluation – A process, usually computerized, that reviews the appropriateness of a drug during the course of therapy. *See also prospective drug evaluation and retrospective drug evaluation.*

concussion – A violent shaking or shock. Most commonly associated with trauma to the head that causes loss of consciousness or other impairment of brain function.

condition – A state of health. Although a person's condition may be normal, the term also applies to any illness, injury, or other changed state of health.

condom – A sheath worn over the penis during intercourse to prevent sexually transmitted diseases or conception. Condoms may be made of sheep intestine (lambskin) or latex. Lambskin condoms are effective for prevention of conception but are too porous to

C

prevent transmission of viruses. Only latex condoms should be used to prevent sexually transmitted diseases.

condylomata acuminata – Genital warts. Condylomata may be contracted during sexual intercourse.

confabulation – A psychiatric symptom where a person fills in gaps of knowledge with fictional, often nonsensical, statements. A person who confabulates is usually convinced that his/her story is truthful and accurate.

confection – A solid or semisolid pharmaceutical preparation made with sugar, syrup, or honey. Seldom used anymore.

confidentiality – The legal or ethical imperative not to disclose details of a person's medical condition.

congenital – Relating to or existing at the time of birth. For example, a congenital heart problem is one that developed during pregnancy and was present at birth. Depending upon the type and severity of the condition, a congenital problem may be detected during pregnancy or may not be discovered until many years later.

congestion – The presence of an unusual amount of fluid or blood.

congestive heart failure (CHF) – *See heart failure.*

conjunctiva – The mucous membrane that covers the exterior of the eye and the inside of the eyelid.

conjunctivitis – Inflammation of the conjunctiva. Conjunctivitis can be caused by mechanical irritation, chemical irritation, allergy, or infection. When caused by bacterial infection, conjunctivitis is often called pink eye.

conservative – In medicine, pertains to a cautious, well-established approach. May apply to diagnostic procedures or treatment methods.

Consolidated Omnibus Budget Reconciliation Act (COBRA) – Legislation whose primary purpose was to fund the federal government. However, one provision of this act requires employers to offer continued health insurance coverage to personnel who

C

leave employment. Individuals who elect to COBRA their health insurance may be required to pay the entire cost of premiums. The act also exempts some categories of employers.

constipated – State of having constipation.

constipation – Infrequent, incomplete, or difficult bowel movements.

consultant physician – A physician with specific expertise who is called in to help evaluate or treat a patient. For example, an internist may ask a surgeon to evaluate and possibly operate on a mass.

contamination – Exposure of a wound or normally sterile field to bacteria. Most traumatic wounds have been contaminated with dirt or other debris; however, contamination is not the same as infection. Contamination is the mere presence of bacteria. Infection relates to the growth and multiplication of virulent microorganisms in a body tissue.

continuing education – A formalized learning process that extends beyond an initial training period. For example, all states require pharmacists to participate in continuing education programs every year. These programs usually involve a teaching experience followed by a test and issuance of a certificate.

continuum of care – The process of passing from one level of care to another. If done properly, patients should be able to transition from one health care facility or organization to another (e.g., from the hospital to home care or from home care to a skilled nursing facility) with minimal disruption. Accrediting organizations examine facilities' processes for assuring that such transfers are performed smoothly.

contra- – Prefix meaning against.

contraceptive – An agent that prevents pregnancy.

contraceptive foam – An aerosolized preparation that prevents pregnancy. Contraceptive foam is instilled into an applicator and then inserted into the vagina. The foam contains a chemical that skills sperm. While use of contraceptive foam reduces risk of pregnancy, it is more effective when used along with a diaphragm or a condom.

C

contraceptive jelly – A spermicidal gel that is used along with a diaphragm to prevent pregnancy. Contraceptive jelly seals the edge of the diaphragm against the vaginal wall so sperm cannot get past the diaphragm.

contraceptive sponge – An over-the-counter product that consists of a sponge permeated with a spermicide. The sponge is introduced into the vagina prior to intercourse and blocks the passage of sperm. Contraceptive sponges reduce risk of pregnancy but are more effective if used along with a condom.

contract – In a health insurance context, a contract is an insured family unit. Health insurance companies may report their size either in terms of members or contracts. A member is an insured individual while a contract is an insured family. A contract may consist of just one person or many persons. A plan with 100,000 members typically has about 43,000 contracts.

contract pharmacy – A pharmacy that has a legal arrangement with a health insurance company where the pharmacy provides service to health plan members for a predetermined rate and mode of compensation. A typical pharmacy contract provides that the pharmacy will serve all plan members who present prescriptions for covered drugs. The pharmacy will collect a copayment from the member and bill the insurance company for any balance due. In return for being listed as an approved pharmacy, the pharmacy charges the insurance company a discounted rate.

contraindication – A medical condition that precludes the use of a particular medication. For example, penicillin is contraindicated for a person who is allergic to the drug. Beta-blockers are contraindicated for people with asthma because they can initiate asthma attacks.

contrast medium – An agent that prevents passage of x-rays. Contrast media are typically injected intravenously at the beginning of a radiology procedure. When x-rayed, the blood vessel or other tissue infused with the contrast medium appears white on x-ray film. This allows the radiologist to see and evaluate any abnormal structures or obstructions.

C

control animal – Nonhuman subjects in a study that form the basis of comparison with the study agent or procedure. In a research study involving animals, control animals are those that are handled in exactly the same way as the experimental animals except that the control animals are not subjected to the experimental intervention. For example, control animals in a drug study eat the same diet, receive the same amount of exercise, live in the same temperature, humidity, etc. as the experimental group. Often the control and experimental animals are of the same age and even from same genetic line. However, when the experimental animals receive the study drug, the control animals either receive no drug or a placebo. After exposure to the study drug, differences between the two groups may be assumed to have been due to the drug rather than to other factors.

control group – Subjects in a study that form the basis of comparison with the study agent or procedure. In most studies, one group of subjects (study group) receives the medication or treatment intended to be evaluated. For comparison, another closely matched group (control group) receives either no treatment or a treatment with known outcome. In most cases, the purpose of such a study is to determine the difference in response between the two groups, and therefore, the differences between the two treatments.

controlled release – A dosage form that discharges drugs over an extended period of time. Most controlled release dosage forms are oral capsules or tablets. In the case of capsules, small beads of medication are specially coated within the capsule so that the medicine dissolves and releases itself more slowly. In the case of controlled release tablets, layers of special coatings within the tablet allow only small amounts of medicine, or minidoses, to be released at any one time. As the controlled release tablet travels through the digestive tract, the tablet eventually releases all of the medication. In most cases, oral controlled release dosage forms release their medications over a period of about 12 hours. Also called sustained release.

controlled study – A research evaluation between two or more groups where variables, with one important exception, are minimized or eliminated.

C

controlled substance – A drug recognized by the Drug Enforcement Agency (DEA) as having abuse potential. The DEA classifies controlled substances in one of five groupings, called schedules. The schedule designation depends upon the drug's clinical value and abuse potential. Schedule I (schedules are designated by Roman numerals) controlled substances have high abuse potential and have no legal clinical use. Marijuana and LSD are schedule I drugs.

Schedule II drugs have clinical value but also have high abuse potential. Schedule II prescriptions cannot be refilled. Examples include morphine and cocaine.

Schedule III and IV drugs have clinical value but less abuse potential. Schedule III and IV prescriptions may be refilled no more than 5 times within 6 months of the date the prescription was written. Examples include tranquilizers, pain relievers, and androgenic steroids.

Schedule V drugs have clinical value but low enough abuse potential that the federal government allows them to be sold without a prescription. Some states, however, do restrict these drugs to prescription-only status. Examples include cough syrups with codeine.

contusion – Blunt trauma to soft tissue. A bruise.

convulsant – An agent that causes a convulsion or seizure.

convulsion – A forceful series of uncontrolled muscle contractions that may affect the arms, legs, trunk, and/or head. The patient may lose consciousness and have no memory of the convulsion. Also known as a seizure.

convulsive – Pertaining to a convulsion.

coordination of benefits (COB) – A provision in health insurance contracts that applies when an insured person has coverage with more than one health plan. In these cases, the involved insurance companies work with each other to coordinate payments for medical service so that no overpayments are made.

copay – *See copayment.*

C

copayment – A fixed charge for health care service paid by the patient at the time service is rendered. Copayments most often apply to pharmacy services (e.g., $5 for a generic prescription and $10 for a brand name drug) and medical appointments.

Copayments serve two purposes. First, they help to reduce costs to insurance companies since the insurer reimburses the provider for the cost of service minus the amount of the copayment. Second, copayments reduce overuse of plan benefits because patients are less likely to see doctors or fill prescriptions for trivial purposes if they have to pay a portion of the cost.

COPD – *See chronic obstructive pulmonary disease.*

copromotion – *See comarket.*

coronary – Pertaining to the heart or the blood vessels supplying the heart.

coronary artery – The blood vessels that provide the blood supply for the heart. These blood vessels are essential for the health of the heart. Obstructions in the coronary arteries, caused either by fatty deposits or blood clots, reduce blood flow to the heart muscle. When blood flow is reduced too much, the heart may radiate pain (angina pectoris) or a section of heart muscle may die (myocardial infarction).

coronary artery bypass – A surgical procedure that splices a transplanted blood vessel into one or more coronary arteries in order to circumvent an obstruction.

coronary artery disease (CAD) – Condition characterized by blockage of the blood vessels (coronary arteries) that supply the heart muscle. In most cases, coronary artery disease is caused by lipid plaques or blood clots that reduce blood flow. Angina pectoris is often the first indication of a problem.

coronary artery spasm – A type of coronary artery disease characterized by sudden contractions of coronary arteries. The spasms temporarily reduce blood flow to the heart muscle and produce symptoms of angina pectoris.

coronary care unit – An intensive care unit specializing in the care of critically ill heart patients.

coronary heart disease (CHD) – Deterioration or occlusion of the blood vessels that supply the heart muscle. Most commonly, coronary heart disease is caused by fat or cholesterol deposits in the coronary arteries.

coronary thrombosis – An obstruction, either a blood clot or a lipid plaque, in a coronary artery.

cortex – The outer layer or portion of an organ. The term is most commonly applied to the kidneys and adrenal glands.

corticosteroid – A steroid that is secreted from the adrenal cortex. The adrenal gland secretes primarily two types of steroids: mineralocorticoids and glucocorticoids. *See steroid, mineralocorticoid, and glucocorticoid.*

cosmetic surgery – A surgical procedure that is not essential for health, but rather, is intended to enhance appearance. Most health insurance companies deny coverage for procedures they perceive to be solely cosmetic. In some cases (e.g., breast reconstruction), however, a health plan may approve a procedure if it can be convinced that the operation will have a positive psychological impact on the patient.

cost-benefit analysis – An assessment of the financial savings or other advantages derived from providing a specific service.

cost containment – A strategy that controls health plan expenses. Cost containment activities may include implementing or tightening a drug formulary, increasing copayments or coinsurance, requiring prior authorization or precertification for certain services, or promoting earlier hospital discharges.

cost effectiveness – The relationship between the cost of providing insurance coverage for a benefit versus the cost of not providing that coverage. For example, a health insurer may wish to examine the cost of covering smoking deterrents versus the cost of treating smoking-related illnesses that could be avoided by promoting smoking deterrents.

cost minimization analysis – A study of various interventions with the intention of finding the lowest cost intervention that provides an acceptable outcome. For example, a cost minimization analysis of drugs for hypertension would seek the least expensive drug that reduces blood pressure to an acceptable level for the majority of patients. These analyses can become quite complex because of related costs. Using an inexpensive drug may require more frequent physician visits or laboratory tests than a more expensive drug.

cost outlier – A patient whose health care expenses are far outside the norm.

cost shifting – A practice of charging some patients more because of discounts given to insurers or government programs. Most managed care companies require health care providers to grant them significant discounts in order to participate in their plans. In some cases, providers increase charges to their other patients (shift costs) in order to make up for the lost revenue.

cough – A sudden expulsion of air from the lungs and through the mouth. Cough is often described as productive or nonproductive. *See nonproductive cough and productive cough.*

cough suppressant – *See antitussive.*

counterdetailing – *See academic detailing.*

counterirritant – A drug that irritates surface nerve fibers when applied to the skin. Depending upon the specific ingredients, counterirritants produce feelings of heat or cold. When they work properly, counterirritants block the nerves trying to transmit sensations of pain or itching.

covered benefit – A service that is paid for by an insurance plan. Covered benefits may have significant limitations or exclusions. For example, many insurance plans provide coverage for prescription drugs in general but do not cover drugs for weight loss.

covered drug – A medication that an insurance plan pays for. While there are exceptions, most health plans only cover prescription drugs.

CPR – *See cardiopulmonary resuscitation.*

C

crab – The crab louse. An insect resembling the appearance of a crab that infests body hair. Crab lice may be transmitted on clothing or by close personal contact.

cramp – A painful muscle spasm. Cramps commonly occur in the muscles of the extremities, uterus, and intestinal tract.

cranial – Pertaining to the head.

cranio- – Prefix relating to the cranium.

cream – A pharmaceutical preparation that combines an oil with water. Creams are usually used topically and may or may not contain medication. Creams are usually dispensed in a tube or jar. Creams differ from lotions in that lotions contain more water and are more fluid.

credential – A person's qualifications for performing a task. Credentials may include university degrees, state licenses, and certificates.

credentialing – The process of determining that a person is qualified for a task or assignment. In a hospital, for instance, the credentialing process verifies that all physicians on staff have graduated from medical school, are licensed by the state, and have completed appropriate residency or fellowship programs.

crisis – An intense attack during the course of a disease. Also, the point during the course of a disease where it becomes apparent whether the patient will survive or not.

critical – Pertaining to a crisis.

critical care – The management of a patient in crisis.

critical care unit (CCU) – A hospital floor specializing in treating patients who are critically ill. Depending upon the size of the hospital, there may be one critical care unit or several specialized units. Examples of specialized critical care units include newborn intensive care units, pediatric intensive care units, burn units, coronary care units, surgical intensive care units, and medical intensive care units.

critical pathway – *See clinical pathway.*

Crohn's disease – A condition of the intestinal tract characterized by patches of inflammation and even ulcer. Symptoms include fever, diarrhea, abdominal cramps and pain, and weight loss.

crossover study – A clinical study where each group in the study receives each treatment. For example, a study may start half of the study population with an investigational drug and half with an inert placebo. Midway through the study the two groups switch (crossover) so that those who started with placebo now take the study drug and vice versa. The purpose of a crossover design is to allow each subject to act as his/her own control.

cross-reactivity – A property where people who have a reaction to one medication have the same reaction to a similar medication. For example, people who have asthma attacks when they take aspirin are likely to have the same reaction (cross-react) if they take ibuprofen.

croup – An inflammation of the airway that produces a hoarse cough and wheezing. Croup is a disorder of children and is usually caused by a viral infection.

cryo- – Prefix pertaining to cold.

cryosurgery – An operation performed using cold. The most common form of cryosurgery is application of liquid nitrogen to remove skin lesions.

CSF – See *colony stimulating factor or cerebrospinal fluid.*

CTZ – See *chemoreceptor trigger zone.*

culture – The cultivation of cells, usually bacteria or viruses, for the purpose of further examination or study. Cultures are commonly employed for the diagnosis of infectious diseases. A specimen (e.g., blood, urine, feces, sputum, tissue scraping) is collected from the patient and a sample is placed in or on a culture medium. As they grow in the culture medium, bacteria can be microscopically or biochemically identified. They can also be exposed to various antibiotics to determine the most effective course of treatment.

culture medium – A nutrient system that promotes the growth of cells, usually microorganisms. Culture media may be either

C

semi-solid or liquid and may be used in petri dishes or test tubes.

cure – A total restoration of health following an illness. Relatively few medical conditions are cured with medication alone. Medicines can cure some skin problems, infections, peptic ulcers, and cancers. Rather than being used as cures, most medicines are employed to control symptoms, slow progression, or improve quality of life. For example, medicines do not cure epilepsy but can reduce the number of seizures. Medicines do not cure depression but can relieve symptoms until the depressive episode passes. Discontinuing medicines for chronic illnesses usually results in recurrence of symptoms.

customary charge – *See usual and customary charge.*

cutaneous – Pertaining to the skin.

cyanosis – Bluish discoloration of the skin. Cyanosis results from decreased oxygen supply to the affected area. Cyanosis may be localized, for example to a finger, when circulation to that area is impaired. Cyanosis may be generalized throughout the body, for example during a cardiac arrest.

cyanotic – Pertaining to cyanosis.

cycle – A repetitive series of events. The cardiac cycle, for example, is the sequence of actions that produce recurring heartbeats.

cyst – An abnormal sac or pouch that most often contains fluid or fat. Fluid cysts can often be reduced by aspirating with a needle and syringe. Fat-containing cysts usually need to be surgically excised. Depending upon its location and size, a cyst may be removed as an outpatient procedure or may require hospitalization.

cystic – Pertaining to a cyst or a bladder.

cystitis – Inflammation of a bladder, usually the urinary bladder.

cystogram – X-ray visualization of the urinary bladder, usually with the help of a contrast medium.

cytology – The study of the anatomy and function of cells.

cytomegalovirus (CMV) – A virus from the herpes family, cytomegalovirus is an opportunistic virus that usually only infects immunosuppressed patients. CMV can affect salivary glands, bone marrow, and the retinas of the eyes. *See also cytomegalovirus retinitis.*

cytomegalovirus (CMV) retinitis – Infection of the retina of the eye caused by cytomegalovirus. This infection rarely occurs in the presence of an intact immune system. However, patients with compromised immune systems (e.g., AIDS, cancer, organ transplant) are at risk of contracting this infection. Untreated, the condition leads to blindness.

cytotoxic – Having properties of a cytotoxin.

cytotoxic drug – A drug that kills cells. Usually used in the context of cancer chemotherapy.

cytotoxin – A drug, chemical, or environmental factor that impairs or destroys cell function.

dacry- – Pertaining to tears, the tear gland, or the tear duct.

dacryo- – Pertaining to tears, the tear gland, or the tear duct.

dacryorrhea – Abnormal and excessive flow of tears.

dactyl- – Pertaining to the fingers.

dactyledema – Swelling of the fingers due to accumulation of fluid.

dactylo- – Pertaining to the fingers.

dander – Minute scales of dead skin tissue not visible to the naked eye. Dander is shed from all skin surfaces. Visible dander shed from the head is called dandruff.

Because of wastes produced by mites that typically live in or on the skin, animal dander has the potential to cause allergic reactions, including asthma, in susceptible individuals. Dog or cat dander is a frequent cause of such problems.

dandruff – Visible flakes of dander, usually on the head. Dandruff by itself is a cosmetic, not a medical problem. Excessive flaking, especially if accompanied by inflammation or itching, may be an indication of a different dermatologic condition.

DAW – *See dispense as written.*

day supply maximum – The upper limit of days of medication the health plan will allow to be dispensed at one time. In general, health plans pay for up to a 34-day supply of medication from a retail pharmacy and a 90-day supply from a mail order pharmacy.

dB – Abbreviation for decibel.

db – Abbreviation for decibel.

D.C. – Abbreviation for doctor of chiropractic. *See chiropractor.*

D.D.S. – Abbreviation for doctor of dental surgery. A dental degree. *See dentist.*

DEA – *See Drug Enforcement Agency.*

deacidification – Removal or neutralization of acid. Seldom used in a clinical context, the term is more often applied to *in vitro* chemical reactions or purification processes.

dead – Lifeless. Having previously been alive, now without life.

Also, without feeling or sensations. For example, a patient may complain that when he sits for prolonged periods his legs go dead.

deaf – Unable to hear.

deafness – Inability to hear or to hear clearly. Deafness may be total, where an individual hears nothing at all, or it may be partial. For example, a person with high frequency deafness is not able to hear high-pitched tones but can adequately hear other sounds.

deaminase – An enzyme that detaches amino groups from carbon bonds.

death – The end of life processes. Formerly, death in humans was associated with the lack of a heartbeat. With cardiorespiratory support, however, a heartbeat can be artificially sustained indefinitely. Brain death, with the cessation of nerve functions in the brain, is now considered to be a better indicator of the end of life.

debility – Weakness, usually caused by aging or a disease process.

debridement – The surgical removal of dead tissue or contamination from a wound. For example, treatment for a decubitus ulcer includes cutting away (debriding) the dead flesh that surrounds the lesion. Debridement exposes living tissue that can begin a healing process.

decalcification – The process of removing calcium. Most commonly used in relation to loss of calcium from bones and teeth.

decant – To pour the liquid off of the top of another substance. Some chemical reactions and pharmaceutical products require that excess fluid be separated from a precipitate. Then either the fluid or the precipitate is saved and used for another purpose.

decarboxylase – An enzyme that removes a carbon dioxide group from an organic molecule.

decarboxylase inhibitor – A class of drug that reduces the effects of the enzyme dopa decarboxylase. This enzyme is responsible for degradation of dopamine, a drug commonly used to treat

Parkinson's disease. The effect of a dopa decarboxylase inhibitor is to increase the effectiveness of dopamine, allowing for lower doses of the drug and fewer side effects.

decay – The decomposition or rotting of organic material.

Also, the change of one radioactive element to another element.

decibel (dB, db) – One-tenth of a bel, a measure of sound intensity.

decompensation – Failure of back-up systems to prevent diminished function. Usually used in the context of heart disease where the course of the illness has progressed to the point where alternative physiologic functions are no longer adequate to control symptoms.

decongestant – A class of drugs that reverses excessive blood flow (congestion) into an area. Decongestants may be taken by mouth or applied directly to the affected area. The most common uses for decongestants are relief of nasal congestion due to infection or allergy and inflammation in the eyes.

decubitus ulcer – An erosion of skin, muscle, and connective tissue caused by the position of a person in bed. Decubitus ulcers (often called decubiti) occur when the weight of the body against a mattress restricts blood flow through the capillaries. If the pressure is not periodically relieved, the tissues in the affected area die due to lack of oxygen and nutrition. Decubiti are difficult to treat and slow to heal. Many cases can be prevented by turning bed-bound patients frequently, by using air mattresses or other pressure-relieving devices, and by practicing good hygiene. Also called pressure sore.

deductible – The money an insurance holder must pay before policy benefits begin. For example, a medical policy may stipulate a $1,000 annual deductible. Such a policy requires that the member pay the first $1,000 of medical expenses each year. Only after the entire deductible is met does insurance coverage begin. In general, a higher annual deductible allows the insurer to charge a lower monthly premium.

deductible carryover credit – Charges incurred at the end of one year that may be applied to the deductible for the following year.

deep vein thrombosis (DVT) – A blood clot in a large blood vessel. DVTs most commonly occur in the legs and are often associated with poor blood flow or lack of exercise. DVTs are usually painful and cause swelling and reddening in the affected area. DVTs are always dangerous since part of the clot may break away and lodge in the blood vessels that supply the heart, lungs, or brain. DVTs are usually treated with anticoagulants until the clot dissolves. Anticoagulant treatment may continue if the patient is at risk of developing more DVTs.

defecation – The process of having a bowel movement.

defensive medicine – The routine of covering all possible contingencies to avoid malpractice suits. Practicing defensive medicine typically causes physicians to order extra diagnostic tests and perhaps to call in additional specialists. These are done in excess of what is ordinarily needed to establish a diagnosis or monitor a patient's progress.

defibrillator – A device that delivers an electric shock for the purpose of correcting an irregular heart rhythm. Traditionally, defibrillators were used only in hospitals, clinics, and emergency vehicles. With advances in technology, some people are able to have small battery-powered defibrillators surgically implanted in their chests. The implanted defibrillator automatically fires a shock into the heart when it detects the presence of a dangerous heart rhythm.

deficiency – Lack of something. Usually used in the context of the lack of an important nutrient or biochemical.

deficiency disease – Any nutritional disorder caused by lack of one or more essential dietary components (e.g., amino acids, fatty acids, vitamins, minerals) or by inadequate calories.

definitive treatment – The therapy administered to treat a specific disorder. By contrast, supportive treatment is intended to relieve symptoms without necessarily treating the cause of the problem. For example, an antibiotic is a definitive treatment for an infection but aspirin, which only reduces pain and fever, is a supportive treatment.

degeneration – A worsening. A degenerative disease, for example, is a medical condition characterized by slow, progressive loss of structure or function of an organ or tissue.

degenerative – Pertaining to degeneration.

degenerative joint disease (DJD) – A slowly developing condition characterized by deterioration of cartilage in joints and over-growth of bone tissue. DJD most commonly affects the weight-bearing joints in the knees and hips, but can also affect the spine, fingers, and any other area where two bones meet. DJD is characterized by pain and stiffness. The condition usually appears first during middle-age and worsens with time. DJD is the most common form of arthritis. Also called osteoarthritis.

degradation – Breakdown of a complex chemical into simpler parts. For example, a drug that is not stored properly degrades, losing its effectiveness and sometimes forming toxic substances.

dehydration – Loss of water. As part of chemical purification process-es, dehydration may be intentional. In living systems, dehydra-tion occurs when fluid loss exceeds fluid intake. Dehydration may occur simply by failing to drink enough fluid. However, dehydration is more likely to occur as a consequence of a dis-ease process such as prolonged vomiting or diarrhea.

delayed hypersensitivity – A type of allergic reaction that takes hours or days to develop. Most allergic skin rashes, for example, are delayed hypersensitivity reactions.

delirium – A short-term state of confusion or disorientation. Delirium usually has an identifiable cause such as anxiety, oxygen starva-tion, drug toxicity, or drug abuse. If not appropriately treated, however, delirium can progress to permanent brain damage.

delivery system – Any dosage form that transfers medication to a liv-ing tissue, organ, or organism. Usually used in the context of a specialized dosage form; for example, a sustained-release tablet or an implanted drug-releasing capsule.

delouse – To remove or kill lice, usually with a topically applied insec-ticide.

delusion – A psychological state characterized by beliefs in things that cannot be true. Persons with delusions of grandeur, for example, are convinced that they have special powers, wealth, or prominence in society, despite evidence to the contrary.

dementia – A long-term deterioration of intellectual function. Unlike delirium, dementia is permanent and irreversible. The most common types of dementia are Alzheimer's disease and multi-infarct dementia. The cause of Alzheimer's disease has not yet been determined. Multi-infarct dementia is the brain damage that results from one or more strokes.

demulcent – An agent that soothes inflamed or irritated tissue, particularly mucous membranes. Most throat lozenges, for example, contain a demulcent. A demulcent is most commonly an oil or a syrup.

denatured alcohol – Alcohol that contains no water or impurities. Also called dehydrated alcohol.

denial of claim – Rejection of payment or reimbursement for an insurance submission.

dent- – Prefix that refers to the teeth.

dental – Pertaining to the teeth.

denti- – Prefix that refers to the teeth.

dentist – An individual who is specially trained to diagnose and treat conditions that affect the teeth and mouth. Dentists earned either a doctor of dental medicine (D.M.D.) or doctor of dental surgery (D.D.S.) degree from an accredited college of dentistry. They must also pass a rigorous examination and be licensed by the state before they can practice their profession.

dentistry – The body of science that deals with the development and health of the mouth and teeth.

dento- – Prefix that refers to the teeth.

dentures – Artificial teeth. Dentures substitute for teeth that have been lost due to trauma or disease.

deodorant – An agent that covers or eliminates a disagreeable odor. Typically used in the context of body odor.

deoxyribonucleic acid (DNA) – A substance primarily composed of a carbohydrate (deoxyribose) and specific purines and pyrimidines (adenine, cytosine, guanine, and thymine). DNA forms long pairs of strands of carbohydrate with pairs of purine and pyrimidine molecules bridging the strands. DNA is found in the chromosomes of the nuclei of cells. Through its arrangement of purine and pyrimidine pairs, DNA carries the hereditary characteristics of the host.

department of insurance (DOI) – The state agency that regulates the insurance industry within that state. Insurers must gain approval from the DOI before they can conduct business in the state or before they significantly change the coverage they provide. Consumers and health care providers may file complaints with the DOI if they feel an insurance company operates inappropriately.

dependent – A person who qualifies for insurance coverage on another person's policy. Dependents are usually the spouses or children of the policy holder.

dependent age limitation – The age at which a dependent's insurance coverage ends. In most cases, the dependent age limitation for a child is 19 years of age. However, coverage may still be provided until age 24 if the dependent is a full-time college student.

depolarizing agent – An agent that blocks muscle contractions and decreases muscle tone by interfering with the electrical aspects of nerve transmission. Depolarizing agents are commonly used in surgery to make muscle tissue flaccid and easier to cut with less residual damage.

deposit – A residue or precipitate. For example, low-density lipoprotein (LDL) may form deposits in blood vessels, obstructing blood flow and increasing the likelihood of a heart attack or stroke.

depot formulation – A preparation that releases drug slowly over a prolonged period of time. The most common application is in the form of depot injections made deep into muscle. Most fre-

D

quently used to administer long-acting hormone therapy, the drug may take several months to be fully absorbed.

depressant – An agent that restricts the function of an organ or tissue. For example, a central nervous system depressant is a drug or other chemical that slows down the rate of nerve cell transmissions.

depression – A psychological state characterized by feelings of doom, lack of self-worth, and the inability to sense pleasure. Depression and anxiety often coexist and are the two most common mental disorders. Medications (antidepressants) are the most frequently used treatments for depression. Other effective treatments include various forms of counseling by trained therapists, exposure to bright lights for specific types of depression, group therapy, and electroconvulsive therapy. Medications are most effective when they are combined with counseling.

Also, a reduced degree of function.

derm- – Prefix indicating skin.

derma- – Prefix indicating skin.

dermabrasion – A procedure that involves scraping away the outer layers of the skin. Dermabrasion may be done with sandpaper, pumice, or other coarse material. The procedure may be done to remove hardened skin, scars, or tattoos.

dermal – Pertaining to the skin.

dermat- – Prefix indicating skin.

dermatitides – Plural form of dermatitis.

dermatitis – An inflammation of the skin.

dermato- – Prefix indicating skin.

dermatographism – A skin condition where hives or welts appear on areas that have been scratched or received pressure. For a person with dermatographism, moving a blunt stylus across the skin often produces a line of hives along the course the stylus traveled. Sometimes called skin writing. Dermatographism usually improves following treatment with an antihistamine.

dermatological – Pertaining to dermatology. Also, a medication used to treat a skin disorder.

dermatologist – A physician who specializes in the diagnosis and treatment of skin disorders:

dermatology – The branch of medicine that deals with the health of the skin.

dermatoses – Plural of dermatosis.

dermatosis – A general term denoting a skin disease or abnormal condition.

dermis – The lowest layer of skin. The dermis is positioned above the subcutaneous fat layer.

desensitization – The process of reducing allergic reactions by exposing the patient to minute amounts of the causative allergens themselves. Usually involves a series of injections of dilute concentrations of allergens. Each injection in the series contains a slightly higher concentration of allergens than its predecessor. The purpose of the injections is to induce the immune system to accept the allergens as a normal part of the body. Colloquially known as allergy shots.

DESI – *See Drug Efficacy Study Implementation.*

desquamation – Flaking or sloughing off of the outer layer of skin. A small amount of desquamation is normal and occurs continuously. However, noxious chemicals and some drug reactions can cause profound, even life-threatening desquamation.

dessicant – A drying agent. Dessicants in the form of sachets or large plastic capsules are often inserted into medicine bottles to absorb humidity. Decreasing the humidity in a medicine bottle usually prolongs the shelf life of the medicine.

detail aid – A sales tool used by a pharmaceutical salesperson.

detail person – A salesperson employed by a pharmaceutical manufacturer. A detail person makes sales calls to pharmacists, physicians, and other drug prescribers to give them the "details" of their products to try to influence their use.

detailing – The sales process used by pharmaceutical salespersons to try to promote use of their products. *See also academic detailing.*

detergent – A chemical that combines with both water and oil. A detergent typically has an area of its molecule that attracts water molecules while another section attaches to lipids. Detergents may be used for cleaning or as emulsifying agents.

detoxification – The process of recovering from the effects of a contaminant, usually a drug or a chemical. While the term is most commonly used in the context of drug abuse treatment, detoxification can also apply to recovery from any type of noxious exposure.

detoxify – To remove or reduce the effects of a contaminant.

dextr- – Prefix meaning right or referring to the right side of something.

dextro- – Prefix meaning right or referring to the right side of something.

dextrorotatory – A chemical capable of deviating a beam of light to the right. Chemicals capable of shifting a beam of light to the left are said to be levorotatory. In the case of some molecules, one isomer is dextrorotatory while another is levorotatory. The ability to rotate light differently indicates that the arrangement of atoms in these otherwise identical molecules is slightly different. In some cases only one of the isomers is pharmacologically active. For example, levodopa is effective for treating Parkinson's disease while dextrodopa is not. Dextroamphetamine is an effective central nervous system stimulant, but levoamphetamine is not.

di- – Prefix indicating two or twice.

diabetes – A condition characterized by an increase in urination. Commonly used in reference to diabetes mellitus.

diabetes insipidus – An endocrine condition characterized by elimination of large amounts of urine with dehydration and extreme thirst. The condition is caused by insufficient production of antidiuretic hormone or by the inability of antidiuretic hormone to control urine formation in the kidneys.

diabetes mellitus – A condition caused by the inability to properly metabolize sugars. Secondarily, the condition also adversely affects metabolism of fats and proteins. The predominant forms of the condition are Type I diabetes mellitus, occurring most often in children and adolescents, and Type II diabetes mellitus, which typically appears in middle age. Poorly controlled diabetes mellitus leads to multiple complications affecting the skin, blood vessels, eyes, and nerves.

Type I diabetes mellitus, formerly called juvenile-onset diabetes mellitus, is characterized by the inability to form insulin. All Type I diabetics must take insulin daily in the form of an injection or by means of an infusion pump.

People with Type II diabetes mellitus, formerly called adult-onset diabetes mellitus, are able to form their own insulin, but the amount of insulin they produce is not sufficient to meet their metabolic needs. Depending upon its severity, this form of diabetes mellitus may be controlled with diet and exercise alone, oral medicines, or insulin injections.

Colloquially referred to as sugar diabetes.

diabetic – Pertaining to diabetes mellitus or a person who has diabetes mellitus.

diabetologist – A physician who specializes in the treatment of diabetes mellitus. Diabetologists are first trained in endocrinology, the area of medicine that deals with glands and hormones. After that, they are further trained in the characteristics of diabetes mellitus.

diagnosis – The process of collecting subjective and objective information in order to identify a disease or other medical condition. The diagnostic process may include questioning the patient or caregiver, physical examination, and/or testing procedures.

diagnosis code – A numeric system for identifying diseases for the purpose of filing claims with insurers. In most cases, the codes used are those published in the *International Classification of Diseases* (ICD). Some mental health facilities use the codes in the *Diagnostic and Statistical Manual* (DSM) as an alternative.

diagnosis-related groups (DRG) – A program that classifies medical conditions to determine reimbursements to hospitals for inpatient care of Medicare patients. The DRG system pays hospitals based on the average cost of treating covered conditions. For example, if a Medicare patient were admitted to a hospital for treatment of a heart attack, Medicare would pay that hospital a set fee, regardless of the costs the hospital actually incurs. If the actual costs of treatment are less than the reimbursement rate, the hospital is allowed to keep the difference. However, if actual treatment costs are higher, the hospital must absorb the loss. Currently, there are nearly 500 DRG categories.

diagnostic – Pertaining to diagnosis.

Also an aid or device used to make a diagnosis.

***Diagnostic and Statistical Manual* (DSM)** – Book published by the American Psychiatric Association that defines the criteria for diagnosing mental illnesses. The value of this book, now in its fourth edition, is that it standardizes the nomenclature of mental health and lists the symptomatology of every disorder. DSM is a standard reference tool used by all psychotherapists and mental health counselors.

dialysis – A process that removes wastes or toxins from the blood. Most commonly used in people who have temporarily or permanently impaired kidney function.

diaphoresis – Sweating.

diaphragm – A thin divider. In the human body, the diaphragm separates the chest from the abdomen.

Also, a female contraceptive device that prevents sperm from entering the uterus.

diarrhea – A condition characterized by frequent, watery bowel movements. While most cases of diarrhea are self-limited and of short duration, uncontrolled diarrhea can lead to dehydration.

diastole – The rest period during the cardiac cycle. The heart ejects blood into circulation during each contraction (systole) and refills with blood during rest periods (diastole). Systole and diastole each last less than a second.

diastolic – Pertaining to diastole.

Also, the lower number of a blood pressure reading. For example, a blood pressure reading of 120/80 indicates a systolic pressure of 120 and a diastolic pressure of 80. The systolic pressure represents the highest pressure the blood reaches, while the diastolic pressure is the lowest.

diet – The nutritional patterns an individual follows. Diets may be routine with no restrictions, or may encourage or discourage certain foods, salts, or nutrients. Diets may be devised to lose weight, to improve health in general, or to treat or prevent a specific disease.

dietary supplement – Originally meant to indicate nutritional enhancements (vitamins, minerals, etc.) to assure a balanced intake of nutrients, dietary supplements now have a new legal definition. Dietary supplements now include virtually any drug extracted from an herb or other natural source. The reason for the redefinition is to exempt these drugs from the safety and efficacy requirements of the United States Food and Drug Administration (FDA). Currently the FDA can regulate these drugs only after they have been proven to cause undue toxicity.

dietetics – The application of principles of nutrition to the prevention or treatment of disease.

dietician (or dietition) – An individual who has graduated from an accredited dietetics program, passed a qualifying examination, and received a license from the state. Dieticians may counsel individuals on their nutrition in order to promote health. Hospital-based dieticians typically work with patients to treat their medical conditions through adjustments to their nutrition.

differential diagnosis – The process of systematically evaluating clinical signs and symptoms to determine which of several possible diseases is the one causing the patient's problems. Elements of a differential diagnosis may include the patient's history of the illness, family history, physical examination, laboratory tests, and x-rays.

digestion – The process of changing food into its simpler constituents prior to absorption. Carbohydrates are converted to simple sugars, proteins to amino acids, and fats to fatty acids. Digestion occurs primarily in the stomach and small intestine.

digestive tract – The organ system primarily responsible for food absorption and elimination of solid waste. The digestive tract consists of the mouth, esophagus, stomach, small and large intestines, pancreas, liver, rectum, and anus. Also called the gastrointestinal tract.

dilation – The stretching or widening of a hollow structure. In the eye, dilation relates to enlargement of the pupil, usually because of diminished light or a medication.

diluent – An agent, most commonly water, used to decrease the concentration of a substance or to dissolve a solid. For example, sterile water is often used as a diluent to solubilize medication prior to injection.

direct-to-consumer (DTC) advertising – Promotional message intended to be broadcast or otherwise distributed to the public. In pharmacy, DTC advertising is the practice of promoting prescription drugs to the general public with the intent of having patients ask their physicians to prescribe the advertised products. DTC prescription drug advertising is funded by the manufacturers of those products.

disallowance – Denial of an insurance claim. A claim may be denied (disallowed) for any number of reasons, including failure to meet a deductible, receiving a service that is not covered by the plan, or billing a fee greater than that allowed for the specific service.

disease – A specific medical problem where at least two of the following apply:

- a recognized cause.

- a consistent pattern of signs and symptoms.

- a consistent pattern of physical changes.

A disease may result from a genetic problem, chemical exposure, infection, poor nutrition, or environmental factors.

disease management – A systematic, comprehensive approach to treating patients with selected chronic illnesses. Most disease management programs are operated by insurance companies. In some cases, insurers may contract this function to outside companies. The purpose of a disease management program is to reduce health costs by preventing recurrence of symptoms, and consequently the expensive treatments and hospitalizations these recurrences might necessitate.

Chronic conditions that disease management programs may focus on include asthma, diabetes mellitus, hypertension, congestive heart failure, osteoporosis, depression, and arthritis.

disenrollment – The process of removing people from a health insurance plan. This is most commonly done when those individuals or families no longer qualify for coverage, for instance after a job change with accompanying change in insurers or failure to pay premiums.

disinfectant – A chemical agent that kills or inhibits growth of microorganisms following physical contact. Usually used in the context of an application to an inert surface. For example, a disinfectant may be used to clean a floor but an antiseptic would be used to clean a wound.

disinhibition – Removal of or blocking of an inhibition. Inhibition of an inhibition. For example, alcohol has disinhibition properties because it diminishes the reservations (inhibitions) people have about certain social behaviors. Many other central nervous system depressants are also disinhibitors.

disorder – An anatomic, physiologic, or physical abnormality. Disorder is a general term often used to describe a wide variety of medical conditions, some of which are very wide-ranging in nature (e.g., emotional disorder) while others are more specific (e.g., generalized anxiety disorder, attention deficit disorder).

dispense – To prepare and distribute prescription medications. During the process of dispensing, a pharmacist may also verify insurance, check for the potential for side effects and drug interaction, and advise the patient.

dispense as written (DAW) – Instruction from a physician to a pharmacist that requires the pharmacist to dispense only the brand of medication prescribed. In these cases, pharmacists are not

D

legally allowed to dispense a generic unless the physician rescinds the DAW instruction.

dispensing fee – The professional fee paid to a pharmacist or pharmacy for the service of filling a prescription, filing an insurance claim, and advising or counseling the patient. Dispensing fees usually substitute for a markup over the cost of the drug.

dissecting aneurysm – A split or tear in the wall of an artery made worse by blood entering the tear and widening it. If not surgically repaired, a dissecting aneurysm will eventually break through the blood vessel, causing hemorrhage. Dissecting aneurysms occur most often in the aorta and cause almost immediate death.

disseminated – Widely spread. A disseminated cancer, for example, is one that has spread from its original site to other locations.

distribution – The part of pharmacokinetics that deals with the dispersal of drug to the organs and tissues of the body. The chemical properties of a drug dictate which tissues will absorb the drug, usually from the blood, and in what concentration the drug reaches those tissues and the cells within them.

diuresis – Formation and passage of urine.

diuretic – A drug that promotes urine formation and elimination. Most diuretics work by causing the kidneys to eliminate more sodium than they ordinarily would. Sodium passing through the kidneys attracts water from the circulatory system and increases the volume of urine.

Diuretics are most often used to treat hypertension and congestive heart failure. In addition, they are used to treat a wide variety of kidney and cardiovascular problems.

diverticulitis – Inflammation of a diverticulum, usually caused by entrapment of feces within the diverticulum. Diverticulitis causes intense abdominal pain.

diverticulosis – Presence of one or more diverticula. Diverticulosis commonly occurs with aging and is not harmful unless a diverticulum becomes inflamed.

D

diverticulum – A pouch or sac protruding from the lining of a hollow organ, usually the large intestine.

DJD – *See degenerative joint disease.*

D.M.D. – Doctor of dental medicine. The degree most dental schools confer on graduating dentists. Alternatively, a dental school may award a doctor of dental surgery (D.D.S.) degree. Both degrees qualify dentists for licensing and clinical practice. *See dentist.*

DME – *See durable medical equipment.*

DNA – *See deoxyribonucleic acid.*

D.O. – Doctor of osteopathy. The degree osteopathic medical schools confer on graduating physicians. *See osteopath, osteopathic medicine.*

doctor – In common usage, a physician.

Also, any person who has received a doctorate degree, including doctor of pharmacy (Pharm.D.), doctor of philosophy (Ph.D.), doctor of dental medicine (D.M.D.), doctor of optometry (O.D.), and many others.

Doctor of Chiropractic (D.C.) – The degree granted to chiropractors. *See chiropractor.*

D.O.H. – Abbreviation for department of health.

DOI – *See department of insurance.*

dopamine – A catecholamine neurotransmitter responsible for transmitting messages within the central nervous system. Dopamine excess in the brain is thought to be responsible for some of the symptoms of schizophrenia. Dopamine deficiency produces symptoms of Parkinson's disease. Dopamine is also responsible for regulating blood pressure and for controlling hormone output from the pituitary gland.

dopaminergic – Pertaining to the effects of dopamine or the nerve fibers that use it as a transmitter.

dope – Colloquial term for any drug of abuse.

dosage – The proper amount of medicine to be taken for a specific problem. For example, the normal dosage of amoxicillin for a

D

mild infection is 250 mg every eight hours. Dosages may be determined by volume (milliliters, teaspoonfuls), by weight (milligrams, micrograms), or by biologic activity (units, international units).

dosage form – The formulation in which a drug is administered. Examples of dosage forms include aerosols, capsules, creams, elixirs, enemas, gels, granules, implants, injections, lozenges, lotions, ointments, powders, shampoos, solutions, suppositories, suspensions, syrups, and tablets.

dose – The amount of medicine to be taken at one time. The term dose is often misapplied in situations where the word dosage is more correct.

double-blind study – A characteristic of a controlled experiment in which neither the patient (subject) nor the health care professionals (investigators) directly involved with the patient knows whether the patient is receiving the study drug or the reference drug. Instead, drugs are identified by coded designations. An individual who does not have direct contact with the patient holds the codes. The purpose of a double-blind study is to eliminate bias on the part of either the subjects or investigators.

douche – The act of washing something with a stream of water. Most commonly applied to the use of water, with or without medication, to cleanse the vagina.

Also, the fluid used to cleanse the vagina.

D.P.H. – Abbreviation for department of public health or doctor of public health.

D.P.M. – Abbreviation for doctor of podiatric medicine. *See podiatrist.*

dram – An apothecary weight that equals 1/96 of an apothecary pound. The term dram is sometimes used in place of the more correct term fluidram. A fluidram is 1/8 of a fluidounce. In the apothecary system of weights and measures, pounds and fluidounces are different than the pounds and ounces of the avoirdupois system commonly used in the United States and Great Britain.

D

Because of difficulty of use and the potential for error, health systems have almost completely replaced the apothecary system of weights and measures with the metric system.

DRG – *See diagnosis-related groups.*

drop – A small amount of fluid that forms a sphere when it falls. A colloquial term for medicines that are administered in drop form (e.g., eye drops).

drug – A synthetic or naturally occurring chemical agent other than food that affects physical or psychological functions. Drugs may be used to treat, prevent, or diagnose disease.

drug abuse – Intentional misuse of a chemical agent to achieve an effect that is not recommended. Drug abuse is intended to produce pleasurable feelings or enhanced physical performance.

drug approval – Formal permission from the United States Food and Drug Administration to market a new drug or a new dosage form.

drug class – A group of therapeutic agents that are similar because of their chemical composition or because of their pharmacological properties.

A single drug may be a member of many drug classes. For example, aspirin belongs to the salicylate drug class because it is a chemical derivative of salicylic acid. Aspirin also belongs to the analgesic drug class because it has the pharmacological property of reducing pain.

Drug Efficacy Study Implementation (DESI) – A program mandated by Congress and administered by the United States Food and Drug Administration (FDA) that evaluated the effectiveness of drugs introduced to the market in the United States between 1938 and 1962.

Currently, pharmaceutical manufacturers must satisfy FDA that their drugs are both safe and effective before FDA approves them for marketing. Prior to 1962, however, manufacturers only needed to prove that their drugs were safe. Proof of effectiveness was not required. As a result of this review, many ineffective products were removed from the market.

Drugs are referred to as DESI drugs if there is insufficient evidence of effectiveness. DESI drugs are allowed to remain on the market but they are not reimbursable under federal programs (e.g., Medicaid). Many managed care programs do not cover these drugs.

Drug Enforcement Agency (DEA) – The bureau within the United States Department of Justice primarily responsible for policing federal laws that concern controlled substances. In addition to investigating the sellers, producers, and smugglers of illicit drugs, the DEA also monitors physician prescribing patterns and pharmacy records.

drug formulary – A list or catalog of drugs approved for use within a managed care plan or a health system such as a hospital. A formulary may be open or closed. In an open formulary, the drug catalog lists the drugs the health system prefers to be used. Drugs not on the formulary (nonformulary drugs) may be prescribed and dispensed without restriction.

In a closed hospital formulary, drugs not listed are not stocked in the hospital pharmacy and special approvals must be sought before a nonformulary drug will be purchased and dispensed. With a closed managed care formulary, nonformulary drugs may be stocked in the pharmacy (because most pharmacies serve more members of many health plans) but the plan will not pay for it without a prior approval from the health plan.

Drugs listed on one organization's formulary may or may not be listed on another's.

druggist – Colloquial term for a pharmacist.

drug holiday – A period of time when a medication is discontinued so the physician may either reduce the patient's exposure to the drug and its side effects or determine whether the patient still benefits from the drug.

drug-induced disease – Any disorder caused by or precipitated by a pharmacologic agent. Drug-induced diseases may be permanent or may remit when the causative agent is discontinued. For example, tardive dyskinesia is in most cases a drug-induced disease caused by long-term treatment with antipsychotic drugs.

drug interaction – The effect two or more drugs have on each other when used concurrently in the same patient. Drug interactions may be intended or not. They may be beneficial or harmful. Interacting drugs may increase the effects of both drugs, decrease the effects of both drugs, or increase or decrease the effects of one drug.

The occurrence of two drugs interacting with each other is often called a drug-drug interaction. Drugs may also interact with laboratory tests or foods. These are referred to as drug-lab test interactions and drug-food interactions, respectively.

drug of abuse – A synthetic or naturally occurring chemical agent whose intended use is to alter physical or psychological functions for the purpose of pleasure. Depending upon the situation, the same drug may be considered to be either therapeutic or a drug of abuse. For example, cocaine is therapeutically used as a local anesthetic for some types of throat surgery. Cocaine is also abused by those who solely seek its stimulant and mood-altering properties.

drug product – A finished pharmaceutical dosage form.

drug product labeling – See *label*.

drug provider – The person or facility licensed to dispense prescriptions. Usually a pharmacy.

drug receptor – The molecular site within or on the surface of a cell where a drug attaches in order to exert its pharmacological effect.

drug selection – Process where a pharmacist determines whether to fill a prescription with a brand or generic drug and, in the case of a generic, which company's product to use.

drug use evaluation (DUE) – An assessment of physicians' prescribing patterns to determine costs and appropriateness of drug therapy. DUE may be performed by a hospital on its inpatients, by a health insurer, or by a pharmacy benefit management company acting under contract with an insurer.

drug utilization review (DUR) – The process of examining drug usage to determine physician prescribing habits and patient usage patterns to manage costs and improve patient safety. DUR may be done before a prescription is written (prospective DUR), at the time a prescription is dispensed (concurrent DUR), or later (retrospective DUR). DUR programs look for duplications of therapy, potential drug interactions, and for optimal drug usage for specific disease states. DUR programs may provide physicians with reports comparing their prescribing practices with those of other physicians who treat the same conditions.

DSM – See *Diagnostic and Statistical Manual*.

DTC advertising – See *direct-to-consumer advertising*.

duct – A tube or channel that allows the flow of a body fluid. For example, the tear ducts conduct tears from the tear glands to the surface of the eye. The bile duct allows bile to flow from the gallbladder to the intestine.

ductal – Pertaining to a duct.

ductless – Having no duct. The endocrine glands are ductless glands, i.e., they do not transport the hormones they secrete by means of ducts. Instead, they secrete their hormones (e.g., estrogen, testosterone, insulin, cortisol, thyroid hormone) directly into the bloodstream. The blood then distributes the hormones to all parts of the body.

DUE – See *drug use evaluation*.

duodenal – Pertaining to the duodenum.

duodenal ulcer – An erosion of the lining of the duodenum. Duodenal ulcer is the most common form of peptic ulcer. Although some individuals never experience significant discomfort, duodenal ulcer typically causes a burning pain that may be temporarily relieved with food or antacids. Treatment usually consists of a combination of antacids and drugs that reduce acid secretion. Antibiotics may also be used if *Helicobacter pylori*, a bacterium often found in association with peptic ulcer, is present. Since effective treatments for this organism have been discovered, patients improve faster and experience fewer relapses.

duodenum – The first ten to twelve inches of the small intestine. The duodenum lies directly beneath the stomach and receives all stomach contents. The duodenum continues the process of digestion, mixing partially digested food with additional acids and enzymes. Absorption of nutrients also begins in the duodenum. Unabsorbed contents pass to the jejunum, the next section of the small intestine.

Contrary to common belief, the stomach does not absorb significant amounts of orally administered drugs. Most drug absorption occurs in the duodenum.

DUR – *See drug utilization review.*

durable medical equipment (DME) – Treatment or convalescent apparatus intended to be used more than a single time. Examples include crutches, wheelchairs, and hospital beds.

In contrast, disposable medical equipment (e.g., needles, syringes) is intended to be used only once.

duration of action – The length of time a single dose of medication continues to exert its pharmacological effect.

DVT – *See deep vein thrombosis.*

-dynia – Suffix denoting pain.

dys- – Prefix meaning bad or difficult.

dyscrasia – A general term applied to any blood disease where the number or physical structure of one or more of the cellular components of blood (red blood cells, white blood cells, platelets) is abnormal. Blood dyscrasias may occur naturally or as the result of exposure to drugs, toxins, or radiation.

dysentery – Severe diarrhea accompanied by blood or mucus in the stool. Dysentery is usually accompanied by pain and the urge to have almost continuous bowel movements. Dysentery is most commonly caused by bacterial or viral infection or by parasitic infestation. If not corrected, dysentery leads to dehydration and may be life-threatening.

dysfunction – An abnormality or impairment of normal activities.

dysfunctional uterine bleeding – Abnormal blood loss from the female genital tract, usually due to hormonal imbalance.

D

dysgeusia – Impaired sensation of taste. Some drugs cause dysgeusia as a side effect.

dyskinesia – Difficulty performing normal muscle movements. Tardive dyskinesia is an example of a movement disorder where individuals experience uncontrollable muscle twitches and facial grimacing. Tardive dyskinesia is usually associated with long-term use of antipsychotic drugs.

dyslipidemia – Abnormally elevated levels of cholesterol, triglycerides, and/or low-density lipoprotein (LDL) in the blood.

dysmenorrhea – Pain during menstruation, often accompanied by cramps.

dyspepsia – Indigestion. Often colloquially called heartburn. Feeling of nausea, fullness, or burning, often occurring shortly after eating. Dyspepsia may be caused by overeating or by gastroesophageal reflux, a condition where stomach acid splashes up and into the esophagus. The esophagus lacks the protective lining of the stomach and intestines and is, therefore, susceptible to burns from acid.

dysphagia – Difficulty swallowing or the inability to swallow.

dysphoria – A psychological feeling of discomfort.

dyspnea – Difficulty breathing. Shortness of breath.

dysrhythmia – Abnormal heart rhythm. *See arrhythmia*.

dystonia – Abnormal tension in a tissue. Most commonly, dystonia refers to muscle tissue. A dystonic muscle may be overresponsive (spastic) or underresponsive (flaccid) in response to a stimulus.

dystonic – Pertaining to dystonia.

dysuria – Pain or difficulty passing urine.

E

EAP – *See employee assistance plan.*

ear – The organ responsible for hearing. The ear receives ambient sound waves and converts them into electronic impulses for transmission to the brain.

The ear is comprised of three parts: the outer ear, middle ear, and inner ear. In addition to processing sounds, the inner ear is also responsible for maintaining balance.

ec- – Prefix meaning out of or away from.

ecchymosis – Blood that has pooled in the skin. Eccymoses (plural form of ecchymosis) are typically large, irregularly shaped, purple patches. They may result from trauma or from a bleeding disorder. Drugs that affect blood clotting may lead to ecchymoses.

ECF – *See extended care facility.*

ECG – *See electrocardiogram.*

echocardiogram – The visual output from echocardiography. The echocardiogram may be viewed on a computer monitor or may be printed.

echocardiography – The use of ultrasonic waves to examine the structures of the heart and major blood vessels. Echocardiography displays the physical appearance of the heart and heart valves as they perform their functions. It is able to detect malformations and dysfunctions.

eclampsia – Seizures in a person with preeclampsia. Eclampsia is a serious complication of pregnancy. *See preeclampsia.*

E. coli – Abbreviation for *Escherichia coli. See Escherichia.*

ECT – *See electroconvulsive therapy.*

-ectomy – Suffix indicating a surgical removal. For example, an appendectomy is the surgical removal of the appendix.

ectopic – Out of proper place. For example, an ectopic pregnancy is one where the fetus implants somewhere other than the uterus. An ectopic heartbeat is one that originates in heart tissue other than the sinoatrial node, the place where heartbeats usually begin.

E

eczema – A chronic skin condition characterized by inflammation, scaling, and often itching. May be due to allergy, exposure to toxins, or unknown causes.

eczematous – Pertaining to eczema.

ED – Abbreviation for emergency department.

edema – Abnormal collection of fluid. Edema may collect in any part of the body due to trauma or poor blood flow. Edema in the ankles or lower legs is often a sign of congestive heart failure.

Pitting edema is a depression (pit) caused by pressure from one or more fingers pressed into the affected area. Pitting edema is often used as a rough measure of the degree of edema present.

edematous – Pertaining to edema.

edentulous – Absence of teeth.

EEG – *See electroencephalogram.*

EENT – Abbreviation for eye, ear, nose, and throat.

effective date – The day an insurance policy or change of premium goes into effect.

effervesce – To bubble, usually from the formation and/or release of a gas from a liquid. Some pharmaceutical dosage forms (e.g., Alka-Seltzer) are formulated to effervesce when mixed with water. The purpose of effervescence is to increase the speed of drug absorption and, therefore, achieve a faster onset of clinical effect.

Products effervesce because they contain both an acid and a base, usually sodium bicarbonate. When mixed with water, the acid and base neutralize each other and produce carbon dioxide, the fizz, as a by-product. Most effervescent products have a high sodium content and may not be suitable for people on low salt diets.

effervescent – Pertaining to the ability to effervesce.

efficacy – The ability of a medication to reliably alter the natural course of a disease or to relieve some or all of its symptoms. Proof of efficacy is one of the two major criteria the United States

E

Food and Drug Administration (FDA) uses to decide whether a drug should be allowed on the market. The other major criterion is safety.

effusion – Leakage of fluid from a blood vessel and into the surrounding tissue. Effusions are usually further defined by their location. For example, a pleural effusion is seepage of fluid from the blood vessels in the lungs into the pleura, the space between the lungs and their outer lining.

egg – The female reproductive cell. Also called an ovum.

ejaculate – The process of discharging semen, the fluid that contains a male's sperm.

Also, the contents of a seminal discharge.

ejaculation – The discharge of semen.

EKG – *See electrocardiogram.*

elasticity – The ability to return to original shape after being stretched or compressed. Because of its elasticity, slightly stretching a healthy muscle causes it to contract with more than normal force. Overstretching, however, causes a muscle to lose elasticity and it contracts with less than normal force.

elective surgery – An operation that does not have to be performed immediately. The patient can elect to have it now or wait for a later time without additional medical problems. Elective is not synonymous with unnecessary; it is just not an emergency.

electro- – Prefix meaning electricity.

electrocardiogram (ECG, EKG) – The graphic representation of the electrical impulses that pass through the heart as it beats. The electrocardiogram may be viewed on a monitor or may be printed.

electrocardiograph – The instrument used to perform electrocardiography. Prior to the procedure, electrodes are attached to the wrists, ankles, and the chest. These electrodes detect electrical discharges in the heart. The electrocardiograph displays this information in an electrocardiogram.

electrocardiography – The process of observing heart rhythms by detecting electrical discharges from the heart muscle. The results of electrocardiography are displayed in an electrocardiogram.

By examining patterns of electrical discharges, a trained observer can diagnose specific arrhythmias and detect the presence of heart damage due to heart attack, congestive heart failure, or other heart diseases. Electrocardiography also offers a means to monitor the beneficial or toxic effects of drugs on the heart.

electroconvulsive therapy (ECT) – A treatment procedure where an electrical current is briefly passed through the brain in order to produce a convulsion. ECT is an effective treatment for depression. It is usually reserved for people who are profoundly depressed or who have not responded adequately to other treatments, such as medication.

ECT has the advantage of reducing symptoms of depression faster than many antidepressant medicines. It has the disadvantage of potentially causing loss of memory of recent events.

electroencephalogram (EEG) – The graphic representation, usually on a strip of paper, of the electrical impulses that pass through the brain.

electroencephalograph – The instrument used to perform electroencephalography.

electroencephalography – The process of observing brain functions by detecting electrical discharges from the brain. The results of electroencephalography are displayed in an electroencephalogram.

The procedure is performed by taping electrodes to the patient's scalp. The patient may or may not be sedated prior to testing. The electrodes detect electrical impulses as they pass among brain structures. A trained analyst may use electroencephalography to diagnosis seizure disorders or other neurological problems. Absence of electrical activity is an indication of brain death.

electrolyte – Chemical ions that allow electricity to pass through a fluid. In a medical context, the primary electrolytes are potassium, sodium, and chloride ions. These electrolytes are necessary for nerve conduction and muscle function.

electronic claim – A computer-to-computer transmission that records a patient-provider encounter and the charges that relate to it.

electronic data interchange – Computerized exchange of information from one organization to another. Although almost any business-to-business transaction may be handled this way, it is an especially convenient way to transmit insurance claims information.

electroshock therapy (EST) – *See electroconvulsive therapy.*

eligibility date – The day an individual qualifies for coverage under an insurance plan.

eligibility verification – The process of checking whether or not an individual is covered by an insurance policy before authorizing a payment or service.

eligibility waiting period – The length of time an individual must be employed before qualifying for insurance benefits. Some companies begin coverage from the first day of employment while others require waiting periods of 30, 60, 90 days, or even longer.

eligible dependent – An individual, usually a spouse or a child, who meets the requirements for coverage under a family insurance policy.

eligible employee – A worker who meets the requirements for coverage under a group insurance policy.

elimination – The process of removing wastes from the body. Elimination products include urine, feces, and carbon dioxide. In some cases, other fluids such as sweat and tears are considered elimination products.

elixir – A pharmaceutical vehicle that consists of water, alcohol, and usually a sweetener and a flavoring agent. Their alcohol content makes elixirs convenient liquid dosage forms for many drugs that are only slightly soluble in water. In these cases, the drug is first dissolved in alcohol and the other elixir components are added.

E

All elixirs contain alcohol. However, some pharmaceutical manufacturers advertise certain products as "alcohol-free" elixirs. This is a misuse of the term that serves only to confuse the public. These so-called alcohol-free elixirs are usually either syrups or solutions.

emaciation – Severe loss of weight, usually due to disease or malnutrition.

embolism – Obstruction of a blood vessel by a plug (embolus).

embolus – A mass that has broken away from the wall of a blood vessel, floated through the bloodstream, and lodged in a smaller blood vessel, obstructing the flow of that vessel.

Most emboli start as either lipid plaques attached to the inside of blood vessels or as part of a thrombus (blood clot). In these cases, a portion of the plaque or thrombus breaks off and floats through the blood.

Once an embolus obstructs a blood vessel, it can cause death of the tissue that vessel normally supplies. Emboli are common causes of heart attacks and strokes.

embryo – An unborn being in the early stages of development. In humans, the embryonic period is considered to be the first two months of life. Thereafter, the developing child is called a fetus.

embryocidal – A drug or procedure that intentionally or unintentionally kills an embryo.

embryotoxicity – Harm caused to an embryo due to exposure to drugs, chemicals, or radiation.

emergency – A sudden occurrence that requires immediate action.

emergency department (ED) – A term some health care facilities use instead of emergency room. *See emergency room.*

emergency medicine – The branch of medicine that routinely deals with the diagnosis and treatment of medical conditions that require immediate intervention.

emergency room (ER) – The area of a health care facility, usually a hospital, intended to evaluate and treat patients with trauma or illnesses that require immediate attention.

E

emergent – Pertaining to an occurrence or situation that requires immediate action.

Also, something that becomes apparent or viewable.

emergent condition – Any medical problem that requires immediate attention in order to sustain life or relieve suffering.

emesis – Vomiting.

emesis basin – A bowl or other vessel intended to catch and contain vomitus until it can be disposed of.

emetic – An agent that causes vomiting. While many drugs are capable of causing vomiting as a side effect, a few are used clinically to specifically produce vomiting. Ipecac, for example, is an emetic drug that is used to treat poisonings. By producing vomiting, ipecac empties the stomach of the poison before all of it can be absorbed.

Emetics can also be abused, primarily by people with anorexia nervosa, to empty the stomach of food for the purpose of losing weight.

-emia – Suffix used to indicate blood.

emollient – A soothing skin preparation that softens skin by restoring water content to it.

emphysema – A lung condition characterized by the destruction of the alveoli and bronchioles. Loss of large numbers of alveoli reduces air exchange with the blood. As the condition progresses, people with this disorder experience increasing shortness of breath following minimal exertion. Inhaling smoke from tobacco products is the most common cause of emphysema. Lung damage from emphysema is usually irreversible, but stopping smoking usually stops or slows the progression of the disease.

Emphysema and chronic bronchitis are the most common components of chronic obstructive pulmonary disease (COPD). *See also chronic obstructive pulmonary disease.*

empirical – Relating to experience rather than scientific information. Drug therapy is said to be empirical when it is started before the diagnosis is firmly established. For example, empirical antibiotic therapy of an infection is that which is started before laboratory tests identify a causative organism. In many cases, patient comfort or safety requires that physicians treat empirically before the diagnosis is complete. The original empiric treatment may be continued or changed once further diagnostic information becomes available.

employee assistance program (EAP) – Counseling services provided by an employer to benefit the workers and, usually, their families. EAP services may include counseling for issues related to the workplace or personal matters. Offerings may include programs for stress, sexual harassment, family and marital problems, child or elder care, finances, legal issues, psychological problems, drug and alcohol abuse. EAP services may be offered on the employer's premises, in a counselor's private office, or at a contracted clinic. They may include classes, group therapy, or individual counseling.

employee contribution – The dollar amount or percentage of an insurance premium paid by the worker.

employer contribution – The dollar amount or percentage of an insurance premium paid by the worker's company.

empyema – Pus in a body space, usually due to an infection.

emulsifier – A chemical agent used to make an emulsion.

emulsion – A pharmaceutical preparation that mixes two agents that cannot ordinarily be mixed. The typical emulsion disperses an oil inside water (oil in water emulsion), although some disperse water inside an oil (water in oil emulsion). Most creams and lotions are emulsions.

Emulsions are prepared by mixing one ingredient with an emulsifier, an agent that forms a thin film around the outside of microscopic droplets of the first ingredient. Once this is completed, the second ingredient is added and mixed thoroughly to complete the product.

encephalitis – An inflammation of the brain. Encephalitis may be caused by either bacteria or viruses.

E

encephalopathy – A general term indicating any disease of the brain.

encounter – Each contact between a patient and a health care provider. For example, a person who has a total hip replacement would experience an encounter with each presurgical physician office visit, admission to the hospital, the surgery itself, each physical therapy appointment, each pharmacy visit, and each follow-up medical appointment. Depending upon the insurance coverage, each encounter could require a copayment or other fee. *Also see episode of care.*

endemic – Native to a geographic area. For example, the organism that causes Rocky Mountain spotted fever occurs naturally in (is endemic to) the American Rocky Mountain states as well as other areas.

endocarditis – Inflammation of the endocardium. Bacterial endocarditis (formerly called subacute bacterial endocarditis) is an extremely serious bacterial infection in this area. Those who survive this infection often have damage to the heart valves and may require valve replacement surgery after recovery from the infection.

endocardium – The lining of the interior structures of the heart and its underlying connective tissue.

endocrine – Pertaining to the ductless glands that secrete hormones directly into the blood.

endocrine gland – A hormone-secreting organ within the endocrine system. *See endocrine system.*

endocrine system – The collective term for the ductless glands that secrete hormones directly into the blood. Glands of the endocrine system include the thyroid, pituitary, pancreas, adrenals, testes, ovaries, and many others. The glands of the endocrine system regulate many of the metabolic functions of the body.

Glands that secrete their metabolic products into ducts are not part of the endocrine system. Examples include the tear, salivary, and mammary glands.

Also see exocrine glands.

E

endocrinologist – A physician who specializes in the diagnosis and treatment of diseases of the endocrine glands.

endocrinology – The branch of medicine that deals with the health and function of the glands of the endocrine system. *See endocrine system.*

endogenous – Pertaining to something whose origin is within the body. For example, endogenous depression is a mental illness that occurs because of chemical deficits within the brain. By contrast, exogenous depression is caused by factors outside of the patient, for example, loss of a job, death of a loved one, etc.

endometriosis – A condition where uterine tissue forms painful cysts outside of the uterus such as the pelvic cavity, intestines, and even the lungs.

endometritis – Inflammation of the endometrium.

endometrium – The mucous membrane that lines the interior of the uterus. The purpose of the endometrium is to provide a nurturing environment for a fertilized ovum.

endorphin – A naturally occurring substance that mimics many of the effects of narcotics. Endorphins are part of the body's pain control system.

endoscopy – Examination of an interior structure by means of a flexible fiber optic tube. An endoscope may be used to examine the esophagus and stomach, the colon, the lungs, and other areas. A light shining down the fiber optic portion of the tube provides visualization for the examiner. Endoscopes usually have a device at the far end to take biopsies for later examination and a camera port at the examiner's end to photograph the site of the examination.

endotoxin – A noxious substance formed by bacteria and retained inside the organisms. Endotoxins are usually not released until the bacteria die.

end-stage renal disease – A deterioration of kidney function to the point where dialysis or a kidney transplant is necessary to sustain life.

E

enema – An infusion of fluid into the rectum. Enemas are most often used to promote bowel movements or to prepare the bowel for x-ray examination. Enemas intended to produce a bowel movement may contain plain water, soapy water, or a laxative. Enemas containing barium sulfate may be used to assist in diagnosing intestinal problems.

In rare cases, an enema may be used to administer a drug other than a laxative or diagnostic aid.

enrollee – A person who is covered by a health insurance plan. An enrollee may be either the policyholder or an eligible dependent.

enrollment – The process of registering people for an insurance plan.

Also, the list of people who are covered by an insurance plan.

enrollment period – The time during which individuals may register for an insurance plan. Most companies allow enrollment at the time of employment and at a designated time each year. The annual enrollment period is usually called an open enrollment period.

ENT – Abbreviation for ears, nose, and throat.

ent- – Prefix meaning inner.

enter- – Prefix meaning intestine.

enteral – Pertaining to the gastrointestinal system. For example, an enteral feeding is food given by mouth or by tube directly into the digestive tract. In contrast, a parenteral feeding is given intravenously.

enteral nutrition – Feedings given into the gastrointestinal system. While normal eating qualifies as enteral nutrition, the term is usually applied to specially prepared liquid feedings.

enteric – Pertaining to the intestines.

enteric coating – A special outside layer applied to certain tablets or capsules to assure that they do not disintegrate until they are past the stomach and into the intestinal tract, usually the lower small intestine or the large intestine. Enteric coatings are usual-

E

ly reserved for drugs that are either irritating to the stomach or are destroyed by stomach acid.

enteritis – An inflammation of the intestine, particularly the small intestine.

entero- – Prefix meaning intestine.

enterocolitis – Inflammation that affects both the large (colitis) and small (enteritis) intestines. Some cases of enterocolitis are caused by antibiotics that irritate the intestinal lining.

enteropathy – A general term indicating any disease of the intestines.

enterospasm – Painful muscle contractions in the walls of the intestines.

enterostasis – A standing still or greatly reduced movement of the intestinal contents.

enterotoxin – A noxious agent, usually produced by infecting bacteria, that acts specifically against the intestinal lining.

ento- – Prefix meaning inner.

enuresis – The inability to retain bladder control. Most often used in the context of nocturnal enuresis, the inability to retain urine at night. Bedwetting.

enzyme – A protein that catalyzes biochemical reactions. In the body, enzymes assist in food digestion, protein formation, drug metabolism, and many other types of reactions. Absence of a single enzyme can lead to serious deficiency diseases. *Also see catalyst.*

EOB – *See explanation of benefits.*

EOI – *See evidence of insurability.*

eosinophil – A white blood cell that gets its name from its characteristic granules that stain red or orange when prepared for microscopic examination. Eosinophils are capable of destroying bacteria and increase in number during allergic reactions.

eosinophilia – An abnormally elevated number of eosinophils in blood. While not a problem itself, eosinophilia may indicate an allergic reaction.

E

epidemic – A disease that affects more people than usual within a prescribed geographic area. For example, during the autumn or winter influenza becomes epidemic in a specific city, county, state, or country when an unusually large number of people contract the illness.

epidemiology – The study of the factors that contribute to the occurrence of a disease. The term is most often applied to studies of patterns of infectious diseases.

epidermis – The outermost layer of skin.

epidural – Pertaining to the area near the dura mater, the tissue that covers and protects the brain and spinal cord. An epidural anesthetic is a local anesthetic infused near the spinal cord for the purpose of pain control. Epidural anesthetics are most commonly used to relieve pain during childbirth.

epigastric – Pertaining to the epigastrium.

epigastric pain – Discomfort that arises from the epigastrium. Epigastric pain is a common symptom of peptic ulcer and a frequent side effect of drug therapy.

epigastrium – The portion of the lower chest that includes the stomach and lower portion of the esophagus.

epilepsy – A disorder characterized by abnormal electrical activity in the brain that causes changes in consciousness, thought processes, and/or involuntary muscle contractions.

Epilepsy manifests itself in many ways, depending upon the location, intensity, and extensiveness of the electrical abnormalities.

epileptic – Pertaining to epilepsy.

Also, a person who has epilepsy.

epileptiform – Resembling epilepsy.

episode of care – The complete course of treatment provided for a specific condition. For example, a single episode of care for a total hip replacement would include presurgical physician office visits, admission to a hospital, the surgery itself, rehabilitation

E

services, prescriptions, and follow-up medical visits. Contrasted with an encounter, which is considered to be each individual contact between a patient and a health care provider. *Also see encounter.*

epistaxis – Nosebleed.

EPS – *See extrapyramidal symptoms.*

ER – Abbreviation for emergency room.

erectile – Pertaining to an erection, usually of the penis.

erectile dysfunction – The inability of a male to achieve or maintain a penile erection until the completion of intercourse. Causes of erectile dysfunction may be physical or psychological. Treatments may involve psychotherapy, surgery, or drug therapy with agents taken by mouth, injections into the penis, or penile suppositories.

Also called impotence.

erection – A normal state where the penis fills with blood and hardens. An erection is necessary for sexual intercourse.

erosion – A tissue or structure whose surface has worn away, decayed, or corroded. In the gastrointestinal tract, gastric or duodenal ulcers usually start as shallow erosions in the protective mucus lining of the affected area.

ERT – *See estrogen replacement therapy.*

eructation – Expulsion of gas from the upper gastrointestinal tract. Belching. Burping.

eruption – Nonspecific term that may be applied to any abruptly occurring lesion on the skin. A drug eruption is a drug-induced skin rash.

erysipelas – An inflamed, painful, edematous skin rash caused by toxins released by streptococcal bacteria. Although caused by a bacterial toxin, erysipelas is not usually contagious.

erythema – Nonspecific term that indicates inflammation and reddening of the skin.

E

erythematous – Pertaining to erythema.

erythr- – Prefix denoting red or redness.

erythro- – Prefix denoting red or redness.

erythrocyte – A red blood cell. Erythrocytes contain hemoglobin, a complex organic compound that binds oxygen from the lungs. As erythrocytes travel through the body, they exchange oxygen for carbon dioxide. Once back in the lungs, the erythrocytes exchange carbon dioxide for oxygen and repeat the cycle.

erythropoiesis – The process of forming erythrocytes in the bone marrow.

erythropoietin – A hormone formed in the kidneys that stimulates red blood cell formation. Erythropoietin is now artificially produced (genetically engineered) and administered to people who have conditions that cause low red blood cell counts. These include some kidney diseases, cancers, leukemias, and the treatments for cancer and leukemia.

eschar – The thickened skin that forms following a thermal or chemical burn.

Escherichia – A genus of bacteria commonly found in the intestinal tract. The most commonly encountered species, *Escherichia coli* (abbreviated *E. coli*), appears commonly in nature, usually due to animal defecation. In humans, most strains of *E. coli* inhabit the intestinal tract without causing problems. Some strains, however, are pathogenic and can cause serious intestinal infections. *E. coli* is the most common cause of urinary tract infections.

esophageal varices – Bulging blood vessels found in the esophagus, particularly in association with liver disease. Esophageal varices are caused by the pressure that occurs when blood flow through the liver is restricted. The most common cause of the condition is cirrhosis of the liver. If one of these varices bursts, there is danger of bleeding to death.

esophagi – Plural of esophagus.

E

esophagitis – Inflammation of the esophagus. Esophagitis most commonly occurs when acid from the stomach splashes up and burns the unprotected esophagus.

esophagoscopy – Examination of the esophagus with an endoscope. *See endoscopy.*

esophagus – A tube-like structure, approximately 12 inches in length, that allows food to pass from the mouth to the stomach.

essential – Pertaining to something that is vital. An essential amino acid, for example, is a constituent of protein that is necessary for life and cannot, in the human body, be made from any other nutrient. Essential amino acids must be ingested in the diet.

Also something that is of unknown cause. *See essential hypertension.*

essential hypertension – High blood pressure that results from an unknown cause. Also called primary hypertension, over 90% of cases of high blood pressure fall into this category. While some factors are known to lead to an increased risk (e.g., family history) or increased severity (e.g., excessive salt intake, tobacco use) of essential hypertension, no single factor or combination of factors has been determined to trigger the sustained elevation of blood pressure.

Most of the known causes of hypertension, called secondary hypertension, relate to kidney disease.

EST – Abbreviation for electroshock therapy, an old term for electroconvulsive therapy. *See electroconvulsive therapy.*

estrogen – The primary female sex hormone. Produced mainly in the ovaries, estrogen is responsible for initiating the menstrual cycle and for the development of secondary sexual characteristics in adult women. These include breast growth, fat deposition on the hips and thighs, and pubic and axillary hair growth.

estrogen dependent – Pertaining to a cancer, usually breast cancer, whose growth is stimulated by the presence of estrogen. Drugs such as tamoxifen block estrogen receptors on these cancer cells, preventing estrogen from stimulating the cancer cells and thereby slowing their growth.

E

estrogenic – Pertaining to estrogen.

estrogen independent – Pertaining to a cancer, usually breast cancer, whose growth is independent of the presence or absence of estrogen. These cancers do not respond to treatment with estrogen receptor blockers such as tamoxifen.

estrogen replacement therapy (ERT) – Hormone treatment intended to substitute for estrogen that is no longer produced due to menopause or surgical removal of the ovaries.

ethanol – Grain alcohol. Ethyl alcohol.

ethical pharmaceutical – A drug that is available only by prescription.

ethical pharmaceutical manufacturer – A company that makes and distributes prescription medicines.

ethics – A moral code of conduct. Medical ethics is the code of conduct that relates to the practice of medicine and the behavior of physicians when they deal with patients or patient-related activities.

etiology – The study of the cause of disease.
Also, the description of the cause of a specific disease. For example, the etiology of congestive heart failure is the weakening of the heart muscle.

eu- – Prefix meaning good or normal.

euphoria – A feeling of well-being, especially emotionally high spirits. Excessive, long-lasting, or inappropriate euphoria may be a sign of a mental illness.

euphoriant – An agent that produces euphoria. Often a drug of abuse.

eustachian tube – An anatomic passageway from the middle ear to the throat. The purpose of the eustachian tube is to equalize air pressure on both sides of the tympanic membrane (ear drum). At times, particularly during an upper respiratory infection, bacteria can migrate up the eustachian tube from the throat to the middle ear, causing otitis media (middle ear infection). This situation occurs most commonly in children.

eutectic mixture – A combination of crystalline materials that, when blended together, change to liquid form. Camphor and menthol are commonly used to make eutectic mixtures. Once camphor and menthol crystals are physically mixed with each other, the crystals slowly liquefy until all that remains is a pool of liquid camphor and menthol.

Eutectic mixtures are pharmaceutical curiosities that are sometimes used to facilitate the preparation of a cream, liniment, or similar product. Otherwise, they are curiosities that have little practical or commercial value.

euthanasia – The act of purposefully causing death to end suffering. Mercy killing. Most states and countries consider euthanasia to be murder; however, cases are not always vigorously prosecuted. The difference between euthanasia and assisted suicide is that assisted suicide involves the active participation of the decedent, while euthanasia is performed entirely by another person.

euthyroidism – The condition of normal thyroid function. Contrasted with hyperthyroidism or hypothyroidism, conditions of excessive or diminished thyroid hormone production, respectively.

evacuant – An agent that induces or facilitates elimination, usually of feces. Laxatives and enemas are examples of evacuants.

evacuate – To eliminate. Usually used in the context of feces. To have or produce a bowel movement.

evidence of insurability (EOI) – Proof that a person is eligible for insurance coverage. This is usually required when an employee or dependent requests insurance coverage outside of the open enrollment period. Depending upon the insurer, the applicant may need to provide documentation of a recent medical examination and/or a listing of all past or current medical problems.

ex- – A prefix meaning out of or away from.

exacerbation – A worsening of a condition or symptom. Typically used in the context of a sudden deterioration in condition.

excipient – An inert substance added to a drug product to give form or consistency. Common excipients include simple syrup to

E

make liquid dosage forms and lactose to provide bulk to fill out a tablet or capsule.

excision – The surgical removal of an organ, tissue, or lesion. Contrasted with incision, the surgical cut itself.

exclusion – A service or condition that is not covered by an insurance policy. In some cases, exclusions may be time limited. For example, pregnancy coverage may be excluded for the first ten months of a new policy's life and then covered thereafter.

excoriation – A scratch, usually one deep enough to cause bleeding.

excretion – The process of elimination. The body excretes fluid wastes in the form of urine, solid wastes as feces, and gaseous wastes as flatus or breath.

excretory – Pertaining to excretion.

exercise-induced asthma – Bronchospasm triggered by any type of strenuous exercise. About 20% of cases of asthma are exercise-induced.

exfoliation – Loss of cells from any tissue surface. Usually applied to conditions of flaking or scaling of skin, especially if the loss of skin is in excess of normal.

exo- – Prefix meaning external.

exocrine glands – The organs whose secretions are transported to the point of use by means of a duct. Exocrine glands include the tear glands, salivary glands, and mammary glands. Unlike the endocrine glands, the exocrine glands do not regulate the functions of other organs nor do their secretions travel in the general blood circulation.

exogenous – Pertaining to something whose origin is outside of the body or organism. *See endogenous.*

exotoxin – A noxious substance formed inside bacteria but released into the outer environment. Unlike endotoxins, exotoxins are continually released by living bacteria and cause symptoms of infection in humans or other host organisms.

E

expectorant – A medication that promotes liquification of mucus in the lungs and facilitates its elimination through coughing.

expectorate – To cough up and spit out or simply to spit.

expedited approval – A procedure followed by the United States Food and Drug Administration (FDA) to allow faster marketing authorization for drugs that show promise in treating life-threatening diseases. Expedited approval can trim months or years off of the normal approval time. This procedure is often applied in the cases of drugs intended to treat cancer or AIDS.

experimental drug – A medication not yet approved by the United States Food and Drug Administration (FDA) for marketing as a prescription product. Before allowing manufacturers to distribute a new drug to pharmacies, it must first be tested in animals. If animal testing indicates that the drug is safe and effective, the FDA approves the drug for human testing, which involves giving the drug to as many as several thousand volunteers. If the FDA decides that the drug is safe and effective for use in humans, it will approve the drug for marketing. At this point it is no longer considered to be experimental.

expiration date – A specific day or month when it is determined that a drug product has lost a significant amount of its potency, usually about 10%. In some cases, expiration dates may be based on the known rate of chemical decomposition. For example, many antibiotic oral suspensions lose significant potency within 14 days of the time they are mixed, and therefore have a 14-day expiration date. In other cases, the assigned expiration date may be arbitrary. Pharmaceutical manufacturers must assign expiration dates to all of their products, even if they do not lose significant potency over many years of storage. In these cases, a drug company may assign an arbitrary expiration date three or four years after manufacture.

expire – To exhale or to die.

explanation of benefits (EOB) – A written statement from an insurer to a covered individual following an encounter or group of encounters. Typically, EOBs indicate charges from the

E

encounter(s), the amount paid by insurance, and the amount the individual owes to the provider.

extended care facility (ECF) – A specially qualified, supervised residential arrangement for individuals who are not capable of living independently, but do not require hospital care. ECFs include skilled and intermediate nursing facilities (nursing homes) and custodial care.

extra- – Prefix meaning outside of.

extracellular – Outside of a cell. For example, extracellular fluid is liquid not found inside a cell. The largest volume of extracellular fluid is the blood.

extract – A drug or other chemical removed from a complex mixture or organism by means of solvents. For example, the active drug ingredients within natural herbal products are usually extracted by grinding the plant into small particles, mixing the plant particles with a solvent such as water, alcohol, or ether in order to selectively dissolve the active drug, and then separating the drug-rich solvent from the plant. Once the solvent evaporates, it leaves behind a highly concentrated drug residue. This residue is the extract.

extrahepatic – Outside the liver. A drug that is metabolized by an extrahepatic pathway is one that is chemically altered within the body, but not in the liver.

extrapyramidal symptoms (EPS) – Neurologic signs indicative of problems with nerve transmissions around the pyramidal tract. EPS are common side effects of the medicines used to treat psychotic disorders. They include tremors, muscle rigidity, difficulty swallowing, difficulty sitting still, and sometimes muscle contortions.

extravasation – A site where blood has leaked into the tissue that surrounds a blood vessel. This most often occurs when an intravenous catheter becomes dislodged from the vein but the intravenous fluid continues to infuse and collects in the subcutaneous tissue.

E

exudate – Any fluid that discharges from an organ or tissue. The term is typically used to describe fluid or pus that forms from an injury or infection.

eyewash – A sterile solution used to cleanse contaminants from the eye or to reduce eye irritation. Eyewashes must be sterile solutions, otherwise they may cause infection.

F

face – The front of the head. Includes the forehead, eyes, nose, mouth, chin, and cheeks. The ears are not considered part of the face.

F.A.C.O.G. – Abbreviation for Fellow of the American College of Obstetricians and Gynecologists.

F.A.C.P. – Abbreviation for Fellow of the American College of Physicians.

F.A.C.R. – Abbreviation for Fellow of the American College of Radiologists.

F.A.C.S. – Abbreviation for Fellow of the American College of Surgeons.

F.A.C.S.M. – Abbreviation for Fellow of the American College of Sports Medicine.

factor – An essential component. Normally used in the context of blood clotting factors, the proteins in the blood that stop bleeding. *See also clotting factor.*

facultative – A term used to describe organisms that are capable of living in more than one type of environment, such as in the presence or absence of oxygen. Typically used to describe certain species of bacteria.

failure – The inability to perform a normal function. For example, congestive heart failure is a condition characterized by the inability of the heart to pump strongly enough to properly circulate blood. Renal failure is the inability of the kidneys to concentrate and eliminate urine.

fallopian tube – The passageway in the female reproductive system that allows an ovum to pass from the ovary to the uterus. The most common form of female sterilization (tube tying) involves closing the fallopian tubes.

false negative – A test result that has reported a normal value when the true value is abnormal. False negative results are problematic because they may obscure or delay proper diagnosis. Because of false negative diagnostic tests, physicians may overlook important signs of disease.

Reasons for false negative results include testing procedures that are not sensitive enough to detect a problem, a drug interaction that interferes with the test, a laboratory error, a patient's failure to follow pretest instructions, or a physician's or technician's misinterpretation of testing data.

Opposite of a false positive.

false positive – A test result that has reported an abnormal value when the true value is normal. False positive results are problematic because they may cause patients and physicians to think a disease is present when it is not. This may cause undue anxiety and unnecessary treatment.

Reasons for false positive results include testing procedures that are too sensitive, a drug interaction that interferes with the test, a laboratory error, a patient's failure to follow pretest instructions, or a physician's or technician's misinterpretation of testing data.

Opposite of a false negative.

familial – Pertaining to a family. A familial disease or disorder is one that is present in several members of a family or in several generations of a family. Familial medical problems may be genetic, environmental, or have other causes that trigger conditions to occur in family clusters.

family deductible – The amount of money that must be paid in order for the entire family to receive full insurance benefits. For example, a policy may require a $1,000 deductible for an individual or a $3,000 deductible for the family. This means that once a specific member of the family incurs $1,000 of out-of-pocket expense, only that family member qualifies for full coverage for the remainder of the year. However, once the members of the family collectively incur $3,000 of out-of-pocket expenses, all members of the family qualify for full coverage. Under a family deductible, all members of a large family may qualify for full coverage even though no one member exceeds the individual deductible.

family membership – An insurance plan that covers the subscribing member and all of his/her qualified dependants.

F

family practice – The medical specialty that focuses on health care of an entire family. *See also family practitioner.*

family practitioner – A primary care physician who treats all age groups and both sexes. Family practitioners prefer to treat all members of the family, enabling them to determine how family dynamics affect the health of each family member. Their training includes adult medicine, geriatrics, pediatrics, obstetrics, and psychiatry. Board eligible family practitioners have completed a three-year residency following medical school.

fat – Any of a wide variety of solid or semi-solid oily or greasy materials found in animal tissue or in plants, particularly their seeds. Chemically, fats are formed by the combination of glycerol with a fatty acid. *See also fatty acid.*

fatal – Pertaining to death or its cause. For example, a fatal drug interaction is a combination of medicines that caused a person's death or could cause death to other persons similarly exposed.

fatigue – The state of being tired. Fatigue can be physical (due to sleeplessness or overactivity) or mental (due to anxiety or other emotional stress).

fatty acid – One of a series of organic acids that have the general formula of $C_nH_{2n+1}COOH$. Fatty acids have an even number of carbon atoms and only one acid combining site (-COOH). Fatty acids have only single bonds between carbon atoms in the main chain, causing each carbon atom to be "saturated" with hydrogen. Several fatty acids are essential for life and must be consumed in the diet.

F.C.A.P. – Abbreviation for Fellow of the College of American Pathologists.

FDA – *See Food and Drug Administration.*

febrile – Pertaining to a fever.

fecal – Pertaining to feces.

fecal impaction – An obstruction in the large intestine or rectum caused by the failure of feces to pass through. Fecal impactions are usually relieved by physically digging the fecal plug out of the rectum. Laxatives or stool softeners may be used prophylactically for those whose medical conditions place them at risk of fecal impactions.

feces – Unabsorbed residue of foods that passes through the intestinal tract and is eliminated through the anus. The solid wastes from digestion are consolidated into a semisolid mass in the large intestine before being discharged as a bowel movement.

Federal Trade Commission (FTC) – The agency of the United States government that regulates advertising, monitors accuracy of advertising, and prosecutes unfair advertising practices. The FTC regulates direct-to-consumer advertising of prescription and nonprescription drugs.

fee – A charge for a professional service. In pharmacy, a dispensing fee is the reimbursement the pharmacy receives for dispensing a prescription. *See also dispensing fee.*

fee disclosure – The practice of informing patients and/or insurers how much they can expect to pay before the service is provided. Patients and insurers may agree or not agree to the fee before service is provided.

fee maximum – The greatest amount a health care provider will be paid for a specified service. *Also see fee schedule.*

fee schedule – A list of payments a health plan or other payer is willing to make for specified professional services. Most contracts with health care providers specify that the plan will pay the provider the lesser of either the fee listed on the fee schedule or the amount the provider bills. If a provider bills the insurer an amount greater than that listed on the fee schedule, the insurer will reimburse only the amount allowed by the fee schedule. If the provider bills a lesser amount, the insurer will pay the lesser amount.

feeding – Giving nourishment. Feedings are usually swallowed but can be given directly into the stomach by means of a tube or can be given intravenously.

fee-for-service – The traditional billing practice where a health care provider bills the patient a usual and customary charge for each

F

professional contact. Fees are usually paid at the time service is provided.

feminization – The development of female features in a male. Feminization can be the result of hormonal problems that develop at puberty or can be artificially induced by treating men with estrogen.

fermentation – A chemical process where a complex organic compound is split into simpler parts, usually with the help of an enzyme. Naturally occurring enzymes and bacterial enzymes in the human intestinal tract ferment complex carbohydrates to form simpler, more absorbable sugars. The major by-products of this fermentation are water, carbon dioxide gas, and methane gas. Better known to most people is the yeast-assisted fermentation of carbohydrates to alcohol.

fertile – Pertaining to the ability to conceive.

fertilization – The union of a sperm with an egg.

In *vivo* fertilization is the combination of a sperm cell with a donor egg within the female reproductive tract. The fertilized egg is later transferred to another woman to sustain the pregnancy.

In *vitro* fertilization is the combination of a sperm cell with an egg in a specially prepared medium outside of the female reproductive tract. Once fertilization is accomplished, the cell is implanted in the uterus.

festination – The characteristic gait of a person with Parkinson's disease. A festinating gait combines a shuffling of the feet with the tendency to pitch the body forward, potentially losing balance. As the condition progresses, a cane or walker may be necessary to assist balance.

fetal – Pertaining to a fetus.

fetid – Pertaining to a foul or putrid odor. The term is often used to describe the smell of decaying flesh.

fetotoxicity – Injury to a developing baby prior to birth. Usually the result of trauma, chemical exposure, or radiation exposure during pregnancy.

F

fetus – An unborn child from the end of the second month of life until the time of birth. During the first two months of life, an unborn child is an embryo.

fever – Body temperature above normal. The average normal body temperature for humans is 98.6° Fahrenheit or 37° Celsius. Normal may vary from one individual to another.

In the usual context, disease-induced elevated body temperature above normal is considered to be a fever, while elevated body temperature due to a normal function, such as exercise, is usually not described as a fever.

Hay fever is neither a fever nor caused by hay. *See allergic rhinitis.*

fever blister – A red, painful lesion on the lip or in the mouth caused by the herpes virus. Fever blisters are most likely to occur in times of physical or emotional stress. *Also see herpes simplex.*

fever reducer – A colloquial term for antipyretic, a drug that reduces fever. *Also see antipyretic.*

feverish – The state of having a fever.

fiber – A threadlike material, for example, nerve fibers or muscle fibers. In common usage, fiber is used as a synonym for bran, the indigestible carbohydrate derived from milling grains or for the indigestible residue of any vegetable or fruit. *Also see bran.*

fiberoptic – Pertaining to fiberoptics.

fiberoptics – The branch of physics that deals with transmission of light and images along a flexible filament. Certain substances (e.g., glass, plastics) are able to conduct light along the course of a strand made of that substance. This allows for transmission of light beams and images around bends and corners. Fiberoptic devices are used extensively in medicine as various types of endoscopes to visualize and biopsy internal tissues and organs. *Also see endoscope.*

fibr- – Prefix designating fiber.

fibric acid derivative – A class of drugs used clinically to lower cholesterol and other blood lipids.

F

fibrillation – Uncoordinated twitching and partial contraction of a muscle. Fibrillation interferes with normal muscle function. The term is most commonly used in the context of atrial or ventricular fibrillation of the heart. Atrial fibrillation is characterized by irregular rhythms of the atrial chambers of the heart. Most cases of atrial fibrillation are self-limited and require no specific treatment. Ventricular fibrillation, however, virtually destroys the ability of the heart to pump blood and is rapidly fatal, requiring immediate cardiopulmonary resuscitation.

fibrin – A protein formed from fibrinogen that forms a net-like structure that allows a blood clot to organize and anchor itself to a blood vessel wall.

fibrinogen – A blood clotting factor responsible for forming fibrin. Without fibrinogen and fibrin, blood would not be able to form the clots necessary to stop bleeding.

fibrinolysis – The enzymatic destruction of fibrin. Once a clot has stopped blood loss and injured blood vessels have healed, fibrin has no further purpose. Enzymes in the blood dissolve the remaining fibrin so normal blood flow can be restored through the injured area.

fibrinolytic – Pertaining to the process of fibrinolysis. Also, an agent that promotes fibrinolysis.

fibro- – Prefix meaning fiber.

fibrosis – Development of connective tissue in an organ or tissue. In its usual context, fibrosis indicates an abnormal state.

filler – An inert substance included in a tablet or capsule to provide enough bulk so that the final dosage form is easier for a patient to take. Most tablets and capsules contain many more ingredients than the drug itself (*see formulation*). As an example, the most commonly prescribed dose of digoxin for heart conditions contains only 0.25 milligrams of digoxin. That amount is too small to see with the naked eye, much less take as a dose of medicine. Consequently, the pharmaceutical manufacturer adds enough filler to the tablets so they are large enough to be handled and swallowed easily.

F

first aid – Immediate medical treatment given at the scene of an injury or sudden illness by a participant, bystander, or witness to the event. The person giving first aid may or may not have training to do so.

first-dollar coverage – An insurance plan that involves no deductible although copayments and exclusions may still apply.

first pass metabolism – The degree to which a drug is chemically altered as it circulates through the liver for the first time. Most orally administered drugs are absorbed into the blood vessels that line the intestinal tract. The blood in these vessels flows directly to the liver, the body's primary site for drug metabolism, before it goes anywhere else in the body. Some drugs are totally destroyed the first and only time they pass through, while other drugs are hardly affected at all.

The oral route of administration is not suitable for most drugs that experience a high degree of first pass metabolism because those drugs are quickly deactivated. Nitroglycerin tablets, for example, are dissolved under the tongue rather than being swallowed because nitroglycerin is completely inactivated during its first pass through the liver.

Also see metabolism.

fissure – A split, crevice, groove, or gap. A fissure may be part of the normal anatomy or may be the result of injury or disease. An anal fissure, for example, is a painful crack in the lining of the anus. Anal fissures are difficult to treat and slow to heal.

fistula – An abnormal passageway from one abscess, cavity, or hollow organ to another or to the surface of the skin. In some cases, fistulas allow abscesses to drain material to the outside of the body, relieving pressure within the abscess. However, fistulas can also allow body fluids to drain into areas that cause even greater problems. For example, a colovesical fistula allows feces from the large intestine to seep into the urinary bladder.

flaccid – Weak or feeble. Most often used in the context of a muscle that no longer contracts with its usual force. Also used to describe a nonerect penis.

F

flare – A reddened area of the skin that spreads out from the point of contact with a toxin or allergen. Often used in the context of a wheal and flare, an allergic reaction that causes a welt surrounded by a reddened area.

flashback – A sudden recall of a past experience. Flashback memories of distressing events are common in post-traumatic stress disorder. Flashback hallucinations are also associated with previous drug abuse, particularly with LSD.

flatulence – The expulsion of excessive amounts of gas from the digestive tract, particularly intestinal gas passed through the anus.

flatus – Gas or air in the digestive tract, particularly in the intestines. Flatus may consist of swallowed air or methane or carbon dioxide formed as a result of digestion and fermentation of carbohydrate.

flavor – The characteristic taste of a substance.

Also, a flavoring agent.

flavoring agent – A material added to a pharmaceutical preparation to improve its taste. Flavoring agents add no medicinal value to the preparation. Common flavoring agents include mint, cherry, and grape extracts.

florid – Flushed with red or pink color. Most commonly used to describe the skin.

flu – *See influenza.*

fluidextract – A concentrated solution of a drug removed from a plant source by mixing ground parts of the plant with a suitable solvent, usually alcohol, and then separating the plant residue from the solvent. Typically, one milliliter (approximately 1/30th of a fluid ounce) contains 1 gram (approximately 1/30th of a dry ounce) of drug.

Fluidextracts are not intended to be administered directly to a patient. Instead, they are used to provide a source of drug in the manufacture of final dosage forms.

fluoridation – The addition of fluoride, usually as sodium fluoride, to the public drinking water supply. Adding one part of fluoride to one million parts of water significantly decreases tooth decay in communities that use fluoridated water. Children who live in areas where the water is not fluoridated may need to take special vitamin products that contain supplemental fluoride.

fluoroquinolones – A group of broad-spectrum antibacterial drugs. Fluoroquinolones are commonly used to treat infections in the skin, respiratory tract, bones, and urinary tract.

flush – To wash with a stream of fluid. Often used in the context of clearing an intravenous catheter with a heparin or saline solution. Depending upon the type of catheter, flushing may be done as often as every few hours. Flushing reduces the risk of infection and irritation to the vein.

Also, to become red in the face due to disease, heat, exertion, or embarrassment.

flutter – Rapid vibration. Atrial flutter is a vibration or twitching of the atrial chambers of the heart resulting in over 250 partial contractions per minute. Atrial flutter is usually not a serious condition and usually resolves without treatment.

focal epilepsy – An electrical disturbance that affects only one specific area of the brain. Focal epilepsy is characterized by seizures that are limited to a specific part of the body, e.g., one hand, one arm, one leg, etc.

folk medicine – The practice of treating illness by means of home remedies that have usually been passed from one generation to the next.

folliculitis – Inflammation of a hair follicle, the sac-like structure where hairs originate. Folliculitis appears as inflamed bumps on the skin that may or may not contain pus.

Food and Drug Administration (FDA) – The agency of the United States government that regulates pharmaceutical products. FDA establishes criteria for judging whether a new drug can be tested in humans and whether it may be released onto the market. FDA also has the authority to recall specific lots of drugs if they

F

are found to have impurities or to rescind its permission to market a drug if it is found to be a danger to the public health. The FDA also regulates foods and medical devices.

Although its authority is wide-ranging, the FDA does not regulate farming (United States Department of Agriculture) or drug abuse (Drug Enforcement Agency of the Justice Department). FDA is excluded by act of Congress from regulating herbal remedies, even though these are legally considered to be dietary supplements.

formula – The recipe or description for compounding a prescription.

Also, the chemical symbols that represent the atoms, their quantity, and positions in a molecule.

formulary – *See drug formulary.*

formulation – All of the ingredients necessary to produce a pharmaceutical preparation. In addition to the drug itself, the formulation includes any fillers, flavoring agents, solvents, binders, suspending agents, coating agents, preservatives, or dissolution agents contained in the final product.

F.R.C.P. – Abbreviation for Fellow of the Royal College of Physicians of England.

F.R.C.S. – Abbreviation for Fellow of the Royal College of Surgeons of England.

freeze drying – A drug manufacturing process that involves freezing a solution of a drug followed by establishment of a partial vacuum in order to force evaporation and removal of the solvent. Freeze dried drugs have longer shelf life than their liquid forms and are easy to redissolve prior to use. Freeze drying is most commonly used in the manufacture of drugs intended for injection.

frequency – The number of times an action occurs in a measured length of time. Often used in the context of urinary frequency, an excessive number of occurrences of urination over a given period of time. Urinary frequency may be a sign of bladder infection, prostate disease, or other urinary tract problem.

F.R.S. – Abbreviation for Fellow of the Royal Society of England.

F

FTC – *See Federal Trade Commission.*

fulminant – Occurring suddenly and with great intensity.

fungal – Pertaining to a fungus.

fungi – Plural form of fungus.

fungicide – A drug or chemical that kills fungi. Medicinal fungicides may be applied to the skin, taken by mouth, or injected intravenously, depending upon the site and severity of fungal infection.

fungoid – Similar in appearance to a fungus.

fungus – A life form that includes yeasts and molds. Fungi are valuable members of the ecosystem, assisting in the decay of dead plants and animals. Some fungi are also capable of infecting living tissue, producing diseases varying in intensity from athlete's foot and diaper rash to pneumonia and meningitis.

G

g – Abbreviation for gram. Previously, gram was abbreviated as gm.

gag clause – A provision in the agreement between a health insurance company and health care providers that prohibits the providers from discussing with plan members the availability of diagnostic or treatment options outside of the plan.

gait – The manner or style of walking. A gait that is markedly different than normal may be a manifestation of disease or compensation for poor balance. For example, a festinating gait (*see festination*) commonly results from Parkinson's disease. A high stepping gait may be a sign of drug toxicity or foot drop.

galactorrhea – A discharge of milk or a milk-like substance from the breasts. Normal lactation for the purpose of breastfeeding is not considered to be galactorrhea. However, milky discharges between sessions of breastfeeding, after weaning, or due to a hormonal imbalance are considered to be galactorrhea.

galenical – A drug derived from a plant source. Also, pulverized medical plants or the extracts made from them.

gallbladder – A hollow organ located next to the liver that acts as the storage place for bile. Bile is formed in the liver to aid in digestion. The bile is then stored in the gallbladder to be released into the intestines as food passes.

gallon – A quantity of fluid in the English system of weights and measures. A gallon is equal to four quarts or 3.785 liters.

gallstone – A solid mass or concretion that forms in the gallbladder or the bile duct. Gallstones are usually formed by the combination of cholesterol and calcium compounds. They can produce intense pain when they block the bile duct, effectively damming the flow of bile and causing painful back-pressure in the gallbladder.

gamete – Any germ cell capable of fertilization. Gametes include sperm cells, ova, and pollen.

gangrene – Death of tissue due to insufficient blood supply. Gangrene may be caused by an infection or bacteria may invade and infect the dead tissue. Gangrene may be limited to a small area, such

G

as a finger or toe, or may involve an entire organ, such as the intestine. Gangrene in the feet or lower legs is a potential complication of atherosclerosis in the elderly or diabetes mellitus.

gangrenous – Pertaining to gangrene.

gargle – A liquid medication intended to rinse the mouth and throat. Gargles may be used for routine oral hygiene or may contain medications to liquefy mucus or relieve a sore throat.

Also, the act of rinsing the mouth and throat whereby the head is tilted back and fluid is allowed to enter the throat. Once in the throat, air expelled from the lungs bubbles through the fluid, making a gurgling sound as it passes.

gas – A material in the vapor state. Some chemical compounds naturally exist as gases at room temperature (e.g., oxygen, carbon dioxide) while others exist as gases only after boiling or evaporation (e.g., water, alcohol). Some medications (e.g., general anesthetics) exist as gases in their natural state and are administered by inhalation.

gastr- – Prefix designating the stomach.

gastrectomy – Surgical removal of part of the stomach. Surgery of this type may be necessitated by a stomach ulcer that does not heal by any other means or by a tumor.

gastric – Pertaining to the stomach.

gastric acid – Hydrochloric acid secreted into the stomach. Hydrochloric acid is a corrosive material that aids in digestion and kills most bacteria that enter the stomach along with food. Acid is secreted when food enters the stomach and stops when the stomach empties. The stomach churns the acid into the food, producing a semisolid material called chyme. The chyme passes into the small intestine where digestion continues.

Special cells that line the interior of the stomach protect it from being burned by the gastric acid. If these cells become damaged or worn away, a gastric ulcer may develop.

gastric ulcer – An erosion of the lining of the stomach. Gastric ulcer accounts for about 10% of cases of peptic ulcer. The most common form of peptic ulcer is duodenal ulcer. Although some individuals never experience significant discomfort, gastric ulcer typically causes a burning pain that may be temporarily relieved with food or antacids. Treatment usually consists of a combination of antacids and drugs that reduce acid secretion. Antibiotics may also be used if *Helicobacter pylori*, (see *Helicobacter pylori*) a bacterium often found in association with peptic ulcer, is present. Since effective treatments for this organism have been discovered, patients improve faster and experience fewer relapses.

gastritis – An inflammation of the mucous membrane that lines the interior of the stomach. Once thought to be a rare occurrence, the increased use of gastroscopy has revealed that gastritis is often present in people with other digestive tract problems, but usually causes few symptoms by itself.

gastro- – Prefix designating the stomach.

gastrocolic – Pertaining to both the stomach and large intestine.

gastrocolitis – Inflammation that affects the interior linings of both the stomach and large intestine.

gastroduodenal – Pertaining to both the stomach and the duodenum, the first portion of the small intestine.

gastroduodenitis – Inflammation that affects the interior linings of both the stomach and the duodenum, the first portion of the small intestine.

gastroenteritis – Inflammation that affects the interior linings of the stomach and the intestinal tract. Symptoms may include loss of appetite, nausea, vomiting, and/or diarrhea. Causes of gastroenteritis include dietary factors, exposure to toxic chemicals, radiation, side effects to drugs, and bacterial or viral infection. Gastroenteritis is the proper term for the condition colloquially known as stomach flu.

gastroenterologist – A physician who specializes in the diagnosis and treatment of diseases of the digestive tract.

gastroenterology – The area of medicine that deals with diagnosis and treatment of disorders of the digestive tract, including the esophagus, stomach, liver, pancreas, and small and large intestines.

G

gastroenteropathy – Any disease of the digestive tract.

gastroesophageal – Pertaining to both the stomach and the esophagus.

gastroesophageal reflux – A condition caused by the regurgitation of stomach contents into the lower portion of the esophagus. Normally, the lower end of the esophagus closes itself off to prevent stomach contents from flowing back into the esophagus. However, if the muscle at the juncture of the esophagus and the stomach is overcome by pressure in the stomach, the stomach's contents can reenter the esophagus. Symptoms of gastroesophageal reflux may range from slight discomfort or a feeling of pressure in the chest or abdomen to intense pain or burning. The symptoms are often colloquially called heartburn.

The pain of gastroesophageal reflux is caused by the acid present in the stomach. While the stomach has a natural barrier to protect it from acid burns, the esophagus does not. The symptoms are the result of acid burns in the esophagus.

gastroesophageal reflux disease (GERD) – A condition where stomach contents frequently or consistently reenter the esophagus due to the inability of esophageal-gastric juncture to close properly or tightly.

Also see gastroesophageal reflux.

gastroesophagitis – An inflammation of both the stomach and the esophagus.

gastrohepatic – Pertaining to both the stomach and the liver.

gastrointestinal (GI) – Pertaining to the stomach and the intestines.

gastrointestinal distress – A nonspecific term that indicates any bothersome symptoms relating to the stomach or intestinal tract. May include nausea, vomiting, abdominal cramps, or diarrhea.

gastrointestinal tract – The digestive system. Includes the esophagus, stomach, pancreas, small intestine, large intestine, rectum, and anus.

gastropathy – Any disease of the stomach.

G

gastroscopy – Use of endoscopy to examine the stomach. *See endoscopy.*

gastrospasm – An intense, often painful, contraction of the muscles in the stomach wall. Gastrospasm often results in vomiting.

gastrotoxic – Pertaining to a substance that is poisonous to the stomach.

gatekeeper – In a managed care setting, a gatekeeper is a physician, usually a primary care physician such as an internist, pediatrician, family practitioner, or gynecologist who is an insured member's first contact for any health care need, other than an emergency. When a need arises, the gatekeeper may either treat the patient himself/herself or refer the patient to a specialist. Under the gatekeeper model, patients who see a specialist without first consulting their primary care physician may be liable for all of the specialists' charges.

The purpose of the gatekeeper model is to control costs by encouraging members to see less costly primary care physicians for the majority of their care and only see specialists when medical needs are beyond the scope of practice of the primary care physicians.

gauge – A scale of measurement used for needles and catheters, whereby the larger the gauge number, the smaller the lumen of the needle or catheter. For example, a 28-gauge needle is extremely fine and is often used for insulin injections. A 16-gauge needle has a large bore and is sometimes used for intramuscular injections.

gauze – A thin, light, loosely woven material used to dress wounds or wrap injuries. Gauze is usually made of cotton and may be sterile or nonsterile.

gel – A jelly-like substance that may be used as a vehicle to administer a topical medication. Some gels have a high alcohol content and can sting if applied to broken skin.

gelatin – A tasteless, odorless protein derived from collagen. Gelatin is the primary ingredient of most capsules. It is ideal for this purpose because it does not dissolve if accidentally exposed to cold

G

water or humidity. However, it dissolves quickly in the warm fluids of the gastrointestinal tract, thereby releasing the capsules' contents.

-gen – Suffix designating production.

gen- – Prefix designating production or precursor.

gene – One of the units along a chromosome that carries hereditary characteristics. Genes are composed of a specific coding sequence within deoxyribonucleic acid (DNA). Genes establish specific traits by determining the structure of proteins or cellular regulators.

general anesthesia – The administration of a drug that causes loss of consciousness and loss of sensation throughout the body.

general hospital – An inpatient health care facility that offers services for a wide range of needs and conditions. Contrasted with special purpose hospitals such as psychiatric hospitals or pediatric hospitals, general hospitals typically offer multiple services that may include general medicine, surgery, pediatrics, obstetrics, and rehabilitation.

generalized – Widely spread through an organism. For example, a generalized seizure is a convulsion that affects the whole body.

general practitioner – A physician who provides medical care to patients of all ages and both sexes. A general practitioner may or may not have formal training in family practice. *Also see family practice.*

general surgeon – A physician who performs surgery on a wide range of medical problems. Contrasted with a specialized surgeon who typically operates primarily on specific organs or tissues; for example, a vascular surgeon operates on blood vessels, a thoracic surgeon operates on organs in the chest, etc.

generator – In nuclear pharmacy, a generator is a column of radioactive material whose decay produces (generates) a desired isotope. For example, technetium-99 is a radioactive nuclide that is commonly used for diagnostic testing. However, technetium-99 has a half-life of only a few hours, far too short to be shipped

G

from a manufacturer. Instead, the pharmacy purchases radioactive molybdenum, which decays to technetium-99. As the molybdenum decays, technetium-99 is collected and prepared for use in testing.

Also a device that converts energy into electricity.

generic – Pertaining to a product or material that is not protected by a patent.

Also, pertaining to a biologic genus.

generic bioequivalent – A generic drug product that has the same pharmaceutical properties as the original trademarked product. In order to be considered bioequivalent, the generic copy must achieve the same blood levels in test subjects as the original. Achieving bioequivalent blood levels is usually interpreted to indicate that both the generic drug and the reference standard provide the same therapeutic effect.

generic drug – A medication that can be produced by any licensed facility after the patent on the medication has expired. When a drug's patent expires, companies other than the originator can make and distribute the same chemical entity. They may not, however, use the trademarked name of the original drug. Generic drugs are typically much less costly than their brand name counterparts.

generic name – The nonproprietary, or nonbrand, name for a drug. Generic names are usually derived from the lengthy chemical name of a drug. Generic names are standardized and approved by the United States Food and Drug Administration for the sake of uniformity. For example, acetaminophen is the generic name of the trademarked product Tylenol as well as for hundreds of other products that use that chemical entity as an ingredient.

generic substitution – The practice of dispensing a generic drug in place of a brand name product. Each state regulates the practice and determines the circumstances under which generic substitution may be done and which drugs may or may not be substituted.

genetic disease – An inherited disorder. A medical condition that is passed from one generation to another because the disease is

G

linked to a specific gene. Examples include diabetes mellitus, sickle cell anemia, and cystic fibrosis.

genetic engineering – A technique where genes from one organism are spliced into the chromosomes of another organism. The purpose of genetic engineering is to alter the function of the recipient cells to make them produce a new substance or to perform a new function.

Production of human insulin is an example of genetic engineering. Prior to genetic engineering, the only insulin available to diabetics was that derived from cattle or swine. The animal insulins were effective in lowering blood sugar but some people had allergic reactions to them because they were not chemically identical to human insulin. Genetic engineering was employed to produce large quantities of insulin identical to that produced by humans. To accomplish this, insulin-producing genes were removed from human chromosomes and spliced into the chromosomes of E. *coli* bacteria. As the bacteria grew and replicated, they began to secrete large amounts of insulin that was chemically identical to that produced by humans. This "human" insulin was harvested and prepared for human use. Genetically engineered human insulin is now the primary source of insulin for diabetics.

A wide variety of human hormones and growth factors are now commercially available because of genetic engineering.

geneticist – A scientist who specializes in genetics. A geneticist may or may not be a physician.

genetic map – The record of the specific locations of genes on a chromosome.

genetics – The branch of biology that deals with the principles of heredity. Medical genetics is the application of genetics to determining the causes and natural outcomes of hereditary diseases.

-genic – Suffix designating production or formation.

genital – Pertaining to the genitalia.

genitalia – The reproductive organs.

genitals – *See genitalia.*

G

genome – The complete set of genes on a chromosome or group of chromosomes. For example, the human genome is the complete set of genes found in a human cell.

genotoxic – A substance that causes damage to DNA and the genes that reside within it.

genus – A classification of plants or animals with common distinguishing characteristics. The genus name may be paired with a species name to identify a specific plant or animal. When written, the genus name is always capitalized and genus and species names are italicized. For example, the genus name for human beings is *Homo*. The combined genus and species name is *Homo sapiens*.

GERD – *See gastroesophageal reflux disease.*

geriatric – Pertaining to old age.

geriatrician – *See gerontologist.*

geriatrics – *See gerontology.*

germ – Colloquial term for bacterium or virus.

Also, the earliest evidence of form or structure within a plant or animal embryo.

germ cell – A reproductive cell. Specifically a sperm or ovum.

germicide – An agent that kills bacteria. Often used synonymously with antiseptic or disinfectant.

gero- – Prefix designating old age.

geront- – Prefix designating old age.

geronto- – Prefix designating old age.

gerontologist – A physician who specializes in the diagnosis and treatment of health problems in the elderly.

gerontology – The specialty within medicine that deals with the health of the elderly.

gestation – Pregnancy. The period of time from the fertilization of an ovum to birth of the child.

G

gestational age – The age of an unborn child, usually expressed in weeks from conception.

GI – See *gastrointestinal*.

gingiva – A gum. The structure in the mouth that provides a foundation for the teeth and the mucous membrane that covers it.

gingivae – Plural form of gingiva.

gingival – Pertaining to the gums.

gingival hyperplasia – An excessive growth of gum tissue. The most common cause of gingival hyperplasia is long-term use of the antiepileptic drug phenytoin. In many cases, the tissue overgrowth must be surgically removed.

gingivitis – An inflammation of the gums characterized by redness, swelling, and bleeding. The most common cause of gingivitis is poor oral hygiene, although conditions such as diabetes mellitus and nutritional deficits can also produce this problem. Gingivitis can lead to tooth decay and tooth loss.

gingivo- – Prefix designating the gums.

gland – A group of cells or an organ that produces secretions. Also see *endocrine glands*, *exocrine glands*.

glandular – Pertaining to a gland.

glaucoma – A condition of increased fluid pressure inside the eye. Glaucoma compresses the end of the optic nerve, and failure to adequately treat the condition leads to blindness. Medications available for treating glaucoma work by either increasing the outflow of fluid from the eye or by decreasing ophthalmic fluid production.

globulin – A class of proteins that circulate in blood. Many of the globulins are essential components of the immune system.

gloss- – Prefix designating the tongue.

glossitis – Inflammation of the tongue.

glosso- – Prefix designating the tongue.

glossodynia – Pain or burning sensations in the tongue.

G

glossopharyngeal – Pertaining to the tongue and the throat.

glossopharyngitis – Inflammation of both the tongue and throat.

glucagon – A hormone produced in the pancreas that increases blood sugar. Glucagon and insulin work opposite of each other to try to regulate blood sugar within a narrow range. If insulin lowers blood sugar too far, the pancreas releases a burst of glucagon. Glucagon triggers a release of glycogen from the liver, which in turn, raises blood sugar. *Also see glycogen, insulin.*

gluco- – Prefix designating glucose.

glucocorticoid – A class of corticosteroid so named because it increases blood sugar levels. Glucocorticoids are mainly used for their anti-inflammatory effect. Clinical applications include arthritis, tendinitis, asthma, and allergic reactions. *Also see corticosteroid.*

glucose – A simple sugar found in fruits and vegetables. In humans, glucose is present in the blood and is the primary source of energy for the body. Blood glucose levels that are too low (hypoglycemia) can lead to dizziness and fainting. Excessive levels (hyperglycemia) may be an indication of diabetes mellitus.

glucosuria – Presence of glucose in the urine. Glucose is not normally eliminated in the urine unless the concentration of glucose in the blood is greatly elevated. The most common cause of glucosuria is diabetes mellitus.

glue sniffing – A form of drug abuse that involves inhaling organic solvents, particularly toluene and xylene. Glue sniffing derives its name from the solvents used in model airplane glue. The practice causes stimulation followed by sedation. Persistent glue sniffing can lead to liver, lung, and nerve damage.

glycemia – The presence of glucose in the blood. *Also see hyperglycemia, hypoglycemia.*

glycemic control – The maintenance of normal levels of glucose in the blood. Most commonly used in the context of controlling blood sugars in diabetes mellitus. In reference to diabetes, good glycemic control means that blood sugars are staying within the

G

normal range. Poor glycemic control means that blood sugar levels are frequently above or below normal.

glyco- – Prefix designating sugar or the amino acid glycine.

glycogen – A starch-like substance composed of linked glucose molecules that acts as an emergency supply of glucose. If blood glucose levels drop too low (hypoglycemia), glucagon causes glycogen molecules to break apart and release glucose into the blood.

glycogenesis – Formation of glycogen from glucose molecules. Glycogenesis occurs when blood glucose is plentiful and continues until either the blood glucose level drops or glycogen storage cells are full.

glycosuria – *See glucosuria.*

gm – Older abbreviation for gram. The currently accepted abbreviation is g.

gold salts – A class of drugs that include gold within their molecules. Most are given by injection into a muscle. Gold salts are primarily used to treat rheumatoid arthritis.

gonad – An organ that produces sex cells. The female gonads are the ovum-producing ovaries. The male gonads are the sperm-producing testes.

gonadal – Pertaining to a gonad.

gonococcal – Pertaining to the gonococcus.

gonococcus – *Neisseria gonorrhoeae*, the bacterium that causes gonorrhea.

gonorrhea – A sexually transmitted disease that typically infects the urethra and may migrate upward to further infect the upper genital tract. Untreated gonorrhea may cause sterility, skin lesions, or arthritis.

gonorrheal – Pertaining to gonorrhea.

good cholesterol – *See high-density lipoprotein.*

Good Manufacturing Practices (GMP) – Guidelines established by the Unites States Food and Drug Administration that apply to

G

the commercial production of drugs. The guidelines, calling for extensive record keeping and quality checks on ingredients and finished products, are intended to assure the purity of products and consistency from batch to batch.

gout – A hereditary form of arthritis characterized by the accumulation of uric acid crystals in joints and other tissues. Gout most commonly affects one or both great toes initially, but can later afflict the knees, fingers, other joints, and muscles.

gouty – Pertaining to gout.

grain – A unit of weight in the English system of weights and measures. Abbreviated gr. A grain is equal to 64.8 milligrams, usually rounded off to 65 milligrams. Although some medication doses are still referred to in grains (e.g., 5 grains in a typical aspirin tablet), grains are generally considered an archaic measurement system.

gram – The basic unit of weight in the metric system. Abbreviated g. There are 31.1 grams in an ounce.

Gram's stain – A method of exposing bacteria to blue (crystal violet) and red (safranin O) dyes to assist in microscopic identification. Bacteria that accept the blue stain are dyed a dark purple and are termed Gram-positive. Bacteria that accept the red stain are dyed pink and are termed Gram-negative.

Bacteria accept dyes differently because of differences in their cell walls. Gram-negative bacteria typically have more complex cell walls and are often more difficult to treat than Gram-positive bacteria.

Gram-negative – Examples of Gram-negative bacteria include *Escherichia coli* and *Neisseria gonorrhoeae*. See *Gram's stain*.

Gram-positive – Examples of Gram-positive bacteria include *Staphylococcus aureus* and *Streptococcus pneumoniae*. See *Gram's stain*.

grand mal seizure – A common form of epilepsy characterized by falling, stiffening, and convulsions throughout the body followed by disorientation and often a deep sleep. This type of seizure may occur with or without warning.

G

granule – A small pill, usually accompanied by many others encased within a gelatin capsule. In most cases, granules within capsules are specially coated to gradually release medication over a period of up to twelve hours.

Also a small grain-like particle within a cell.

granulo- – Prefix designating a granule.

granulocyte – A white blood cell that contains granules within its cytoplasm. Granulocytes are capable of ingesting and digesting bacteria and other foreign proteins in blood. Consequently, they play an important role in the body's defenses against infection. Neutrophils, eosinophils, and basophils comprise the granulocytes.

granulocytopenia – Low numbers of granulocytes in the blood. Granulocytopenia is a potentially serious condition because it leaves the body with an impaired ability to fight infection.

granulocytosis – An abnormally high number of granulocytes in the blood. Granulocytosis is often an indication of infection since the body typically responds to infection by releasing large numbers of granulocytes into the blood. Granulocytosis may also be a sign of some forms of leukemia.

-graph – A suffix designating a visual display. Examples include electrocardiographs and electroencephalographs. Graphs may be recorded on paper or electronic media or may be displayed on a monitor.

-graphy – A suffix designating a process that results in a graph.

Graves' disease – A condition characterized by excessive release of thyroid hormone. Common manifestations include tremors, rapid heartbeat, protruding eyes, weight loss due to increased metabolic rate, and fatigue. Treatment may include thyroid suppressant drugs, surgery, or radiation to the thyroid gland.

gravid – Pregnant.

grievance procedure – In the context of insurance, the process by which a plan member may formally complain about the conduct of the insurance company or appeal denial of coverage.

G

Grievance procedures may be internal within the insurance company or external, for example with the state department of insurance (DOI). *Also see department of insurance.*

grippe – Colloquial term for influenza.

group – In the context of health insurance, a group is a set of people who have a common link. Most insurance groups are organized by common employer. However, a group may be determined by a common trade union, profession or trade, or fraternal organization.

group contract – An agreement for insurance coverage for a defined set of people with a common link (*see group*). The group contract details the premiums, eligibility, benefits, and exclusions of coverage.

group insurance – An insurance plan in which the members are all covered by one plan.

group practice – A formal association of physicians, usually located in the same office or building, who share staff, overhead expenses, medical and business records, and equipment.

group purchasing organization (GPO) – A company that negotiates procurement contracts on behalf of its members. GPO members are typically engaged in closely related businesses (e.g., hospitals, nursing home pharmacies, home infusion pharmacies, etc.). The GPO uses the collective buying power of its members to negotiate discounts from manufacturers, wholesalers, and other suppliers.

growth factor – A hormone that stimulates cell production and/or maturation. Commercially available growth factors stimulate bone marrow to produce red and white blood cells and platelets.

growth hormone – A protein produced in the pituitary gland that stimulates growth in children. Deficiency of growth hormone causes short stature. In adults, growth hormone builds muscle mass and is sometimes used to treat diseases that cause muscle wasting. Growth hormone is sometimes abused by athletes to help build strength. Sometimes called human growth hormone.

G

gtt – Abbreviation commonly used on written prescriptions for the Latin *guttae* meaning drops.

guaiac – A reagent used to test for blood that is not visually apparent. Most commonly, guaiac is used by clinical laboratories to detect traces of blood in feces. A positive finding of blood in stool may indicate the presence of a bleeding ulcer or colon cancer.

gut – The intestines. Also, a colloquial term for the abdomen.

GYN – *See gynecology.*

gyn- – Prefix pertaining to a woman or female sex.

gyne- – Prefix pertaining to a woman or female sex.

gyneco- – Prefix pertaining to a woman or female sex.

gynecological oncologist – A physician who specializes in the diagnosis and treatment of cancers that affect the female reproductive system.

gynecologist – A physician specializing in the health care of women, especially the diagnosis and treatment of diseases and conditions that occur exclusively in women.

gynecology (GYN) – The medical specialty that deals with the health of women and diagnosis and treatment of conditions that occur in the female reproductive system.

gynecomastia – Englargement of the breast in a male. Gynecomastia may be caused by excessive production of estrogen or by estrogen treatment. Short-term gynecomastia is common in puberty.

gyno- – Prefix pertaining to a woman or female sex.

gynopathy – Any disease exclusive to women.

H

h – Abbreviation for the Latin *hora*, meaning hour. The abbreviation is frequently used in the directions portion of written prescriptions.

H$_2$ antagonist – *See histamine-2* (H$_2$) *receptor.*

habituation – The process of performing repetitive acts, usually to satisfy a psychological need. Most commonly used in the context of drug habituation, the repetitive abuse of a legal or illegal pharmacological agent for the purpose of achieving an altered state of mind. Persons who exhibit drug habituation may or may not be physically addicted to the drug(s) used.

Haemophilus influenzae – A gram-negative bacterium that commonly causes otitis media in children. Also the most common cause of bacterial meningitis in children. *Haemophilus influenzae* was originally thought to be the cause of influenza (flu) and thus the species name. Most cases of *Haemophilus influenzae* can be prevented with vaccination.

hair follicle – The sac-like indentation from which hair grows. Hair follicles are found in all areas of external skin, even though some may no longer produce hair, as in baldness.

half-life – The amount of time it takes for half of a substance to disappear or change form. The term is frequently applied in two aspects of pharmacy: nuclear pharmacy and drug elimination.

Nuclear pharmacy: The principles of nuclear physics apply when dealing with the radioactive medications that are sometimes used for diagnostic testing. In this context, half-life is the amount of time it takes for 50% of a radioactive element to change or decay into another element. *See the definition of generator for one example of how this principle is applied.* The half-lives of different radioactive substances range from milliseconds to millennia. With each passing half-life, half of the existing amount of radioactive element decays. If an element has a half-life of one year, 50% of the element will decay in one year. When another year passes, 50% of the material present at the beginning of the second year decays, and so forth.

H

Drug elimination: Most drugs have elimination half-lives similar to the example above. For example, if a drug has a half-life of four hours, 50% of the drug will be either inactivated or excreted from the body in four hours. Another 50% of the remaining drug will be inactivated or excreted over the next four hours. After four half-lives (16 hours in this example) only 6.25% of the original amount of drug remains.

halitosis – Bad breath. Usually due to bacteria in the mouth or throat. Most cases of halitosis are eliminated with daily oral hygiene but chronic cases may require antibiotic therapy to eliminate the causative bacteria.

hallucination – The apparent perception of sights or other sensory perceptions when no physical stimulus is present. Hallucinations are often symptoms of mental illness or drug abuse. Hallucinations may be auditory (e.g., hearing voices), visual (e.g., seeing colors, patterns, or people), olfactory (e.g., smelling odors), or tactile (e.g., feeling touch). Auditory and visual hallucinations are the most common. Although there are many exceptions, visual hallucinations are usually due to drug toxicity or neurological problems and auditory hallucinations are usually due to mental illness.

halogen – The family of chemical elements that includes fluorine, chlorine, iodine, astatine, and bromine.

halogenation – The chemical process of adding a halogen atom to a molecule.

Hamilton Depression Scale – A commonly used psychological test to determine the presence and severity of depression. This test, often abbreviated as Ham-D, is a standard means of comparing the effectiveness of antidepressant drugs in clinical studies.

hand surgeon – A physician who specializes in treating injuries to or diseases of the hands.

hardening of the arteries – *See atherosclerosis.*

hashish – The resin from the flowers and sprouts of the marijuana plant. Hashish contains a high concentration of cannabinols, the active chemicals in marijuana.

H

hay fever – *See allergic rhinitis.*

HCFA – *See Health Care Financing Administration.*

HCFA 1500 – A universal claim form developed by the Health Care Financing Administration (HCFA) for Medicare billings and frequently used by health care providers to bill insurers. Retail pharmacies normally use a different universal claim form to bill insurance companies for prescriptions. However, pharmacies operating in nontraditional settings such as home care often bill their services by means of HCFA 1500 forms.

HDL – *See high-density lipoprotein.*

headache – Pain in the head. Headache has many different manifestations depending upon its cause. *Also see cluster headache, migraine headache, tension headache.*

heal – To return to health.

healer – A person who restores health to another person. A healer may practice traditional medicine in the sense of a medical doctor or may practice alternative medicine.

health – The absence of disease or the presence of normal physical and mental function. More commonly, the term is used in the context of good health or bad health where bad health is considered to be the presence of disease or less than optimal function.

health and beauty department – The section of a discount or department store where cosmetics and health-related products are sold. Health-related products may include nonprescription drugs, herbal remedies, vaporizers, toothbrushes, and similar products. If the store has a pharmacy, it is usually located nearby.

health care coalition – An alliance of insurers, buyers, and consumers of health services that work in concert to try to improve the quality of medical care while containing its cost. Participants in health care coalitions may include HMOs, self-insured employer groups, and trade unions.

health care consumer – An individual who receives medical care. A health care consumer may receive services from an individual or an institution. Individual providers include physicians, dentists, nurses, pharmacists, or other health care providers. Institutions include hospitals and clinics.

health care delivery system – Collectively, all the organizations, facilities, and personnel that provide health care.

Health Care Financing Administration (HCFA) – The agency of the United States government that is responsible for administering the Medicare program and supervising states' Medicaid programs.

health care industry – The businesses that either directly or indirectly provide medical services to consumers. The health care industry includes hospitals, clinics, pharmacies, insurance companies, health care professionals, pharmaceutical manufacturing companies, and medical equipment retailers and manufacturers.

health care professional – An individual who has successfully completed a prescribed course of study, usually at a college or university, and passed a certification or licensing examination administered by the state. Health care professions include pharmacy, medicine, nursing, dentistry, physical therapy, psychology, and many others.

health care provider – A person, institution, or business that provides medical care directly to a patient. Health care providers include pharmacists, physicians, nurses, hospitals, and clinics.

health care worker – Any individual employed in the health care industry. A health care worker can be a licensed professional (e.g., physician, pharmacist, etc.) or an unlicensed person (e.g., housekeeper, nurse's aide, delivery person, etc.).

Health Employer Data and Information Set (HEDIS) – A set of performance measures originally developed by large employer groups to evaluate and compare the performance of health plans. HEDIS data allow health insurance purchasers to determine the value they are likely to receive for their health insurance premiums. They may use these data to negotiate insurance

H

rates or as tools to help them decide among the plans competing for their business.

health insurance – A contract agreeing to pay the costs of specified medical and related expenses. Health insurance may be purchased by individuals or by employers as part of the employee benefit package.

health maintenance organization (HMO) – A form of health insurance in which members prepay, usually by means of a monthly premium for health services, and which generally includes inpatient and ambulatory care. Advantages to the patient include no required deductible, no insurance claim forms to file following physician visits or other contacts, and only a small copayment for certain specified services.

According to federal law, an HMO must satisfy each of the following requirements:

- Establish an organized system for providing health care in a geographic area,

- Establish a set of basic and supplemental treatment services, and

- Assure that all HMO members are voluntarily enrolled.

Originally, HMOs directly employed physicians and operated medical office buildings that housed the physicians' offices, examining rooms, and treatment areas. These buildings typically included a pharmacy and other necessary health care services. Over time, it became more common for physicians as individuals or groups to contract with HMOs to provide care in their own practices.

health plan – The medical insurance package offered by an employer to its employees. Health plans typically cover hospitalizations, medical office visits, and diagnostic tests. They may or may not cover prescriptions, glasses and contact lenses, dental visits, and mental health.

Also, the medical insurance company itself.

health record – The clinical documentation relating to a patient's

H

care. A health record may be written on paper or stored in an electronic medium. Typically, a health record contains demographic information, insurance information, laboratory test values, and health care workers' notations regarding the patient's specific problems, treatments given, and changes in status.

hearing aid – An electronic device inserted into the ear canal or placed nearby in order to assist the wearer to perceive sound.

heart – A muscle in the chest consisting of four hollow chambers (right and left atrium, right and left ventricle) that is responsible for pumping blood through the body. Blood is received from the systemic circulation into the right atrium during the period when the ventricles contract (systole). When the ventricles relax (diastole), the atria contract and eject blood into the ventricles. During its systole, the right ventricle pumps blood into the blood vessels of the lungs where the blood exchanges carbon dioxide waste for fresh oxygen and then returns to the left atrium. During diastole, the left atrium ejects blood into the left ventricle. When the left ventricle contracts, it pumps freshly oxygenated blood into general circulation.

The rhythmic contraction and relaxation of the chambers of the heart is controlled and coordinated by a series of electrical impulses. Any disruption of these impulses can lead to a cardiac arrhythmia. *Also see arrhythmia.*

heart attack – *See myocardial infarction.*

heartbeat – A complete cycle of heart contraction and relaxation. Most resting adults have 70 to 80 heartbeats per minute (slightly more in women and slightly fewer in men) but this frequency is highly variable.

heartburn – Colloquial term for gastroesophageal reflux. *See gastroesophageal reflux.*

heart block – A type of cardiac arrhythmia caused by obstructed passage of electrical impulses through the heart. Heart block may be treated with medications or a cardiac pacemaker.

heart failure – The inability of the heart muscle to contract with enough force to properly circulate blood. The most common

H

form of heart failure is often referred to as congestive heart failure because of the characteristic collection of fluid (congestion) in the lungs and extremities. Heart failure may be treated with a variety of drugs that include digoxin, diuretics, and ACE inhibitors.

heart-lung machine – An apparatus that circulates and oxygenates blood. During heart surgery, the surgeon must stop the heart from beating in order to make accurate incisions and repairs. While the heart is stopped, the patient's blood is diverted from the heart to the heart-lung machine. The device acts as a temporary pump, continuing to circulate blood while the heart is incapacitated. The machine also exchanges waste carbon dioxide for fresh oxygen. Once the surgeon is finished with the heart, it is restarted and the heart-lung machine is disconnected.

heart rate – The speed with which the heart beats. *Also see heartbeat.*

heatstroke – Potentially fatal brain damage caused by exposure to excessive heat. Symptoms of impending heatstroke may include headache, dizziness, increased heart rate, confusion, dry skin, and increased body temperature. Appearance of more than one of these symptoms requires immediate cooling, preferably in an air-conditioned environment, and emergency medical treatment.

heaves – Colloquial term for vomit or vomiting. Dry heaves is retching that produces no material from the stomach.

HEDIS – *See Health Employer Data and Information Set.*

Helicobacter pylori – A bacterium often found in the stomachs and duodenums of patients with peptic ulcer disease. Usually abbreviated H. *pylori*. Most patients with ulcers are now tested for this organism. If present, a course of antibiotic therapy is normally prescribed along with traditional antiulcer medicines. Presence of these bacteria is actually a good sign because these ulcers typically heal faster than those that form in the absence of H. *pylori*.

hem- – Prefix designating blood.

hema- – Prefix designating blood.

hemarthrosis – Blood in a joint, usually due to trauma. Hemarthrosis is a common complication of hemophilia where, following a bump or a fall, blood collects in an injured joint. In hemophiliacs, repeated episodes of hemarthrosis can be disfiguring and crippling.

hematic – Pertaining to blood.

hematinic – Improving the condition of the blood, particularly a vitamin and mineral product that is intended to raise blood cell counts.

hematocrit – The relative percentage of the volume of red blood cells to total blood volume. The hematocrit usually ranges between 43% and 49% in men and 37% to 43% in women. A lower than normal hematocrit may be an indication of anemia.

hematologist – A physician who specializes in the diagnosis and treatment of blood disorders. Hematologists are usually also trained in oncology, the diagnosis and treatment of cancer.

hematology – The medical specialty concerned with the blood and the tissues that form blood.

hematoma – Blood loss into a tissue, organ, or other confined space. Hematomas may compress nearby organs, causing pain and impairing their function. Hematomas are most common after trauma or as a side effect of anticoagulant medications. In many cases, hematomas must be surgically drained.

hematopoiesis – *See hemopoiesis.*

hematuria – The presence of blood or blood cells in the urine. Most commonly a sign of kidney disease.

hemi- – Prefix designating half.

hemiplegia – Paralysis of one side of the body. Hemiplegia is a common complication of stroke.

hemisphere – One half of a ball-shaped object. Frequently used in the context of one side of the brain.

hemochromatosis – Disorder caused by deposition of hemosiderin in the tissues of the body. Hemochromatosis can cause cirrhosis of

H

the liver, destruction of the pancreas, and heart failure. The most common cause of hemochromatosis is long-term intake of excessive amounts of iron. Iron is unique in that the body has no natural way to eliminate it except through bleeding. Daily iron supplements are safe only for actively growing children, women who have menstrual cycles, and those with a diagnosed iron deficiency. Adult men and postmenopausal women should take iron supplements only if advised to do so by a physician.

hemoconcentration – Higher than normal percentage of red blood cells in the blood (elevated hematocrit). Hemoconcentration is characteristic of dehydration, adjustment to living at a high altitude, and polycythemia vera. Opposite of hemodilution.

hemodialysis – The process of filtering blood through a kidney machine for the purpose of removing toxins. Hemodialysis may be performed to sustain life in patients with kidney failure or to remove toxins from the blood following a poisoning.

hemodilution – Reduced concentration of red blood cells in the blood (reduced hematocrit). Normally used in the context of overly aggressive hydration, resulting in replacing too much fluid in the vascular system and, therefore, diluting the concentration of blood cells, electrolytes, and proteins.

hemodynamic – Pertaining to the physics of blood flow.

hemoglobin – The protein within red blood cells that accounts for those cells' ability to exchange carbon dioxide and oxygen. Each red blood cell contains as many as 300 molecules of hemoglobin, each capable of transporting one molecule of carbon dioxide or oxygen.

Normal values of hemoglobin in blood (grams of hemoglobin per milliliter of blood) range from 13.5–18 g/100 ml in men to 12–16 g/100 ml in women. Low hemoglobin values usually indicate iron deficiency anemia.

hemoglobinemia – The presence of hemoglobin floating free in blood, not as part of a red blood cell. Hemoglobinemia is often a sign of hemolytic anemia.

H

hemoglobinopathy – A collective term denoting one of several hereditary diseases characterized by the presence of abnormal hemoglobin in blood.

Different types of hemoglobin are designated by a letter or the name of the laboratory or individual who first identified it. Hemoglobins A and F are the normal forms of hemoglobin where A (adult hemoglobin) is that typically present in children and adults and F (fetal hemoglobin) is that seen in fetuses and babies.

Examples of abnormal hemoglobins include hemoglobin S (abbreviated Hb-S), the hemoglobin typically found in people with sickle cell anemia, and hemoglobin Kansas, a hemoglobinopathy characterized by the impaired ability of red blood cells to bind oxygen.

hemoglobinuria – The presence of hemoglobin in the urine. Hemoglobinuria is often found in association with hemolytic anemia.

hemolysis – The abnormal destruction of red blood cells resulting in release into the blood of the contents of those cells, including hemoglobin.

hemolytic – Pertaining to hemolysis.

hemolytic anemia – A condition characterized by premature destruction of red blood cells. Hemolytic anemia may be due to a drug reaction, toxins, or inherited disease.

hemopathy – Any disease of the blood-forming tissues.

hemophilia – An inherited disease characterized by the inability of blood to clot properly. Hemophilia is caused by insufficient amounts of clotting factors, proteins that normally circulate in blood. Bleeding normally initiates a sequence of events where the clotting factors (13 are currently known, designated by Roman numerals I through XIII) act in concert to stop blood flow through a broken blood vessel. If just one clotting factor is missing, the blood cannot form a functional clot. The most common causes of hemophilia are deficiencies of either factor VIII or factor IX. Treatment consists of transfusions of missing clotting factors.

H

hemophilia A – Deficiency of clotting factor VIII. *See hemophilia.*

hemophilia B – Deficiency of clotting factor IX. *See hemophilia.*

hemophiliac – A person with hemophilia.

hemophilic – Pertaining to hemophilia.

hemopoiesis – The process of formation of blood cells. Most blood cells are formed in the marrow of long bones such as the legs, the sternum, and the pelvis.

hemopoietic – Pertaining to hemopoiesis.

hemopoietic stem cell – A type of cell found in bone marrow that is the common origin of all blood cells formed in the marrow. Stem cells differentiate themselves into different cell lines depending upon the body's needs at the time. A stem cell may eventually become a red blood cell, white blood cell, or platelet.

hemorrhage – Bleeding. Hemorrhage is often described in relation to the area of the bleeding or the physical characteristics of the bleeding. For example, cerebral hemorrhage is bleeding into the cerebrum, the largest part of the brain. Petechial hemorrhage is bleeding into the skin that appears as pinpoint spots of blood.

hemorrhoid – A bulging blood vessel in the anus. Hemorrhoids are often painful and may bleed. Most hemorrhoids appear and disappear spontaneously. They may be treated with topical anti-inflammatory drugs, particularly hydrocortisone, astringents, topical anesthetics, or lubricants. Stool softeners often relieve the irritation of feces passing over a hemorrhoid. In some cases, surgical removal (hemorrhoidectomy) may be necessary.

hemorrhoidal – Pertaining to hemorrhoids.

hemorrhoidectomy – Surgical removal of a hemorrhoid.

hemosiderin – An insoluble iron-containing protein formed when red blood cells are destroyed.

hemostasis – The body's mechanism for controlling bleeding. Normal hemostasis involves the proper functioning of the platelets and clotting factors.

H

hemostat – A drug, chemical agent, or surgical instrument capable of stopping bleeding.

hepat- – Prefix designating the liver.

hepatic – Pertaining to the liver.

hepatic artery – The major blood vessel that supplies blood to the liver.

hepatico- – Prefix designating the liver.

hepatitic – Pertaining to hepatitis.

hepatitis – Inflammation of the liver. Hepatitis may be caused by a drug or chemical toxin, but more commonly is caused by a viral infection. Many forms of viral hepatitis are highly communicable and epidemics may be prevented by the use of vaccines. Means of spreading hepatitis are diverse and include eating or drinking virus-contaminated food or water, sexual intercourse, and shared use of contaminated needles and syringes. Some forms of hepatitis are self-limited and resolve without residual damage but others may progress to the point of liver failure and death. Characteristic signs of hepatitis include itching, enlargement of the liver and lymph nodes, headache, nausea and vomiting, clay-colored stools, and yellow or orange coloration in the skin and eyes.

hepato- – Prefix designating the liver.

hepatobiliary system – The liver, gallbladder, and bile duct. The hepatobiliary system produces (liver), stores (gallbladder), and delivers (bile duct) bile for digestion.

hepatocyte – A parenchymal liver cell. These are cells that perform the liver's vital functions, including metabolism and bile formation. The cells that provide structure to the liver or cover the organ are not considered to be hepatocytes.

hepatoenteric – Pertaining to both the liver and intestine.

hepatogastric – Pertaining to both the liver and stomach.

hepatologist – A physician who specializes in the diagnosis and treatment of diseases of the liver.

hepatology – The branch of medicine that specializes in diseases of the liver.

hepatoma – A malignant tumor that originates among the functional cells of the liver.

hepatomegaly – Enlargement of the liver, usually due to liver disease, leukemia, or lymphoma.

hepatopathy – A nonspecific term denoting any disease of the liver.

herb – A plant or part of a plant that is used as a drug, seasoning, or flavoring. Examples of plants that are used as drugs include spearmint (indigestion), foxglove (heart failure), periwinkle (leukemia), and ginkgo biloba (aging). Hundreds of prescription drugs in current use are extracted from herbs.

herbal remedy – According to the Dietary Supplemental Health and Education Act of 1994, herbal remedies are nutritional supplements, not drugs. Consequently, the United States Food and Drug Administration (FDA) does not have the legal authority to require manufacturers of herbal remedies to prove that their products are safe and effective before selling them to the general public. Nor can the FDA require herbal remedy manufacturers to submit evidence that their products actually contain the amount of medicine indicated on the package label. The FDA can only take action against a specific herbal product once it has shown itself to be toxic when used in the general population.

hereditary – Pertaining to transmission from one generation to a subsequent generation. Hereditary traits are thought to be passed via genes.

heredity – The transmission of characteristics from parents to children or grandchildren by means of genes in the chromosomes.

heroic – An extreme treatment measure that in itself may be dangerous for a patient. Heroic treatments are invoked when more conservative treatments are likely to fail. For example, a bone marrow transplant may be considered heroic because complications of the procedure itself may prove fatal. However, the underlying disease, usually a cancer, will probably continue to advance if the transplant is not done.

herpes – See *herpes simplex virus* (HSV).

herpes genitalis – A red, painful, highly contagious lesion on the genitals caused by the herpes virus. Herpes genitalis lesions are most likely to occur in times of physical or emotional stress. The infection is most likely to be spread by sexual contact when the lesion is apparent. However, it may also be passed even when the lesions are quiescent. Herpes genitalis is most often caused by herpes simplex virus 2, but may also be caused by herpes simplex virus 1. Colloquially known as genital herpes.

herpes labialis – A red, painful lesion on the lip or in the mouth caused by the herpes virus. Herpes labialis is most likely to occur in times of physical or emotional stress. Herpes labialis is most often caused by herpes simplex virus 1, but may also be caused by herpes simplex virus 2. Colloquially known as fever blister.

herpes simplex virus (HSV) – A virus of the herpesvirus group. Herpes simplex may infect either the area around the mouth (herpes labialis) or the genitals (herpes genitalis).

herpesvirus – A group of five related viruses that include herpes simplex virus 1, herpes simplex virus 2, varicella-zoster virus, Epstein-Barr virus, and cytomegalovirus.

herpes zoster – An infection caused by the varicella-zoster virus, the same virus that causes chickenpox. Persons who have previously had chickenpox continue to harbor the varicella-zoster virus in their nervous systems. The virus may emerge during times of physical stress or when the immune system is impaired. When the virus reactivates, it inflames nerves in the trunk and abdomen, causing blisters and severe pain. Colloquially known as shingles.

herpetic – Pertaining to herpesvirus.

herpetiform – Resembling a herpes lesion.

hesitancy – Delay or inability to begin urination. Hesitancy is most often a sign of a prostate problem.

heter- – Prefix designating other or different.

hetero- – Prefix designating other or different.

heterogeneous – Composed of unrelated or dissimilar pieces or parts.

hgb – Abbreviation for hemoglobin.

hiccough – *See hiccup.*

hiccup – A spasm of the diaphragm causing a sudden inspiration of air and a characteristic sound. Prolonged hiccuping can occur with some chronic diseases and leads to exhaustion. Prolonged hiccuping sometimes responds to treatment with sedating drugs.

hidr- – Prefix designating sweat or sweat glands.

hidro- – Prefix designating sweat or sweat glands.

hidrosis – Sweat production and secretion.

hidrotic – Pertaining to sweat.

high blood pressure – *See hypertension.*

high-density lipoprotein (HDL) – A blood molecule composed in part of protein and in part of fat. HDL is often colloquially referred to as "good" cholesterol. Its function is to carry cholesterol from the blood to the liver or glands where it is either stored or converted into other vital biochemicals, such as hormones and red blood cell walls. HDL levels can be increased through regular exercise and cessation of smoking and alcohol consumption.

Hippocratic Oath – Ceremonial professional oath administered by some medical schools as part of the graduation ceremony. Attributed to the fifth century B.C. Greek physician Hippocrates of Cos, the oath has formed the ethical framework for the practice of medicine since that time. Following is the oath in its entirety.

"I swear by Apollo the physician, by Aesclepius, Hygeia, and Panacea, and I take to witness all the gods, all the goddesses, to keep according to my ability and my judgement the following Oath:

H

"To consider dear to me as my parents him who taught me this art; to live in common with him and if necessary to share my goods with him; to look upon his children as my own brothers, to teach them this art if they so desire without fee or written promise; to impart to my sons and the sons of the master who taught me and the disciples who have enrolled themselves and have agreed to the rules of the profession, but to these alone, the precepts and the instruction. I will prescribe regimen for the good of my patients according to my ability and my judgement and never do harm to anyone. To please no one will I prescribe a deadly drug, nor give advice which may cause his death. Nor will I give a woman a pessary to procure abortion. But I will preserve the purity of my life and my art. I will not cut for stone, even for patients in whom the disease is manifest; I will leave this operation to be performed by practitioners (specialists in this art). In every house where I come I will enter only for the good of my patients, keeping myself far from all intentional ill-doing and all seduction, and especially from the pleasures of love with women or with men, be they free or slaves. All that may come to my knowledge in the exercise of my profession or outside of my profession or in daily commerce with men, which ought not to be spread abroad, I will keep secret and will never reveal. If I keep this oath faithfully, may I enjoy my life and practice my art, respected by all men and in all times; but if I swerve from it or violate it, may the reverse be my lot."

hirsutism – Excessive growth of hair, especially in a woman, in a typical male pattern. May be the result of a hormonal imbalance or drug therapy.

histamine – A naturally occurring chemical that has multiple functions, including:

- dilation of capillaries, which may cause congestion and a drop in blood pressure;

- contraction of smooth muscle, including the bronchioles in the lungs, which may cause wheezing and difficulty breathing;

- increased stomach acid secretion;

H

- increased heart rate; and

- initiation of allergic reactions.

histamine receptor – The cellular sites where histamine interacts.

histamine-1 (H_1) receptor – A site on a cell surface that mediates the allergic response to histamine. The H_1 receptor may be blocked with antihistamine drugs.

histamine-2 (H_2) receptor – A site on a cell surface that mediates the stomach acid-stimulating effects of histamine. The H_2 receptor may be blocked with H_2 antagonist drugs such as cimetidine (Tagamet), famotidine (Pepcid), ranitidine (Zantac), and nizatadine (Axid).

histamine H_2 receptor antagonist – A drug that blocks the functions of the histamine-2 (H_2) receptor.

See histamine-2 (H_2) receptor.

histo- – Prefix designating a relationship to tissue.

histocompatibility – A state of similarity between tissues from two different people. Histocompatibility is necessary to reduce the risk of tissue rejection following an organ or tissue transplant.

histoincompatibility – A state of dissimilarity between tissues from two different people. Histoincompatibility increases the risk of tissue rejection following organ or tissue transplant.

histologist – A scientist who specializes in histology.

histology – The study of the cellular structure, composition, and function of tissues.

HIV – *See human immunodeficiency virus.*

HMO – *See health maintenance organization.*

Hodgkin's disease – A malignant cancer of the lymph nodes that occurs most commonly between the ages of 15 and 34, although it has been known to occur as late as age 50. The first signs of Hodgkin's disease are usually hard, swollen glands in the neck,

H

armpits, or groin. Hodgkin's disease is usually highly curable if caught early and treated aggressively with chemotherapy and radiation.

holistic – Pertaining to the entire body. For example, holistic medicine recognizes that disease affects the whole body and, consequently, it addresses both the physical and emotional aspects of health.

home care pharmacy – A specialized area of pharmacy oriented to treating patients in their own homes, usually coordinated with nursing or other home care services. Most home pharmacy services involve the use of intravenous drugs. Types of drugs commonly provided by a home care pharmacy include intravenous antibiotics, narcotics, cancer chemotherapy, hydration fluids, and enteral and total parenteral nutrition.

home health agency – A company that provides home health services. A home health agency may be a nonprofit or for-profit company. It may be a local, independent enterprise, part of a nationwide corporation, or a department of a hospital. Most states require home health agencies to be licensed and inspected periodically.

home health care – Health services supplied or delivered in a patient's private residence. Home care is usually employed when a patient is medically stable enough to be treated outside of a hospital but is unable to travel to a health care facility for care or when it is impractical to do so. Home care services may include nursing care, drug therapy, physical therapy, respiratory therapy, occupational therapy, counseling, hospice care, and the use of durable medical equipment.

home infusion therapy – Intravenous fluids or medications administered in a patient's private residence.

Also see home care pharmacy.

homeo- – Prefix designating the same or alike. Opposite of hetero-.

homeopathic – Pertaining to homeopathy.

homeopathic physician – A medical practitioner of homeopathy.

H

homeopathy – A system of treatment based on the "law of similars," a theory that like cures like. The law of similars holds that a substance known to cause toxic symptoms in a healthy person may be curative when given in minute doses to a person whose disease exhibits those same symptoms.

The law of similars works when applied to vaccination, where a small dose of killed or attenuated microorganisms is given in order to stimulate the immune system to destroy similar infecting microorganisms. Otherwise, the effectiveness of homeopathy is highly controversial.

homeostasis – The normal state of balance of functions in the body. Numerous nerves and hormones exist within the body that oppose the effects of each other. In some cases these checks and balances allow the body to respond to emergencies and other stresses and then to return back to normal function once the emergency has passed. In other cases, homeostatic mechanisms regulate routine functions throughout the day. For example, the pancreatic hormone insulin facilitates transfer of glucose from blood into the cells where it is burned as fuel. In so doing, insulin lowers the blood sugar levels. If these levels fall below a safe level, another pancreatic enzyme, glucagon, is released. Glucagon stimulates the liver to release stored glucose. The interaction between these two opposing hormones helps to maintain homeostasis.

homo- – Prefix designating the same or alike. Opposite of hetero-.

hormone – A chemical produced in an endocrine gland and secreted into the blood that helps to regulate the functions of one or more other organs or tissues. Examples of hormones include thyroid hormone, antidiuretic hormone, cortisol, growth hormone, erythropoietin, and the sex hormones estrogen, progesterone, and testosterone.

hormone replacement therapy (HRT) – Treatment with an exogenous chemical regulator to substitute for that which is missing or produced in insufficient quantity. The most common form of hormone replacement therapy is estrogen during menopause. *Also see estrogen replacement therapy.*

hormonogenesis – The formation of hormones.

hospice – Originally a facility, usually within a hospital, intended to care for the terminally ill, particularly by providing physical comfort to the patient and emotional support and counseling to the patient and the family. Currently, hospice organizations continue to offer the same type of support services but in the patient's home rather than in an institution. Hospitalizations are reserved for times when the patient's condition is temporarily or permanently beyond the capabilities of home care or when the family needs a brief respite from the stresses of caring for a dying loved one.

hospital – A facility where the sick or injured may seek medical care. In addition to physicians, hospitals utilize the services of a wide variety of health care professionals. Depending upon the type and mission of an individual hospital, it may provide the services of nurses, pharmacists, dieticians, dentists, physical therapists, laboratory and radiology technologists, and many others.

Patients may be admitted to a hospital (inpatient services) for periods ranging from a few hours to several days, weeks, months, or even years or they may receive diagnostic and/or treatments services and leave the same day (outpatient services).

hospital affiliation – A business arrangement or an ownership situation where a hospital cooperates with another entity to the benefit of both parties. For example, a hospital may affiliate with a medical school, providing a training site for medical students while receiving the benefit of the faculty's medical expertise. A hospital may contract with another hospital to share services, thereby decreasing the costs of these services. A hospital may also contract with an insurance company to become an approved provider in the insurer's network. Hospitals that are part of the same ownership group commonly pool resources to negotiate favorable contracts with suppliers or insurers.

hospitalization – The state of being confined in a hospital.

hospitalization insurance – Colloquial term for health insurance.

host – Any organism upon or within which another organism (parasite) depends for nourishment and/or reproduction. Humans act

H

as unwilling or unwitting hosts for a wide variety of microorganisms. Some of these microorganisms may infect their human hosts, causing disease. Others provide vital metabolic functions, such as digestion of foods, to their hosts.

house officer – A graduate of a medical school who receives additional medical training while working as an employee of the hospital. An intern or resident.

H. pylori – *See Helicobacter pylori.*

HRT – *See hormone replacement therapy.*

h.s. – Abbreviation for the Latin *hora somni*, meaning the hour of sleep or bedtime. The abbreviation is frequently used on prescriptions.

HSV – *See herpes simplex virus.*

human clinical study – An experiment performed using human beings as subjects. Such studies may test the effectiveness of various types of equipment, techniques, or drugs. While most testing is initiated with animals, at some point potential treatments have to be tried in human volunteers. The United States Food and Drug Administration closely regulates human testing of experimental products and must give formal approval before they can be marketed.

human genome project – A research study that is attempting to map the location of every human gene. The purpose of this project is to provide researchers with basic information about human genes in order to develop means of altering gene behavior in hereditary diseases.

human growth hormone – *See growth hormone.*

human immunodeficiency virus (HIV) – The virus that causes acquired immune deficiency syndrome (AIDS). Formerly called HTLV-III (human T-cell lymphotrophic virus type III), LAV (lymphadenopathy-associated virus), and ARV (AIDS-related retrovirus). *See acquired immune deficiency syndrome.*

humectant – An agent that provides moisture. Sometimes used synonymously with expectorant. *Also see expectorant.*

H

humor – Any clear fluid in the body. The term is most commonly applied to the aqueous and vitreous humors of the eye. These fluids fill the eyeball and allow it to maintain a consistent shape. Excessive aqueous humor can lead to glaucoma. *Also see glaucoma.*

hydr- – Prefix designating water or hydrogen.

hydration – The process of increasing water content. The term is most commonly applied to the act of giving water by mouth or intravenously to treat or prevent dehydration. *Also see dehydration.*

hydro- – Prefix designating water or hydrogen.

hydrocarbon – A type of organic chemical compound that consists solely of hydrogen and carbon.

hydrochloric acid – A caustic material that consists of one atom of hydrogen and one atom of chlorine. Hydrochloric acid, abbreviated HCl, is widely used in chemistry. In medicine, it is the primary secretion of the stomach and aids in digestion of food and kills many of the bacteria ingested with food. Under certain circumstances, hydrochloric acid can lead to peptic ulcers and esophagitis. *Also see peptic ulcer, gastroesophageal reflux.*

hydrogenation – A process whereby hydrogen is added to oils or fats to convert them to solids. Hydrogenation of unsaturated fats reduces the health-promoting effects of unsaturated oils. *Also see fat.*

hydrophilic – A chemical substance that attracts water molecules or is easily dissolved in water. Most hydrophilic substances are easily absorbed from the digestive tract.

hydrophobic – A chemical substance that repels water molecules or is difficult or impossible to dissolve in water. Fats and oils are examples of hydrophobic materials. Hydrophobic substances need the assistance of bile to be absorbed from the digestive tract.

hydrotherapy – Treatment with water. Formerly, hydrotherapy was used extensively as a treatment for schizophrenia. It was felt that extended bathing in water soothed the emotional distresses of the disease. Currently, hydrotherapy is used in physical therapy and sports medicine in the form of whirlpool baths to relieve muscle stiffness.

hydrothorax – Abnormal leakage of fluid into the pleura, the space between the lungs and their outer, membranous lining. Hydrothorax is often due to congestive heart failure.

hygiene – Cleanliness. Hygiene may encompass the body as a whole or specific areas of the body, such as dental hygiene.

hyper- – Prefix designating excess or beyond normal.

hyperacidity – Excessive secretion of hydrochloric acid into the stomach. Symptoms often attributed to hyperacidity (e.g., stomach pain and burning, heartburn) are more likely due to gastroesophageal reflux. *Also see gastroesophageal reflux.*

hyperactivity – Abnormally increased movement or other action on the part of an organ, tissue, or entire organism. Often used to describe the increased physical activity of children with attention deficit disorder.

hyperalgesia – A state of increased sensitivity to pain or increased perception of pain.

hyperalimentation – Ingestion or overadministration of nutrients in excess of that needed to sustain life. Typically used in the context of parenteral hyperalimentation, the administration of intravenous feedings to patients who are not able to take feedings by mouth or by means of a feeding tube.

Parenteral hyperalimentation is more commonly referred to as total parenteral nutrition. *See also total parenteral nutrition.*

hypercalcemia – Excessive levels of calcium in blood. Hypercalcemia may be an indication of parathyroid gland disease, Paget's disease, osteoporosis, or a bone tumor.

hypercalciuria – Presence of an abnormally high concentration of calcium in the urine. Hypercalciuria is often a sign of parathyroid or bone disease.

hyperchlorhydria – Excessive amount of hydrochloric acid in the stomach. Symptoms often attributed to hyperchlorhydria (e.g., stomach pain and burning, heartburn) are more likely due to gastroesophageal reflux. *Also see gastroesophageal reflux.*

hypercholesterolemia – Excessive amount of cholesterol in the blood. Ideally, blood cholesterol levels should be below 200 mg/100 ml of blood. Levels between 200 and 230 mg/100 ml are considered borderline elevated and should be managed with improvements in exercise and diet. Levels above 230 mg/100 ml are considered high and require intervention with diet, exercise, and possibly cholesterol-lowering medication.

Hypercholesterolemia is considered a risk factor for future heart disease.

hyperemesis – Excessive vomiting. Normally used in the context of hyperemesis gravidarum, vomiting during pregnancy that is far in excess of typical morning sickness. Women who experience hyperemesis gravidarum are at risk of serious dehydration. Treatment is conservative use of antiemetic drugs to stop or reduce the vomiting and intravenous fluids to replace lost liquids.

hyperemia – Presence of an increased amount of blood in a tissue or organ. Hyperemia is usually caused by a localized increased blood flow due to allergy, fever, inflammation, or other causes of vasodilation.

hyperemic – Pertaining to hyperemia.

hyperesthesia – Increased sensory perception. Hyperesthesia may manifest itself as increased pain perception, or heightened sense of taste, touch, or smell.

hyperextension – Movement of a limb or joint beyond its normal range. Hyperextension injuries may be painful and temporarily debilitating. Treatment usually includes rest and anti-inflammatory drugs.

hyperglycemia – A blood glucose level in excess of 110 mg/100 ml of blood. Hyperglycemia is a normal occurrence after a meal or snack. However, blood glucose levels that remain elevated two or more hours after eating may be a sign of diabetes mellitus.

H

hyperglycosuria – Persistent presence of large amounts of glucose in the urine. An extreme form of glucosuria. *Also see glucosuria.*

hyperhidrosis – Excessive sweating.

hyperhydration – Excessive amount of body fluids. The term is most commonly applied to conditions produced by overly aggressive use of intravenous fluids.

hyperinsulinism – Abnormally high levels of insulin in the blood due to either excessive secretion of insulin by the pancreas or by decreased metabolism of insulin.

hyperkalemia – Elevated concentration of potassium in the blood. Hyperkalemia may indicate metabolic disease or kidney problems. Hyperkalemia can potentially cause heart arrhythmias.

hyperkaluresis – Excessive loss of potassium in the urine. Most commonly caused by treatment with diuretic drugs.

hyperkeratosis – Thickened condition of the outermost layer of skin. Hyperkeratosis is usually treated with emollient lotions. Severe cases may require topical corticosteroids.

hyperkinesis – Abnormally increased movement. Often used to describe the increased physical activity of children with attention deficit disorder.

hyperkinetic – Pertaining to hyperkinesis.

hyperlipemia – Excessive levels of triglycerides in the blood. Hyperlipemia may be due to dietary factors or metabolic diseases such as diabetes mellitus.

hyperlipidemia – General term indicating excessive levels of any specific fat or fats in general in the blood. Includes excess cholesterol, triglycerides, or low-density lipoprotein (LDL).

hyperlipoproteinemia – Excessive levels of fat-protein complexes in the blood. The term is typically used to indicate elevated levels of low-density lipoprotein (LDL) and very low-density lipoprotein (VLDL).

hypermenorrhea – Excessive amount of menstrual flow or prolonged period of menstruation.

H

hypermetabolism – An accelerated metabolic state. Hypermetabolism commonly occurs in persons with excessive secretion of thyroid hormone.

hypernatremia – Excessive concentration of sodium in the blood. Often due to dehydration.

hyperparathyroidism – Overactivity of the parathyroid glands with excessive secretion of parathyroid hormone. Hyperparathyroidism causes loss of bone calcium, increases levels of calcium in blood and urine, and increases absorption of calcium from the digestive tract. Hyperparathyroidism is usually treated by surgically removing parathyroid tissue.

hyperphagia – Overeating.

hyperpigmentation – Excessive deposition of pigment in a tissue or organ. Hyperpigmentation can occur in internal organs, but is most commonly observed in the skin. Hormonal changes during pregnancy or long-term use of corticosteroids can lead to hyperpigmentation.

hyperpituitarism – Overactivity of the pituitary gland, especially the portion that produces growth hormone. Hyperpituitarism can lead to excessive height or elongation of the extremeties in a growing child.

hyperplasia – An overgrowth of normal cells in a tissue or organ. Hyperplasia is not cancerous. Hyperplasia of tissue of the gums is called gingival hyperplasia and that in the prostate gland is called benign prostatic hyperplasia. *Also see benign prostatic hyperplasia, gingival hyperplasia.*

hyperplastic – Pertaining to hyperplasia.

hyperpnea – More rapid or deeper breathing than normal. Hyperpnea may occur during exercise, times of emotional stress, or as a result of metabolic disease.

hyperprolactinemia – Excessive secretion of the hormone prolactin. Hyperprolactinemia can produce galactorrhea in either men or women. *Also see galactorrhea.*

hyperpyrexia – Extremely high fever.

H

hypersensitivity – Overreaction of the body to a foreign material. Hypersensitivity reactions are produced by an inappropriate response of the immune system to a material it senses to be a threat to the organism. Synonymous with allergy.

hypersomnia – Excessively long periods of sleep. While awake, a person with hypersomnia is fully alert and rested and unlikely to spontaneously fall asleep, as in narcolepsy.

hypertension – Elevated blood pressure, usually considered to be above a reading of 140/90. Essential or primary hypertension occurs without known cause and accounts for over 90% of cases of high blood pressure. Secondary hypertension is elevated blood pressure due to a known cause, usually kidney disease. Malignant hypertension is a rapidly advancing form of high blood pressure that causes serious damage to internal organs and is quickly fatal if not controlled.

Untreated or inadequately treated hypertension leads to a wide variety of problems including congestive heart failure, angina pectoris, and heart attack. Optimal treatment includes an exercise program, weight loss, reduction of salt in the diet, stress reduction, and medications. A wide variety of medicines are currently available to treat hypertension.

hypertensive – Pertaining to hypertension.

Also, a person who has hypertension.

hypertensive crisis – A suddenly elevated blood pressure, usually in excess of 200/120. Untreated hypertensive crisis can be fatal. Hypertensive crisis is most likely to occur in people who have never been treated for high blood pressure or who have stopped taking their antihypertensive medicines.

hyperthermia – Elevated body temperature caused intentionally or unintentionally by therapy. Malignant hyperthermia is a rare condition characterized by rapidly rising body temperature caused by an anesthetic.

hyperthyroidism – Abnormally increased function of the thyroid gland with excessive secretion of thyroid hormone. Symptoms include anxiety, tremor, weight loss, hunger, agitation, and increased heart rate. Hyperthyroidism may be temporarily treated with thyroid suppressing drugs. Longer-lasting treatments such as surgery or radiation are used to destroy all or part of the thyroid gland.

hypertrichosis – Excessive hair growth. The hair growth may affect the whole body or only specific areas.

hypertriglyceridemia – Excessive levels of triglycerides in the blood, usually above 250 mg/100 ml of blood. Hypertriglyceridemia may occur due to dietary factors or metabolic diseases such as diabetes mellitus.

hypertrophy – *See hyperplasia.*

hyperuricemia – Excessive levels of uric acid in the blood. Hyperuricemia is most commonly due to gout. Hyperuricemia may also occur when large numbers of white blood cells suddenly die, as with the initial dose of chemotherapy for leukemia.

hypervitaminosis – Excessive levels of vitamins in the blood. Usually caused by overuse of commercial vitamin preparations. Most vitamins are capable of causing side effects in high doses, but vitamins A and D are particularly toxic in high doses.

hypervolemia – An abnormally increased volume of blood. Usually caused by overly aggressive administration of intravenous fluids or kidney or heart disease.

hypn- – Prefix designating sleep.

hypno- – Prefix designating sleep.

hypnotic – A drug that causes sleep. Colloquially called a sleeping pill or sedative.

hypo – Colloquial term for hypodermic injection.

hypo- – Prefix designating beneath or below.

hypoallergenic – Pertaining to a substance that is less likely to cause allergic reactions. Normally used in the context of skin creams and lotions that have had potentially irritating substances removed.

hypocalcemia – Low level of calcium in the blood.

hypodermic injection – An inoculation into the fat layer beneath the skin. A subcutaneous injection.

hypodermic syringe – A hollow device intended to inject a drug or withdraw fluid from beneath the skin. A hypodermic syringe must have a hollow-bore needle attached in order to pierce the skin and deliver medications.

hypodermoclysis – An infusion of fluids into the subcutaneous space under the skin. Hypodermoclysis is sometimes used to infuse large volumes of fluid to treat or prevent dehydration. The procedure is normally reserved for individuals who cannot drink enough fluid and whose veins cannot tolerate sustained infusion of fluids.

hypogammaglobulinemia – Decreased levels of the blood protein gammaglobulin. Gammaglobulin is an important component of the immune system. Low levels predispose to infections or increased difficulty fighting existing infections.

hypogastric – Pertaining to the hypogastrium.

hypogastrium – The area in the center of the abdomen starting a few inches below the umbilicus and extending to the genitals. The pubic region.

hypoglycemia – Abnormally low blood sugar. The most common causes of hypoglycemia are insulin rebound following a high carbohydrate meal or snack, an excessively high dose of antidiabetic medication, or failure to consume enough calories after taking a dose of antidiabetic medication. Symptoms include hunger, dizziness, and potentially fainting or coma.

hypoglycemic – Pertaining to hypoglycemia.

hypogonadism – Failure of sexual organs to develop normally, particularly in regard to producing reproductive cells and sex hormones. Hypogonadism usually results in short stature and slowed sexual development.

hypokalemia – Low blood potassium levels. Hypokalemia occurs most often as a side effect of diuretic therapy although it may also occur as a result of prolonged diarrhea. Symptoms include muscle weakness, cramps, and irregular heart rhythms. Hypokalemia may be treated or prevented by using a so-called potassium-sparing diuretic instead of or along with the causative diuretic, potassium supplements, or increased intake of potassium-rich foods such as bananas and citrus.

hypokinesia – *See hypokinesis.*

hypokinesis – Abnormally slowed movement. Hypokinesis may be a sign of neuromuscular disease such as Parkinson's disease or drug toxicity.

hypomagnesemia – Low blood levels of magnesium. Hypomagnesemia may cause nausea, vomiting, muscle weakness, and possibly seizures. Hypomagnesemia may be caused by overly aggressive diuretic therapy, prolonged total parenteral nutrition, and breastfeeding. Hypomagnesemia is prevented by taking magnesium supplements via a multiple vitamin and mineral product.

hypomania – A condition of less than full-blown mania in a person with bipolar affective disorder (manic-depressive illness). The term is often misinterpreted to mean only a mild form of mania. While indeed milder than mania, persons in a hypomanic state may still exhibit psychotic delusions and behaviors and may require hospitalization to prevent them from harming themselves or others. In some cases, the appearance of hypomania indicates a recurrence of illness and the opportunity for early intervention.

hyponatremia – Low level of sodium in the blood. Hyponatremia may be due to excessive sweating. Dilutional hyponatremia is a condition where fluids have been replaced by mouth or intravenously without sufficient amounts of sodium in the solution.

hypoparathyroidism – A condition distinguished by reduced secretion of hormone from the parathyroid gland.

hypoperfusion – Decreased or insufficient blood flow through an organ or tissue. Hypoperfusion may be due to heart failure or vascular disease.

hypoplasia – Lack of development of an organ or tissue. Usually due to a decrease in the number of cells.

hypoplastic anemia – Deficiency of red blood cells due to an insufficient number of precursor cells in the bone marrow.

hypopnea – Abnormal decrease in the rate or depth of breathing.

hyposalivation – Diminished ability to form saliva. Dry mouth. Hyposalivation is a side effect of many drugs. It may also result from dental disease, radiation treatments to the mouth, Sjögren's syndrome, or rheumatoid arthritis.

hypotension – An abnormally low blood pressure. The normal blood pressure is considered to be 120/80; however, some individuals consistently maintain blood pressures significantly below that value. This is not considered hypotension if these individuals experience no adverse symptoms of low blood pressure. People who normally maintain low blood pressures may be at lower risk of future cardiovascular disease.

Symptoms of hypotension include weakness, dizziness, and fainting. Hypotension may be due to blood loss, dehydration, or overly aggressive use of antihypertensive drugs. Some antihypertensive drugs also cause a condition known as postural hypotension or orthostatic hypotension. This is a condition where standing up from a lying or sitting position causes a precipitous drop in blood pressure that can cause dizziness or even fainting.

hypotensive – Pertaining to low blood pressure or an agent that lowers blood pressure.

hypothermia – A body temperature significantly below normal. Hypothermia is most often due to prolonged exposure to a cold environment. Some drugs, such as the antipsychotic drugs, are capable of making patients more susceptible to hypothermia.

hypothyroidism – A condition characterized by reduced levels of thyroid hormone in the blood. Hypothyroidism slows the body's metabolic rate and causes lack of energy, sleepiness, and weight gain.

hypotrichosis – Lack of hair on the head or body.

hypovitaminosis – A deficiency of one or more vitamins.

hypovolemia – A decreased amount of blood in the cardiovascular system.

hypovolemic shock – Precipitous drop in blood pressure due to low blood volume. Hypovolemic shock is usually caused by excessive blood loss.

hypoxemia – Low concentration of oxygen in the blood. Hypoxemia is usually caused by poor pulmonary function.

hypoxia – Low concentration of oxygen in a tissue. Hypoxia may be the result of poor pulmonary function or inadequate blood circulation.

hypoxic – Pertaining to hypoxia.

hyster- – Prefix designating the uterus.

hysterectomy – Surgical removal of the uterus. In most cases the ovaries are left intact to prevent the sudden onset of menopausal symptoms.

hystero- – Prefix designating the uterus.

hysteropathy – Any disease of the uterus.

hysteroscope – An endoscope specially designed to examine the interior lining of the uterus. *See endoscope.*

hysteroscopy – Examination of the interior lining of the uterus.

hysterotomy – Surgical incision into the uterus.

I – Chemical symbol for iodine.

-ia – Suffix designating a condition. Examples include the mental conditions of phobia, mania, and schizophrenia as well as anemia, hemophilia, and many others.

iatro- – Prefix designating a condition caused by a physician.

iatrogenic – Pertaining to a disease or condition caused by a physician's treatment. For example, side effects of drugs are sometimes referred to as iatrogenic conditions.

-ic – Suffix designating similar to or pertaining to; for example, hyperglycemic (pertaining to a high concentration of glucose in blood), genetic (pertaining to genes).

In chemistry, an ion with a higher valence than another ion of the same element' for example, sulfuric acid (vs. sulfurous acid), ferric sulfate (vs. ferrous sulfate).

ICD – *See International Classification of Diseases.*

ICF – *See intermediate care facility.*

ichthyosis – A congenital skin condition characterized by dryness, cracking, and fish-like or alligator-like scaling.

ictal – Pertaining to a stroke or seizure.

icteric – Pertaining to jaundice.

icterus – Jaundice. *See jaundice.*

ICU – *See intensive care unit.*

IDDM – *See insulin-dependent diabetes mellitus.*

idio- – Prefix meaning characteristic of or peculiar to.

idiopathic – Pertaining to a disease or condition of unknown cause.

idiopathic disease – A medical condition where the causative factors are not known.

idiopathic thrombocytopenic purpura – A blood condition of unknown cause characterized by low platelet counts with the risk of serious bleeding complications. Patients with this condition

I

need to avoid the use of aspirin and other drugs that may compromise the function of the few platelets they still have.

idiosyncrasy – A behavior, habit, or symptom peculiar to an individual or a group.

idiosyncratic – Pertaining to an idiosyncrasy.

Ig – *See immunoglobulin.*

ileitis – An inflammation in the ileum section of the small intestine.

ileostomy – A surgically implanted passageway that connects the ileum to an opening on the outside of the body. Ileostomies are performed to allow elimination of feces for patients with inflammatory bowel disease or cancer that affects intestinal function.

ileum – The last part of the small intestine, about 12 feet in length. The ileum connects the middle portion of the small intestine (jejunum) with the first portion of the large intestine.

ileus – An intestinal obstruction. Ileus may be caused by fecal material, by a tumor that blocks the flow of intestinal material, or by failure of intestinal smooth muscle to contract properly and, therefore, not move material through the entire intestine.

illness – A change from a normal state of health.

I.M. – Abbreviation for intramuscular. Normally used in the context of an injection of medicine into a muscle.

i.m. – Abbreviation for intramuscular. Normally used in the context of an injection of medicine into a muscle.

IM – Abbreviation for intramuscular. Normally used in the context of an injection of medicine into a muscle.

IM – Abbreviation for internal medicine.

im- – Prefix designating within, into, on, or inside.

imaging – Creation of a picture. Normally used in the context of a radiologic image of an internal organ or tissue such as an x-ray, CT scan, or radionuclide scan.

I

imaging agent – A dye or other radiopaque substance that allows an organ or other internal structure to be viewed on an x-ray or other type of radiographic test.

imbalance – A condition marked by inequality of factors. For example, a nutritional imbalance is a condition where food components (e.g., proteins, fats, carbohydrates) are either not ingested or absorbed in proper proportions.

immiscible – Unable to mix together in solution in the natural state. For example, oil and water are immiscible fluids unless they are both bonded to an emulsifier.

immune – Pertaining to the state of being resistant to an infectious disease due to the presence of antibodies against that disease.

immune complex – The large molecule formed when an antibody protein attacks and combines with an antigen. This reaction is intended to neutralize the invading antigen.

immune system – The organized collection of mechanisms the body uses to protect itself from invading microorganisms. The immune system includes white blood cells, phagocytic cells in the liver and other organs, and the immunoglobulins.

immunity – The state or condition of being resistant to invading microorganisms. Immunity is normally acquired either by contracting a disease and then developing immunity to it or by being vaccinated with proteins from the causative agent. For example, a person with a normal immune system who contracts rubella (German measles) develops a lifelong immunity to the disease. Alternatively, a person may be vaccinated with dead rubella viruses in order to acquire immunity. In each case, the immune system responds to proteins in the virus and develops a "memory" for it. The next time the person is exposed to the live virus, the immune system "remembers" its past exposure and attacks and kills the virus before it can cause an infection.

immunization – The procedure for conferring immunity. Immunization is most commonly performed by giving an injection. However, some immunizations are given by mouth (e.g., polio) and some may someday be given by means of nasal sprays or drops.

I

immunocompetence – The ability to produce a normal immune response to antigens, such as those produced by invading microorganisms.

immunocompromised – *See immunodeficiency.*

immunodeficiency – The inability to produce a normal immune response to antigens, such as those produced by invading microorganisms. Immunodeficient persons are usually unable to produce sufficient quantities of immunoglobulins. This may be due to inherited disease, immunosuppressant drug therapy (e.g., corticosteroids, cancer chemotherapy), or infections such as AIDS.

immunoglobulin (Ig) – A group of proteins in the blood that functions as part of the immune system. All antibodies are immunoglobulins.

Immunoglobulins identify and attempt to destroy potentially harmful proteins and other substances that are foreign to the body. In some cases, immunoglobulins overreact, causing uncomfortable and sometimes fatal allergic reactions.

The five types of immunoglobulins are classified as immunoglobulin A (IgA), immunoglobulin D (IgD), immunoglobulin E (IgE), immunoglobulin G (IgG), and immunoglobulin M (IgM). About 80% of the immunoglobulins circulating in the blood are IgG, also known as gammaglobulin.

immunologist – An individual who specializes in immunology. An immunologist may or may not be a physician.

immunology – The study of the immune system, including resistance to disease and allergic reactions.

immunosuppressant – An agent that reduces the effectiveness of the immune system. Immunosuppression may be intended or a side effect of treatment. For example, corticosteroids such as prednisone and hydrocortisone are immunosuppressant drugs that are often used to treat allergic reactions and reduce inflammation. Most cancer chemotherapy drugs have the unfortunate side effect of immunosuppression because they impair the body's ability to form immunoglobulins. Consequently, cancer chemotherapy often increases patients' susceptibility to infection.

I

immunosuppression – Inhibition of the normal function of the immune system. Immunosuppression may be caused by treatment with certain drugs (see immunosuppressant) or exposure to toxic chemicals or radiation.

impairment – A disorder that interferes with the function of an organ, organ system, or organism.

impermeable – Unable to be crossed or penetrated. For example, extremely fine filters are sometimes used to sterilize fluids because the filters allow fluids to pass through but are too fine for bacteria to pass. These filters are impermeable to bacteria.

impetigo – A bacterial skin infection most commonly seen in, but not totally limited to, children. Impetigo is highly contagious and spreads rapidly in schools where children have physical contact with each other during athletics or playtime. Impetigo initially appears as a fluid-filled blister that may burst, leaving a crusty margin around the lesion. The condition often causes intense itching that may help to spread the infection. Impetigo is usually treated with both oral and topical antibiotics.

implant – An insert or a graft. The best known implants are those inserted during breast augmentation surgery. However, drugs may also be implanted in some cases. For example, one form of female contraception involves surgically inserting hormone-containing rods (e.g., Norplant) beneath the skin of the forearm. Once implanted, the rods slowly and consistently secrete enough hormone to prevent conception. The rods may be removed if the woman wants to reestablish fertility. If left in place, the implants are effective for up to five years.

implantation – The attachment of a fertilized ovum to the wall of the uterus. Implantation occurs approximately seven days after conception.

impotence – Inability of a physically mature male to initiate and maintain a penile erection to the completion of intercourse. *Also see erectile dysfunction.*

impregnate – To make pregnant.

Also, to diffuse, saturate, or mix with another substance. For example, a gauze pad may be impregnated with antiseptic before applying to a wound.

in- – Prefix designating within, into, on, or inside.

inactivate – To destroy the functional capacity of an agent or organism. For example, the liver inactivates many drugs as a result of metabolism. Most of these drugs are no longer functional following this process. As another example, excessive heat may inactivate microorganisms.

inactivation – The process of destroying the function of an agent or organism.

inactive ingredient – A substance added to a pharmaceutical dosage form that does not directly cause the therapeutic effect. *See excipient.*

incentives – Inducements, usually financial, given to health care providers to encourage them to control the costs of the care they provide. Typically, incentives are offered to physicians for reducing costly services such as hospital stays, emergency room visits, excessive laboratory or other diagnostic tests, and unnecessary referrals to specialists.

incidence – The number of new cases of a disorder or problem that occur in a specified period of time. For example, a side effect that occurs in 10 of every 100 patients who take a given drug is said to have an incidence of one in ten cases or 10%. Contrasted with prevalence, which is the number of cases of a problem or disorder that exist at any point in time.

incision – A surgical cut into an organ or tissue.

incompatibility – A state or condition of being incompatible.

incompatible – Not able to be mixed without causing an undesirable change. Two drugs are said to be incompatible when they cannot be combined without causing a harmful reaction. While drugs that interact with each other inside the body may be considered to be incompatible, the term is normally applied to drugs that

I

chemically react with each other when they are physically mixed in a prescription or an intravenous solution.

incompetence – Inability to function at a normal level. For example, a heart valve is said to be incompetent if it is unable to keep blood from flowing backwards through it. Incompetent heart valves decrease the efficiency of the heart and can be detected as murmurs.

incontinence – Inability to control body wastes. For example, a person who is incontinent of urine is unable to keep from leaking large or small amounts of urine. This may be the result of a bladder problem or an aftereffect of prostate surgery.

incubation period – The time between exposure to an infecting organism and the onset of symptoms of illness.

incurable – Pertaining to a medical condition whose progress cannot be reversed despite treatment.

IND – *See investigational new drug.*

indemnity plan – A type of health insurance policy where the policyholder (the patient) is responsible for all health care bills after the service is rendered. The policyholder, in turn, sends receipts and claims forms to the insurance company. The insurance company then pays either the health care provider or the policyholder, minus any applicable deductible amounts, depending upon terms of the insurance contract. Indemnity plans typically do not employ cost containment tools. Rather, they pay costs as billed as long as those costs are within the plan limits. If the policy limits do not fully cover providers' fees, the policyholder may be responsible for the difference.

independent pharmacy – A drugstore that is owned by an individual or a family rather than a large corporation. Most independent pharmacies exist either as a single entity or as one of just a few commonly owned pharmacies. Opposite of chain pharmacy.

indication – The reason for using a treatment. For example, pneumonia is an indication for using penicillin. The United States Food and Drug Administration (FDA) establishes the approved indications for every prescription drug distributed in the United States.

I

While physicians may legally prescribe any drug for any purpose they feel is appropriate, drug manufacturers may not promote their drugs for any use (indication) not approved by the FDA. The approved uses for a drug may be found in the "Indications" section of its package insert.

indigestion – Colloquial term for a digestive problem that includes symptoms of stomach fullness, belching, burning, sharp pain, or pressure. Indigestion may be caused by overeating or gastroesophageal reflux. *See gastroesophageal reflux.*

indirect costs – Expenses incurred as part of doing business but not directly related to providing a specific service. Indirect costs include utilities, rent, insurance, cleaning, and equipment purchases and maintenance.

individual contract – *See individual plan.*

individual deductible – The amount of money a single insurance holder must pay before policy benefits begin. *Also see deductible, family deductible.*

individual membership – An insurance policy held by one person independent of any other group. For example, persons who are over 19 years old and not full-time students may not be covered by their families' insurance policies but may qualify for individual memberships in an insurance plan.

individual plan – An insurance policy issued to a single person or a family that is not a member of any other group.

induction – The process of causing something to occur. For example, induction of labor is attempted by administering drugs and hormones that stimulate the uterus to contract.

Also, the period of time between the beginning of administration of a general anesthetic and the point at which the patient has achieved the desired level of unconsciousness.

inebriant – A drug or chemical that causes a state of intoxication. Most commonly used in the context of alcohol intoxication.

inebriation – The state of being intoxicated by a drug or chemical. Most commonly used to describe alcohol intoxication.

I

in extremis – At the point of death.

infant – A young child. Some consider infancy to be the first 12 months of life. Others consider it to be the period from birth to the time when the child can assume an erect posture, usually 12 to 14 months. Still others consider infancy to be the first 24 months of life.

infantile – Pertaining to an infant.

infantile paralysis – *See poliomyelitis.*

infarction – Dead tissue caused by a sudden interruption of blood flow to an area. Most commonly used in the context of myocardial infarction (heart attack) or cerebral infarction (stroke). *Also see myocardial infarction.*

infect – The process of microorganisms invading an organ or tissue.

infection – Growth and multiplication of parasitic microorganisms inside a tissue or organ. Viruses and bacteria cause most infections. When conditions are favorable, infecting organisms are able to multiply and spread within the organism. Some infections are said to be self-limiting when the organism is able to contain and then eradicate the infecting organism without medical treatment. The common cold is an example of a self-limited infection.

Mixed infections are those caused by more than one species of microorganism.

Opportunistic infections are those that occur because the host is in a weakened state. For example, cytomegalovirus is a herpesvirus that quietly resides in most adults. If the immune system becomes impaired, as in AIDS or persons treated with immunosuppressant drugs, cytomegalovirus may attack the host and cause blindness.

infectious arthritis – Pain in one or more joints caused by invasion of microorganisms. Causes include gonorrhea, tuberculosis, and syphilis.

infectious disease – A medical condition caused by the growth and multiplication of parasitic microorganisms inside a tissue or organ.

I

infectious disease specialist – A physician who focuses on the diagnosis and treatment of diseases caused by microorganisms.

infectious waste – Rubbish that is contaminated with pathogenic microorganisms. Infectious waste must be handled carefully to prevent trash handlers from being exposed to potentially dangerous microorganisms. In a hospital, for example, all infectious waste is placed in red containers and kept separate from all other trash. Infectious waste is usually destroyed in an incinerator.

inferior – Pertaining to a lower surface of an organ. For example, the inferior aspect of the liver refers to the lower portion of the liver.

Also, when two anatomic structures are located one above the other, the inferior structure is the lower of the two.

Opposite of superior.

infertility – The inability to conceive a child. Most cases of infertility are treatable. Treatments may include surgery, supplemental hormones, or *in vitro* fertilization.

infestation – Presence of a parasite on the external surface of the skin and skin structures, although some parasites (e.g., mites, scabies) may burrow into the skin. Contrasted to an infection where parasites invade tissues and organs. For example, head lice attach themselves to the scalp and hair shafts (infestation), while bacteria may invade the structures inside and beneath the skin (infection).

infiltration – The process of diffusing a fluid into tissue. In some cases, infiltration is intended as when a local anesthetic medicine is injected into tissue to deaden the sensations of a minor surgical or dental procedure. In other cases, infiltration is not intended, as when an intravenous fluid or medication leaks from the vein into the surrounding tissue.

infirmary – A clinic or small medical facility, most commonly operating in a school, university, or factory.

inflammation – A natural response on the part of the body to injury or infection. As part of the inflammatory process, the organism attempts to isolate the affected area from the rest of the body in an attempt to prevent the injury or infection from spreading

I

elsewhere. Inflammation is characterized by any or all of the following: reddening of the affected area, local heat production, swelling, pain, and temporary loss of function in the affected area.

In some cases, the inflammatory response may be misapplied and do more damage than good. Examples include rheumatoid arthritis and asthma.

Inflammation may be limited by local application of cold packs or by administration of anti-inflammatory drugs such as corticosteroids, salicylates, or nonsteroidal anti-inflammatory drugs (NSAIDs).

influenza – A viral infection of the upper respiratory tract causing fever, chills, extreme lethargy, headache, muscle ache, and/or cough. Influenza is temporarily debilitating and secondary infection is common. Colloquially known as flu.

Intestinal influenza or stomach flu is actually not a form of influenza. Most often it is a form of gastroenteritis caused by a different family of viruses.

informed consent – A requirement of any ethical human clinical study whereby potential study subjects are informed, orally and in writing, of all the known medical benefits and risks of participating in the study. After they have been so informed, they may consent to participate in the study or they may refuse to participate. Even individuals who consent to participate in the study may revoke their consent and withdraw at any time.

infusion – The slow administration of a fluid other than blood and by a route other than oral. Infusions may be used to administer fluids by themselves or in combination with drugs, vitamins, minerals, or other nutrients.

Also a process for extracting drugs from herbs whereby the herbs, usually previously crushed to prepare them for extraction, are soaked in hot or boiling solvent. Water is the most common solvent used for infusion. When steeped in hot or boiling solvent, the active constituents of the herbs dissolve in the solvent, the solvent is drained away, and the active drug-solvent solution is further processed.

I

ingestion – The process of swallowing food, beverages, drugs, or other substances. Ingested materials enter the stomach and continue through all or part of the digestive tract.

ingredient cost – The cost of the medication(s) in a prescription. The price of a prescription is comprised of ingredient costs, the pharmacist's professional fee or markup, and any applicable taxes.

ingrown hair – A hair that either did not emerge properly from the hair follicle and grew beneath the skin or did emerge from the hair follicle and turned back into the skin. Hairs often ingrow because of constricting clothing or equipment, for example, an elastic waistband or the chinstrap of a helmet.

inhalant – A medicine or other agent that is breathed in through the nose or mouth.

inhalation – The processes of introducing a gas, vapor, or fine particle to the respiratory system by breathing it in through the nose or mouth.

inhalation anesthesia – A type of surgical anesthesia administered by having the patient breathe a combination of anesthetic drug and oxygen. Alternative routes of administration of surgical anesthesia include intravenous injection and infusion into the spinal fluid.

inhaled medicine – A therapeutic agent administered by having the patient breathe a gaseous or aerosol form of the drug. Inhaled medications are often used to treat respiratory conditions such as asthma.

inhaler – A device used to allow medicines to be administered in aerosol form through the mouth or nose. Inhalers are commonly used to deliver asthma medications to the lungs.

inhibition – The arrest or restraint of a process normally performed by a molecule, cell, tissue, or organ.

inhibitor – A drug or other agent that impedes the normal function of a molecule, cell, tissue, or organ. For example, the angiotensin converting enzyme (ACE) inhibitors are drugs that lower blood pressure by blocking the functions of the enzyme that forms

I

angiotensin II, a biochemical that causes blood vessels to constrict.

injectable – A material, usually a drug, suitable for injection.

injection – The act of forcing a fluid beneath the skin or into a body cavity, usually by means of a syringe and hollow needle.

Also, the material injected through a syringe.

Injections may be made into a wide variety of tissues. These include into a vein (intravenous injection), into an artery (intra-arterial), between layers of the skin (intradermal), beneath the skin (subcutaneous), into a muscle (intramuscular), beneath the membrane that covers the spinal cord (intrathecal), or into the eye (intraocular).

injector – A device other than a syringe that can be used to inject a drug. Most injectors shoot fluid at a pressure high enough to pierce the skin without the use of a needle. They are most commonly used to vaccinate large numbers of people in a short period of time.

injury – Damage to the body caused by trauma.

innervation – The supply of nerve fibers to an area.

Also, the degree of nerve stimulation to an area.

in-network – A diverse group of health care providers (e.g., pharmacies, physicians, hospitals, dentists) contracted with a health insurance plan to provide professional services to the plan's members.

innocuous – Harmless.

innovator drug – The first trademarked version of a pharmaceutical product. An innovator drug is protected by patent and the manufacturer has exclusive marketing rights for 17 years from the time the patent is granted. After the patent expires, other companies can make and distribute exact copies (generic forms).

inoculate – To vaccinate.

Also, the process of introducing live microorganisms into a laboratory culture medium for the purpose of further study.

I

inoculation – Vaccination. The process of injecting antigens from viruses or bacteria in order to promote immunity.

inoculum – The microorganisms introduced into a laboratory culture medium.

inoperable – Unable to surgically treat. Often used in the context of a tumor that has spread to such a great extent that surgical excision is not an option.

inorganic – Not formed by a living creature.

In chemistry, any molecule that does not contain at least one carbon atom.

inotrope – A drug that causes an inotropic effect.

inotropic – Pertaining to the force of muscle contraction. Most commonly used in relation to the heart where an inotropic drug is one that causes the heart muscle to contract harder.

inpatient – A person who is admitted to a hospital for a stay of at least 24 hours.

inpatient care – Medical and related care given to a patient during a course of hospitalization.

insanity – A colloquial term typically used to describe a mental condition characterized by loss of contact with reality. Psychosis.

insecticide – A chemical agent that kills insects. Includes the topical agents that are used to treat skin infestations of lice and scabies.

insemination – The process of depositing semen into the vagina, usually during intercourse. In artificial insemination, however, a semen specimen is collected from a man and is instilled into the uterus by a health care professional.

insidious – Functioning in a slow or not easily apparent manner. An insidious disease is a condition that manifests itself at such a slow pace that its presence or significance is easily overlooked for a time.

in situ – Pertaining to being in the normal or natural place. For example, a tumor *in situ* is a growth that has not metastasized or invaded other tissues.

insomnia – The inability to sleep normally. Insomnia includes inability to get to sleep in an appropriate amount of time, unnatural waking during the night, or waking earlier than normal with the inability to get back to sleep.

insomniac – A person who experiences insomnia.

inspiration – The act of breathing air into the lungs.

inspirometer – An instrument used to measure the amount of air that can be inhaled into the lungs. Inspirometers may be used to monitor progression of respiratory illnesses or to measure the response to respiratory medications.

inspissation – Drying or thickening of a fluid, particularly the mucus in the respiratory tract. Inspissation is often a complication of bronchial asthma.

instillation – The act of administering a fluid by means of drops. Most commonly, instillation refers to administration of eye drops or ear drops.

institutional pharmacy – A pharmacy that operates as part of a hospital, clinic, nursing home, or health maintenance organization.

institutional providers – Facilities that deliver health care services to patients. Institutional providers include hospitals, clinics, skilled nursing facilities, etc.

institutional review board (IRB) – A group of health care professionals and laypersons from the community who review protocols for human research studies. The IRB is responsible for assuring that the proposed study is ethical, safe for the participants, and scientifically valid. The IRB may approve the study in question, deny permission to conduct the study, or defer a final decision until changes are made to the protocol. IRBs may be organized by hospitals or by universities.

insufficiency – The inability of an organ to perform at a normal level of function. The term is often used in reference to a diseased heart that can no longer pump with normal force. It is also applied to respiratory conditions such as chronic obstructive pulmonary disease where the lungs are unable to adequately exchange oxygen and carbon dioxide.

I

insulin – A hormone produced by the pancreas that lowers blood sugar by allowing the cells of the body to absorb glucose from the blood. Cells use this glucose as their primary fuel and cannot live long without it. Insulin is normally released in greater amounts following a carbohydrate-containing meal or snack. Insulin also raises levels of fat in the blood.

insulin-dependent diabetes mellitus (IDDM) – Type I diabetes mellitus. IDDM is characterized by the inability to form insulin. All persons with IDDM must take insulin daily in the form of an injection or by means of an infusion pump.

The term insulin-dependent diabetes mellitus is sometimes used inappropriately to describe persons with type II diabetes (also called noninsulin-dependent diabetes mellitus—NIDDM) who no longer respond to oral medicines and must begin to take insulin injections. The difference is that persons with IDDM produce virtually no insulin of their own and must satisfy all of their insulin needs by injecting the drug. In contrast, persons with type II diabetes still produce their own insulin; however, that insulin production is not sufficient for their total insulin needs.

insult – Damage or injury to an organ or tissue.

insurance – A form of protection against financial loss due to unforeseen or unpredictable events. The underlying premise is to collect small amounts of money (premiums) from a large number of people to build a large pool of funds. Insurable events are paid from the money pool so that no individual is personally responsible for a devastatingly large claim. An actuary determines the amount of premiums that needs to be collected to accumulate a sufficiently large pool. *Also see actuary.*

insurance carrier – A business entity that provides insurance coverage and administers premiums, claims, and payments.

insured – A person who is covered by an insurance policy.

intensive care unit (ICU) – A hospital floor specializing in treating critically ill patients. Depending upon the size of the hospital, there may be one general intensive care unit or several specialized units. Examples of specialized intensive care units include newborn intensive care units, pediatric intensive care units, burn units, coronary care units, surgical intensive care units, and medical intensive care units.

inter- – Prefix designating between or among.

intercostal – Between the ribs. For example, intercostal pain is discomfort that originates from the space between two ribs.

interferon – A group of blood proteins that have antiviral effects. The genes that produce some of the interferons have been isolated and those interferons are now commercially produced by means of genetic engineering. The drugs are given by injection and are used to treat infections such as viral hepatitis and some cancers.

intermediate – A substance formed as part of chemical reaction that is itself changed during a subsequent reaction. In a sequence of reactions, all of the chemicals formed as part of the reaction, except for the last product, are intermediates. In the body, some drugs have intermediate metabolites that may or may not be pharmacologically active.

intermediate care facility (ICF) – A health care organization that provides a level of residential care of an intensity between that of a skilled nursing facility (a typical nursing home) and an assisted living facility.

intermittent claudication – A condition characterized by pain in one or both legs during walking or other physical activity involving the legs. The pain remits when the leg is at rest and returns again with activity. Intermittent claudication is usually an indication that blood flow to the painful area is insufficient.

intern – A trainee or apprentice. In medicine, an intern is a graduate physician in the first year of post-medical school practice. Medical interns are not eligible for licensure until completion of the internship.

In pharmacy, an intern is a student or graduate pharmacist who either is not yet eligible for or has not yet achieved licensure but works in a pharmacy under a licensed pharmacist's supervision.

internal medicine – That area of medicine that deals with diagnosis and nonsurgical treatment of diseases primarily affecting the

I

internal organs. Internal medicine has many subspecialties, including cardiology, gastroenterology, oncology, endocrinology, and rheumatology.

Internal medicine is considered a primary care specialty, along with pediatrics, family practice, and in some cases, obstetrics-gynecology.

internal medicine specialist – *See internist.*

International Classification of Diseases (ICD) – A reference book that lists medical conditions, disorders, and diseases along with a coding number. The ICD, now in its tenth edition and often referred to as ICD-10, provides a standardized nomenclature and numeric code for the purpose of filing medical insurance claims.

international unit (IU, I.U.) – The amount of a drug that produces a specific, measurable response in an animal, as defined by an international body, such as the World Health Organization. International units are often used to designate the strength of a product when the mass (milligrams, grams, etc.) of the product produces an unreliable clinical effect. For example, drugs such as insulin, heparin, and vitamin E are often standardized by their units of activity rather than their milligram strength because the potency of a milligram of each of these drugs varies depending upon the animal or plant source from which it was derived.

internist – A physician who specializes in internal medicine in adults.

interstitial fluid – The liquid that fills most of the spaces between the cells and tissues of the body. Interstitial fluid is similar in chemical composition to the plasma of the blood.

intertrigo – Inflamed skin that occurs in skin folds and crevices. Intertrigo is often caused by heat and collection of sweat in these areas. Fungal infections are common with intertrigo. The condition is usually treated with drying agents and topical antifungal drugs.

intervention – An imposed interference or disruption in a condition. For example, a therapeutic intervention is the administration of a treatment intended to improve the course of an illness.

intestinal flora – The microorganisms that normally live in the intestinal tract. The intestinal flora aid in food digestion and secrete vitamins and other nutrients. In some cases, they assist with drug metabolism. The bacteria, viruses, and fungi of the intestinal flora normally hold each other's growth in check. However, if the balance is upset, as sometimes occurs with antibiotic therapy, one species may become temporarily dominant and cause diarrhea or other intestinal problems.

intestinal obstruction – A blockage in the intestinal tract that impairs the movement of nutrients or waste. Causes include impacted feces, tumor, hernia, or narrowed intestines due to inflammation. Signs and symptoms may include pain, vomiting of feces, dehydration, and low blood pressure.

intestine – The lengthy, tube-like lower portion of the digestive tract that runs from the stomach to the anus. The intestines are composed of the small intestine, intended primarily for food digestion and nutrient absorption, and the large intestine, whose main role is disposal of digestive waste.

intolerance – A sensitivity or allergy to a substance or treatment. Most commonly used to describe foods or nutrients that a person cannot digest properly. For example, lactose intolerance is the inability to properly digest the primary sugar in milk (lactose). Lactose intolerance may cause severe intestinal gas, bloating, and diarrhea.

intoxicant – An agent that causes poisoning. The term is most commonly applied to alcohol.

intoxication – A state of poisoning. The term is most commonly applied to a state of physical and mental dysfunction caused by alcohol.

intra- – Prefix designating within.

intracellular – Pertaining to the inside of a cell.

intracerebral – Pertaining to the tissue of the brain.

intracoronary – Pertaining to the inside of a coronary artery or the heart.

I

intracranial – Within the skull.

intracranial aneurysm – A bulging blood vessel inside the brain. *Also see aneurysm.*

intracranial hemorrhage – Bleeding that occurs inside the brain.

intractable – Unrelenting. Resistant to treatment.

intractable pain – Discomfort that is not alleviated by the usual treatment methods. The term is most often applied to pain caused by advanced cancer. This type of pain is usually successfully treated with higher than normal doses of narcotic analgesics. These drugs may need to be administered by some combination of oral, sublingual, subcutaneous, intravenous, or dermal routes.

intradermal – Between the layers of the skin.

intradermal injection – A dose of an agent administered between the layers of the skin. The tuberculin skin test for exposure to tuberculosis is the most common type of intradermal injection.

intrahepatic – Pertaining to something inside the liver.

intramuscular (IM, I.M., i.m.) – Inside a muscle. Normally used in the context of an injection given into a muscle. The intramuscular site is usually a good place for drug absorption. These injections have the disadvantages of pain at the site of injection and the difficulty of teaching a family member to administer medicines in this fashion.

intranuclear – Inside the nucleus of a cell. For example, most of a cell's DNA is intranuclear.

intrathecal – Pertaining to the inside of the sheath that covers and protects the spinal cord.

intrathecal injection – Administration of a drug into the intrathecal space. For example, some patients with leukemia are given intrathecal injections of chemotherapy in order to kill leukemic cells that may have invaded the brain.

intrauterine – Within the uterus.

I

intrauterine device (IUD) – A contraceptive appliance that is inserted into a woman's uterus. IUDs prevent implantation of fertilized eggs in the uterus. IUDs are inserted in a physician's office and may remain in place for months or years. In most cases, the devices must also be removed in a physician's office. Some IUDs secrete hormones that assist in the contraceptive effect.

intravasation – The entry of foreign material into a vein.

intravascular – Pertaining to the inside of blood vessels.

intravenous (IV, I.V., i.v.) – Into a vein. Most commonly used in the context of an injection given directly into a vein. Intravenous injection is usually the fastest way to deliver a medicine to its site of action or to replace large amounts of fluid to the cardiovascular system.

intravenous fluids – Solutions of water and electrolytes, sugars, lipids, and/or amino acids that are administered directly into a vein. Intravenous fluids may also have drugs added to them.

intraventricular – Inside the hollow spaces in the brain or heart.

intravesical – Within the urinary bladder. In some cases, antibiotic irrigations may be instilled into the urinary bladder to fight infection in the bladder's lining.

intrinsic – Located within an organ, tissue, or organism.

intubation – Insertion of a hollow tube into an organ or space. Normally used to describe the process of passing a tube through the nose, mouth, or a surgical opening in the trachea until it reaches a lung. The tube may be used to supply anesthesia during surgery or to oxygenate the lungs during a medical emergency.

in utero – Within the uterus. Normally used to describe an unborn child.

invasion – The beginning of a disease, especially an infection.
Also the spread of a cancer into a new area.

invasive – Pertaining to an invasion. Disruptive. Normally used in the context of a diagnostic test or treatment that requires inserting an instrument, needle, or catheter through the skin or into an

I

orifice. In general, invasive methods are reserved for situations where less uncomfortable procedures are not effective.

inventory – The stock of medications a pharmacy keeps immediately on hand. Like most businesses, pharmacies strive to keep their inventories as small as reasonable in order to control overhead costs. This may lead to pharmacies not stocking brand name drugs when generics are available or not stocking drugs that are not commonly prescribed in their local area. In most cases, however, pharmacies can obtain these medications in one or two days if the need arises.

investigational new drug (IND) – An experimental pharmaceutical agent that has not yet been approved for use by the United States Food and Drug Administration (FDA).

investigator – A researcher who organizes, conducts, or assists with the performance of clinical research study. Investigators may be physicians, pharmacists, nurses, physical therapists, dentists, or other health care professionals.

in vitro – Literally meaning "in glass" or "in a glass," the term is most commonly applied to processes, tests, or procedures that take place outside of the body. For example, an *in vitro* drug study is performed in a laboratory setting with tissue specimens or artificial media. Opposite of *in vivo*.

in vivo – Literally meaning "in life," the term is applied to a function or experiment that takes place within a living organism. For example, an *in vivo* study may examine the effects of an experimental drug when it is administered to a living human. Opposite of *in vitro*.

involuntary – Not done consciously or of free will. Tics and tremors are examples of involuntary muscle movements because they occur spontaneously without the willful intent of the individual.

ion – An electrically charged atom. Ions are chemically unstable and seek to either combine with or pair with an ion of an opposite charge.

ionic – Pertaining to an ion.

I

IRB – *See institutional review board.*

irides – Plural form of iris.

iris – A diaphragm in the eye that separates the two chambers within the eye. The iris is the portion of the eye that gives the eye its color and controls the amount of light that enters the eye.

iritis – Inflammation of the iris.

iron deficiency anemia – A low red blood cell count caused by an insufficient amount of iron in the blood and bone marrow. Iron deficiency anemia is most common in children and menstruating women.

The disorder can be prevented with sufficient dietary intake of iron, particularly from meats and fish, or by taking iron supplements. Vegetables are usually poor sources of absorbable iron.

Iron deficiency anemia is usually treated with oral iron supplements. Severe cases may require iron injections or blood transfusions.

irradiation – Exposure of a tissue to external radiation. Often used in the context of radiation therapy of cancer where the tumor is exposed to (irradiated with) a beam of radiation energy.

irreversible – Unable to be changed back. Permanent.

irrigation – Washing of an area with a large volume of water. For example, wounds are often irrigated to flush out dirt, bacteria, and blood.

irritable bowel syndrome – Increased activity of the lower intestinal tract, usually precipitated by emotional stress. Signs and symptoms include abdominal pain, cramps, and diarrhea. Irritable bowel syndrome is sometimes called spastic colon.

irritant – An agent that inflames a tissue.

ischemia – A temporary reduction of blood supply to an organ or tissue due to obstruction of a blood vessel. For example, myocardial ischemia is an obstruction of blood flow, usually due to a thrombus or lipid plaque, that produces the pain of angina pectoris during physical exertion.

ischemic – Pertaining to ischemia.

I

-ism – Suffix designating a condition caused by another factor. For example, plumbism is a toxic condition caused by ingestion of lead. Hyperthyroidism is a condition caused by excessive secretion of thyroid hormone.

isolation – Separation from others. Hospitals use a variety of isolation techniques to prevent the spread of infectious diseases from one patient to a visitor or another patient, from patients to staff, or from staff to patients. Depending upon the specific infection and its means of transmission, isolation techniques may include meticulous handwashing with disinfectant soap, and use of gloves, masks, gowns, hair covers, or shoe covers.

isotonic – Pertaining to a solution that exerts the same concentration of solute as another solution.

Also see isotonic solution.

isotonic solution – A fluid that exerts the same concentration of solute as a reference standard, usually blood plasma. Most intravenous fluids, irrigating fluids, and eye drops are isotonic solutions. Solutions that are hypotonic (less than the concentration of blood) cause blood cells to swell and burst while hypertonic (greater than the concentration of blood) solutions cause blood cells to crinkle and die. While some clinical situations require the use of hypo- (less concentrated than plasma) or hypertonic (more concentrated than plasma) solutions, most solutions used on sensitive tissues are isotonic. Isotonic eye drops, for example, cause less stinging when applied.

isotope – One of two or more forms of the same chemical element. Isotopes of an element all have the same number of protons and electrons, but they have a different number of neutrons. Isotopes may or may not be radioactive.

itch – An irritating, mildly painful feeling in the skin that is often satisfied by scratching.

-itides – Suffix that is the plural form of –itis.

-itis – Suffix designating inflammation. For example, dermatitis is an inflammation of the skin.

I.U. – *See international unit.*

I

IU – *See international unit.*

IUD – *See intrauterine device.*

i.v. – *See intravenous.*

I.V. – *See intravenous.*

IV – *See intravenous.*

J

jaundice – Yellowing of the skin and the white portion of the eyes. Jaundice is caused by the presence of bilirubin and bile pigments in the skin and is usually a sign of liver disease.

JCAHO – *See Joint Commission on Accreditation of Healthcare Organizations.*

jejunectomy – Surgical removal of all or part of the jejunum.

jejunum – The middle portion of the small intestine. The jejunum lies between the duodenum and the ileum. The jejunum is approximately eight feet long.

jelly – A semisolid pharmaceutical dosage form. Jellies are most commonly used to administer drugs to mucous membranes. Contraceptive jellies, for instance, contain a spermicide and are intended to temporarily seal a diaphragm to the vaginal wall.

jet lag – A fatigue syndrome caused by passing quickly through multiple time zones. Most commonly associated with air travel.

joint – The place where two or more bones come together. Most joints are constructed so that movement of both bones is possible. Examples of moveable joints include the knees, ankles, elbows, shoulders, and knuckles. Examples of immovable joints include the junctures of the bones in the skull.

Also, a colloquial term for a marijuana cigarette.

Joint Commission on Accreditation of Healthcare Organizations (JCAHO) – A nonprofit organization that reviews the quality of care provided by a wide variety of health care facilities and determines whether to award or deny its endorsement (accreditation). The Joint Commission evaluates hospitals, home care companies, hospices, mental health facilities, ambulatory care facilities, infusion centers, skilled nursing facilities, and others. Licensing bodies (e.g. state regulatory agencies) do not require health care facilities to be accredited, but many health insurance carriers decline to contract for services with nonaccredited organizations. Joint Commission accreditation is difficult to achieve and is highly valued. Being unable to attain Joint Commission accreditation may exclude an organization from taking care of some insurers' patients and is also a potential source of embarrassment within the organization's local community.

juvenile – A child or adolescent.

    Also, pertaining to a child or adolescent.

juvenile rheumatoid arthritis – An inflammatory and painful disease of the joints that affects children under the age of 16.

juvenile-onset diabetes mellitus – *See diabetes mellitus.*

K

K – Chemical symbol for the element potassium.

kaluresis – The presence of excessive amount of potassium in the urine. Most commonly caused by treatment with a diuretic drug.

Kaposi's sarcoma (KS) – A skin cancer that most commonly appears in people with damaged immune systems, particularly those with acquired immune deficiency syndrome (AIDS). KS may also occur in elderly men, diabetics, and persons with other types of cancer. Kaposi's lesions appear as purple or blue patches or nodules that grow in size and appear in various parts of the body. They may eventually metastasize to lymph nodes and internal organs.

kcal – See *kilocalorie.*

keratin – The tough protein that forms the basis for most skin structures, including hair, nails, and horns of animals.

keratinization – A process where environmental factors cause the skin to form a keratin layer to protect itself. Keratinization may be caused by factors that include chemical irritation, mechanical friction, ultraviolet radiation exposure from the sun or tanning beds, and lack of humidity.

keratitis – Inflammation of the cornea of the eye.

keratopathy – Any noninflammatory medical condition of the cornea of the eye.

keratosis – Any skin lesion that is surrounded by hard, thickened skin.

kernicterus – A serious form of jaundice seen in some newborn babies. In some cases, kernicterus can occur when the mother takes a sulfa drug late in pregnancy.

ketoacidosis – An acidic state of the blood where ketone bodies are also present. Ketoacidosis is a life-threatening condition most commonly seen in type I diabetics who miss doses of insulin. The acid and ketones are waste products that accumulate in blood in the absence of insulin.

ketosis – The accumulation of ketone bodies in the blood. Ketosis is most commonly seen in diabetes (*see ketoacidosis*) and in starva-

K

tion. Ketones are formed when the body has to burn fats for energy in the absence of glucose.

kg – See *kilogram*.

kidney – One of two bean-shaped organs located in the lower back. The primary function of the kidneys is to filter wastes and excess water from the blood and to form them into urine. In addition, the kidneys also secrete hormones that stimulate production of red blood cells and control blood pressure.

kilo- – Prefix designating 1,000.

kilocalorie (kcal) – A measure of heat energy that is equal to the amount of heat necessary to raise one kilogram (2.2 pounds) of water 1° Celsius. A kilocalorie is 1,000 times greater than a simple calorie. The "calories" attributed to foods are actually kilocalories.

kilogram (kg) – A unit of mass that equals 1,000 grams. A kilogram is approximately 2.2 pounds.

knee – The joint that connects the bones in the upper and lower legs. The knee is a commonly affected joint in persons with osteoarthritis (degenerative joint disease).

knuckle – The joint that connects the bones in the fingers. The knuckles are commonly affected in rheumatoid arthritis and osteoarthritis (degenerative joint disease).

KS – See *Kaposi's sarcoma*.

kyphosis – A hunched deformity of the back. Kyphosis is common in osteoporosis.

kyphotic – Pertaining to kyphosis.

L

l – *See liter.*

L – *See liter.*

label – The information attached to a container that identifies the contents of the container. For example, the label for a bottle of regular-strength aspirin would identify the contents as aspirin, 325 mg.

The United States Food and Drug Administration (FDA) requires that manufacturers include extensive information as part of a drug product's label, especially for prescription drugs. Since the FDA requires far more information than can be printed on a bottle label, the agency requires drug manufacturers to list this information on papers that are inserted into or attached to the container. These labels, commonly called "package inserts," contain information that includes the drug's chemistry, intended uses, pharmacology, side effects, drug interactions, normal dose, warnings, precautions, contraindications, and how it is supplied. In some cases, a package insert can contain many pages of information.

labia – Plural of labium.

labial – Pertaining to a labium.

labile – Unstable. Given to changes in intensity. For example, labile hypertension refers to blood pressure with frequently changing readings.

labium – A lip or lip-like formation. The term can apply to the lips of the mouth (more properly called the labia oris), the outer folds of skin on the outside of the vagina (labia majoris), or the smaller, inner skin folds at the opening to the vagina (labia minora).

labor – The uterine contractions that lead to the birth of a baby and expulsion of placenta. Labor may be stimulated by use of hormones and prostaglandins or may be slowed or stopped by use of beta-agonists or intravenous alcohol.

laboratory – A facility equipped to perform scientific experiments. The work of a clinical laboratory may include chemical analysis of the contents of blood and other body fluids and tissues, blood cell counts, and identification of tumors and microorganisms.

L

labyrinth – A structure in the inner ear.

labyrinthitis – An inflammation of the labyrinth of the inner ear. Labyrinthitis often leads to vertigo.

laceration – A jagged cut or wound in the skin.

lacrimal – Pertaining to tears.

lacrimal gland – A fluid-secreting organ located in the corner of each eye, near the nose. The purpose of the lacrimal gland, also called a tear gland, is to secrete a protective and lubricating fluid (tear fluid) onto the surface of the eye. Insufficient tear production leads to irritation of the eye. In extreme cases, it can lead to dehydration and subsequent ulceration of the eye surface.

lacrimation – The secretion of excessive amounts of tear fluid.

lact- – Prefix designating milk.

lactase – An intestinal enzyme necessary for digestion of lactose. Lactase converts each molecule of lactose into one molecule each of the simple sugars galactose and glucose, which are easily absorbed.

lactase deficiency – A condition where an individual produces insufficient amounts of the enzyme lactase for proper digestion of dairy products. Depending upon the severity of the deficiency, persons with this condition may experience mild intestinal discomfort following ingestion of milk products or may have severe diarrhea, gas formation, or abdominal bloating. Lactase deficiency becomes more common with aging and is also more common in people of Asian or African descent.

Also known as lactose intolerance.

lactation – The process of formation and secretion of milk. Lactation is necessary for successful breastfeeding.

lacti- – Prefix designating milk.

lacto- – Prefix designating milk.

lactose – A sugar commonly found in milk. Lactose is a disaccharide, meaning it is composed of two simple sugars. The sugars in lactose are galactose and glucose.

L

lactose intolerance – See *lactase deficiency*.

laminar flow hood – A cabinet-sized device that pushes room air through a high efficiency particulate air (HEPA) filter. The pores in the HEPA filter are so fine that they filter out bacteria, producing sterilized air. Pharmacists use laminar flow hoods to provide a bacteria-free environment for compounding intravenous solutions and other sterile prescription products.

lance – To pierce or cut into a structure or lesion.

lancet – An instrument used to cut into a structure or lesion. For example, a specially designed lancet is typically used to draw a drop of blood for simple blood tests.

laparo- – Prefix designating the abdomen.

laparoscope – An instrument designed to be inserted through a small incision through the abdominal wall. Laparoscopes may be used to view the inside of the abdomen for diagnostic purposes or may be used to surgically treat abdominal conditions. For example, laparoscopic removal of the gallbladder or appendix has become the preferred method for removal of those organs, usually making laparotomy unnecessary.

laparotomy – Surgical incision into the abdomen. Laparotomy usually involves a long incision down the center of the abdomen and requires a lengthy convalescent period.

lapse – The termination of an insurance contract due to the failure of the insured party to satisfy his/her obligations. The most common cause of such termination is failure to pay the premiums.

large calorie – See *kilocalorie*.

laryng- – Prefix designating the larynx.

laryngeal – Pertaining to the larynx.

laryngitis – Inflammation of the mucous membranes in and around the larynx. The primary symptom is hoarseness or total loss of voice. Laryngitis is most often due to either voice strain or a viral infection. Antibiotics are typically of no value in treating laryngitis. Treatment usually centers on resting the voice, humidifying the air, and using demulcent throat lozenges.

laryngo- – Prefix designating the larynx.

laryngology – The medical specialty that deals with diagnosis and treatment of diseases of the throat. Laryngology is normally part of the practice of otolaryngology, the medical specialty that deals with conditions of the ears, nose, and throat.

larynx – The portion of the throat responsible for voice. The larynx forms the protrusion in the throat commonly called the Adam's apple.

laser – An instrument that concentrates lights into a narrow, high energy beam. Laser is an acronym for "light amplification by stimulated emission of radiation." In some cases, light beams from a laser can be used for surgical procedures, including surgery on the eyes and gums.

latent period – The amount of time between exposure to a toxin, especially radiation, and the appearance of symptoms. Depending upon the nature of the toxin and the extent of exposure, the latent period may range from minutes to weeks.

LAV – Abbreviation for lymphadenopathy-associated virus. Now, more commonly referred to as human immunodeficiency virus (HIV).

lavage – The process of washing out an organ by first instilling, then removing, large amounts of fluid. The organs most commonly lavaged include the urinary bladder (sometimes called bladder irrigation), the bowels (enema), and the stomach. The most common reason for stomach lavage is the removal of poisons. Stomach lavage is more commonly called stomach pumping.

law – In science, a sequence of events that has been observed to occur with unvarying uniformity when conditions remain the same. Examples include the law of gravity and Newton's laws.

At times the term is misused to imply that a theory has better scientific acceptance than it actually has. The so-called law of similars is one such example.

law of similars – The basic principle supporting the practice of homeopathy. The law of similars holds that "likes cure likes" or "let likes be cured by likes." In other words, a chemical agent that produces side effects or symptoms of toxicity in healthy individ-

L

uals can, in minuscule doses, relieve those same symptoms when they are caused by a disease. *Also see homeopathy.*

laxative – A chemical agent that promotes bowel movements. Various types of laxatives work by softening the feces, drawing water into the feces, stimulating the bowel to expel feces, lubricating the intestinal tract, or providing extra bulk to facilitate passage of feces.

LDL – *See low-density lipoprotein.*

legend drug – A medication available only by prescription. A pharmaceutical whose distribution is limited to a prescription written by a legally authorized person. Depending upon state law, legal prescribers may include physicians, dentists, nurse practitioners, podiatrists, and others. Legend drugs are so named because they formerly had the following "legend" on their labels: "Caution: Federal law prohibits dispensing without a prescription." Legend drugs may or may not be controlled substances. Pharmacists who dispense legend drugs without a valid prescription risk losing their licenses.

Legionella pneumophilia – The genus and species name of the organism that causes legionella, more commonly known as Legionnaire's disease. *Legionella pneumophilia* thrives in water and causes pneumonia when air containing the organism is breathed. One common source of this infection is contaminated water in air conditioning cooling towers.

Legionnaire's disease – A form of pneumonia that causes death in about 20% of untreated cases. Symptoms include high fever, chills, cough, muscle ache, headache, chest pain, and diarrhea. The condition usually responds to treatment with antibiotics.

lentigines – Plural form of lentigo.

lentigo – Large brown patch on the skin, similar to a freckle but much larger. Lentigines are more common in aging, where they are sometimes called liver spots. Solar lentigines are associated with long-term sun exposure.

-lepsy – Suffix indicating seizure; for example, epilepsy.

L

lesion – A visible wound, injury, or disease-related change in a tissue or organ.

lethal – Pertaining to death. A lethal drug interaction, for example, is a combination of drugs that can kill the recipient. A lethal dose is an amount of drug that can cause death when ingested.

lethargic – Pertaining to lethargy.

lethargy – A state of drowsiness, sluggishness, or indifference.

Also, stupor or coma caused by a disease or drug overdose.

leuk- – Prefix designating white.

leukemia – A cancer of the tissues that form blood cells, causing a large increase in the number of leukocytes (white blood cells). Leukemia is characterized as either acute or chronic and also by the type of white blood cell primarily affected.

Acute leukemia is an aggressively growing form of the disease that, without treatment, can be fatal within a few weeks or months after diagnosis. Common signs and symptoms of acute leukemia include fatigue, infections, and unusual bleeding or bruising. Chronic leukemia is a slowly advancing type of leukemia that presents few signs or symptoms other than high white blood cell counts. Late in the course of the disease, chronic leukemia may undergo a conversion to an acute form, and death may quickly ensue. Persons with a chronic form of leukemia may live with the disease for years before it converts to an acute stage.

In addition to acute or chronic, leukemia is also named for the white blood cells or precursor cells that are primarily affected. For example, acute lymphoblastic leukemia, abbreviated ALL, is an aggressively growing form of leukemia that primarily affects lymphoblasts. Lymphoblasts are lymphocyte precursors. ALL is the most common form of leukemia in children and has the highest cure rate of all of the leukemias. Other types of leukemia include promyelocytic, granulocytic, and myeloblastic leukemia.

leukemic – Pertaining to leukemia.

Also, a person who has leukemia.

leuko- – Prefix designating white.

L

leukocyte – A white blood cell. Five types of white blood cells circulate in human blood: neutrophils, basophils, eosinophils, lymphocytes, and monocytes.

Neutrophils, basophils, and eosinophils are called granulocytes because they all contain granules in their cytoplasm. The agranulocytes (no granules in the cytoplasm) are the lymphocytes and monocytes.

leukocytosis – An abnormally large number of white blood cells in the blood. The most common cause of leukocytosis is the body's response to a bacterial infection.

leukopenia – An abnormally low number of white blood cells in the blood. Causes of leukopenia may include overwhelming infection, drug toxicity, radiation poisoning, or acute leukemia. Leukopenia increases the risk of contracting an infection and makes fighting an infection more difficult.

levorotatory – *See dextrorotatory.*

Li – Chemical symbol for the element lithium.

libido – The desire for sex. The sex drive.

lice – Plural of louse.

licensed health care professional – An individual who must pass a state-administered examination prior to practicing his/her health-related profession. Licensed health care professionals include pharmacists, nurses, physicians, dentists, dieticians, chiropracters, and psychologists.

licensed practical nurse (LPN) – An individual trained in basic patient care who works under the supervision of a registered nurse or a physician. The LPN training program is typically one year, compared to a minimum of two years for a registered nurse. In some areas, these individuals are called licensed vocational nurses (LVN).

licensed vocational nurse (LVN) – *See licensed practical nurse.*

lichen – A flat, scaly skin lesion that is similar in appearance to moss-like plants that grow on rocks.

L

lichenification – The appearance of lichens on the skin. Lichenification is most commonly due to long-term irritation or inflammation of the skin or by repeated scratching.

life – The essential property of organisms that allows them to consume food, derive energy from food, adapt to their surroundings, and reproduce.

lifetime maximum – The upper limit of health-related expense an insurance company will pay over the lifetime of an insured member. When this applies, the lifetime maximum is typically in the area of $1 million. Lifetime maximums usually do not apply to pharmacy benefits; however, they often do apply to patients who receive drugs by means of home infusion therapy.

ligament – A fibrous band that connects two or more bones or cartilages to each other. Ligaments are slightly elastic. Ligaments are often confused with tendons, bands of connective tissue that allow a muscle to connect to a bone.

limb – An extremity that branches off the trunk of the body. An arm or a leg.

limbic system – The group of structures in the brain that are responsible for emotions. Anxiety, depression, fear, pleasure, and sexual arousal are thought to be functions of the limbic system.

limitations – Conditions or situations under which an insurer is not obligated to pay claims. Limitations must be written into the insurance policy at the time it is sold. Limitations to or exclusion of specific pharmacy benefits often involve injectable drugs, appetite suppressants, anabolic steroids, and birth control.

lingual – Pertaining to the tongue. For example, sublingual is the area under the tongue. Some medications, particularly nitroglycerin tablets, are dissolved here for better absorption into the bloodstream.

liniment – A liquid medication intended for external application. Most liniments are counterirritants intended to treat muscle or joint pain.

lipemia – The presence of larger than normal amounts of fat in the blood.

L

lipid – An organic chemical that consists of fat or has properties similar to those of fat, such as greasiness to the touch. Lipids are not soluble in water but may dissolve in other lipids, oils, ether, chloroform, or alcohol. Lipids include fatty acids, fats, oils, and waxes.

lipid membrane – A covering or wall over a cell or a tissue that is composed to a large extent of fatty materials. Lipid membranes prevent the passage of water-soluble drugs and toxins.

lipid soluble – A substance that can be taken into solution in a lipid, oil, ether, chloroform, or alcohol.

lipidemia – The presence of larger than normal amounts of fat in the blood.

lipodystrophy – A condition characterized by improper fat metabolism.

lipoid – Pertaining to a lipid.

lipoma – A benign tumor that consists of fat and adipose tissue.

lipophilic – Able to dissolve fats or to be dissolved by fats. Lipophilic compounds possess strongly nonpolar atomic groups.

lipoprotein – A class of blood chemicals whose molecules are comprised of a lipid portion and a protein portion.

Also see high-density lipoprotein, low-density lipoprotein.

liquifaction – The process of changing from a solid to a liquid. Liquifaction may occur due to melting or decay of organic tissue.

liter (L, l) – The volume of one kilogram (approximately 2.2 pounds) of water at 25° Celsius. A liter consists of 1000 milliliters or 1.057 quarts.

lith- – Prefix designating stone.

lithiasis – Formation of a stone, particularly a kidney or gall stone.

litho- – Prefix designating stone.

litholysis – The breakup or dissolution of kidney stones.

L

lithotripsy – A procedure where kidney or gall stones are destroyed, most commonly by using ultrasound.

livedo – A bluish, patchy discoloration of skin.

liver – The largest gland in the body and an organ that performs over 500 functions within the body. Among these functions, the liver produces bile to assist in digestion, metabolizes drugs, removes damaged blood cells from circulation, stores and secretes glucose, stores vitamins, minerals, fats, and amino acids, synthesizes proteins, and clears the blood of toxic metabolic by-products.

liver spot – *See lentigo.*

loading dose – An initial quantity of medicine administered with the intent of bringing the blood level of the drug up to a therapeutic level in the shortest amount of time possible. Drugs typically need to be administered repeatedly in order for their blood levels to accumulate to the extent needed for a full therapeutic effect. A loading dose consists of a large, single dose of medication that accomplishes the same effect but in a much shorter amount of time. Loading doses are most commonly used in emergency situations.

local – Limited to a specific area.

local anesthetic – A drug applied to a specific area of the body with the intent of temporarily eliminating all sensations from the application area. Local anesthetics are frequently injected prior to dental procedures or medical procedures where it is not otherwise necessary for the patient to be rendered unconscious. Depending upon the administration technique used, local anesthetics may be used to suture a laceration, extract a tooth, perform major surgery, or deliver a baby.

lock-in – An insurance contract provision that requires members to receive all of their health care from providers who are contracted with or employed by the health plan. Services received from health care practitioners outside of this network may not be reimbursed by the insurance plan.

L

loop diuretics – Medications that inhibit sodium reabsorption from urine in the loop of Henle. The loop diuretics are the most potent diuretics available. They are used to remove excess water from the body and are useful in treating heart failure, hypertension, and kidney diseases.

loop of Henle – A structure in the kidneys that is involved in urine production.

lotion – A pharmaceutical preparation intended for external application that typically contains water and an oil. Lotions may or may not contain medications. The most common use for a lotion is to treat or prevent dry skin.

lot number – A number printed by the drug manufacturer on each bottle of medicine that identifies the batch that this particular medication came from. Lot numbers are important in case of a recall of a defective product. As part of the recall, manufacturers notify pharmacies of all affected lots and advise pharmacists of the proper actions to take.

Lou Gehrig's disease – *See amylotrophic lateral sclerosis.*

louse – A small parasitic insect that typically infests hairy areas of the body. Lice survive by biting their hosts and sucking their blood. Bites often cause extreme itching. Lice are usually treated with a pediculocide, a specially formulated insecticide that is safe to use on the skin.

low-density lipoprotein (LDL) – A chemical in blood whose molecules consist of a fat component and a protein. LDL contains high concentrations of triglycerides and cholesterol. It is commonly implicated as a cause of or risk factor for lipid deposits on the inside of arteries.

lower esophageal sphincter – A muscle at the junction of the esophagus and stomach that relaxes to allow food and fluids to pass into the stomach but then contracts to prevent them from regurgitating back into the esophagus. Gastroesophageal reflux occurs when this sphincter is not properly functioning. *Also see gastroesophageal reflux, gastroesophageal reflux disease.*

L

lower respiratory tract – The portion of the respiratory system that includes the lungs and the structures within the lungs. Also see *upper respiratory tract.*

lower respiratory tract infection – Invasion of viruses or bacteria into one or more of the structures of the lungs. Bronchitis and pneumonia are examples of lower respiratory tract infections.

LPN – *See licensed practical nurse.*

lucid – Pertaining to clear, rational mental faculties.

lumbago – A nonspecific term that describes pain in the middle or lower back. Lumbago may have many causes, including muscle strain or spasm, osteoarthritis, or a herniated disk.

lumbar – The area of the back or sides of the body between the ribs and the pelvis.

lumen – The channel formed by a hollow, tube-like anatomic structure or piece of equipment. These structures include blood vessels, intestines, and hypodermic needles.

lung – One of a pair of organs in the chest that are responsible for providing oxygen to the blood and for expelling carbon dioxide waste. As air enters the lungs it travels through the ever-narrowing passages and branches of the bronchi and bronchioles, eventually ending in the alveoli. In the alveoli, hemoglobin in the oxygen-poor blood returning from the general circulation picks up fresh oxygen in exchange for carbon dioxide. The newly oxygen-enriched blood continues through the circulation while the lungs expel the carbon dioxide during expiration. The oxygen-for-carbon dioxide cycle repeats itself continually.

lupus – A commonly used term for systemic lupus erythematosis. Systemic lupus erythematosis, abbreviated SLE, is an inflammatory disease that affects the connective tissue in nearly every organ in the body. SLE may cause skin rash, weakness, fatigue, hair loss, anemia, kidney failure, inflammation of heart tissue, and nerve damage. SLE is treated with anti-inflammatory drugs but is often fatal. SLE affects four times as many women as men.

LVN – Abbreviation for licensed vocational nurse. *See licensed practical nurse.*

L

Lyme disease – An inflammatory disease caused by a virus transmitted by ticks. Symptoms include fever, chills, headache, skin rash, and arthritis. Without treatment, Lyme disease can persist for years. Lyme disease is treated with anti-inflammatory drugs and antibiotics.

lymph – A clear fluid of slightly yellowish color that is produced by many organs of the body and circulated through special vessels that connect to lymph nodes. Lymph eventually drains into the bloodstream. Lymph typically contains a few blood cells but otherwise is similar in content to the plasma portion of blood.

lymph- – Prefix designating lymph.

lymph node – One of many bean-sized structures organized into clusters and located primarily in the axilla (armpits), neck, mouth, lower arm, and groin. The main function of the lymph nodes is to filter bacteria and other cells out of the lymph. Lymph nodes may swell during infections and some types of cancer, particularly breast cancer. Swollen lymph nodes are often the first indication of a lymphoma such as Hodgkin's disease.

lymphadenopathy – Any disease that affects one or more lymph nodes.

lymphatic – Pertaining to lymph fluid, a lymph vessel, or a lymph node.

lymphatic vessels – A network of channels similar to blood vessels that transport lymph throughout the body.

lympho- – Prefix designating lymph.

lymphoblast – An immature lymphocyte.

lymphocyte – A type of white blood cell that normally comprises 25% to 33% of the white blood cell count. Lymphocytes perform a vital role in the immune system, secreting chemicals that destroy foreign proteins.

lymphocytic – Pertaining to lymphocytes.

lymphocytopenia – A deficiency of lymphocytes.

lymphocytosis – An unusually large concentration of lymphocytes in blood. Lymphocytosis is often seen during allergic reactions or infections.

lymphoid – Pertaining to the tissue in the lymphatic system.

lymphoma – A malignant cancer of the lymphatic system. Lymphoma normally appears first as a single, painless, enlarged lymph node, usually in the neck. Later signs and symptoms include fever, weight loss, weakness, and anemia. The disease may spread to the liver, spleen, gastrointestinal tract, and bones.

Lymphomas are usually categorized as Hodgkin's or nonHodgkin's lymphomas. With early treatment, Hodgkin's lymphoma is usually cured. The prognosis for nonHodgkin's lymphoma is generally not as optimistic.

lymphomatous – Pertaining to a lymphoma.

lymphopathy – Any disease of the lymphatic system.

lyophilization – A drug manufacturing process that involves freezing a solution of a drug followed by establishment of a partial vacuum in order to force evaporation and removal of the solvent. Lyophilized drugs have longer shelf life than their liquid forms and are easy to redissolve prior to use. Lyophilization is most commonly used in the manufacture of drugs intended for injection.

lysis – The destruction of a cell, often by the actions of drug, enzyme, or other chemical.

m – Abbreviation for meter.

MAC – *See maximum allowable cost list or maximum allowable cost program.*

MAC – *See Mycobacterium avium complex.*

maceration – Softening of tissue after prolonged exposure to a liquid. Maceration often occurs to skin under an adhesive or occlusive bandage if the bandage is left in place too long. The liquid necessary for maceration to occur is provided when the bandage traps water that would normally evaporate from the skin. The water saturates the skin and softens it.

macr- – Prefix designating large or long.

macro- – Prefix designating large or long.

macrobiotic – Pertaining to long life.

macrobiotic diet – A nutritional therapy intended to provide longevity. Extreme macrobiotic diets are sometimes employed by non-licensed health advisors in the treatment of advanced cancer. Many of these diets are deficient in essential nutrients and lack scientific validity.

macrocyte – An abnormally large red blood cell.

macrocytosis – A condition characterized by large numbers of macrocytes in the blood. Examples of conditions that cause macrocytosis include pernicious anemia due to vitamin B_{12} deficiency and megaloblastic anemia, caused by folic acid deficiency.

macrolide – A class of antibiotic whose molecules include large ring structures. Erythromycin is the best known example of a macrolide antibiotic.

macronutrient – One of the food substances required in the largest amounts. Carbohydrates, proteins, and fats are macronutrients.

macrophage – A large phagocytic cell produced in the bone marrow and initially released from the marrow as a monocyte. Macrophages are widely distributed through the body. Macrophages may lodge in the walls of blood vessels or in connective tissue. Macrophages also produce immunoglobulins.

M

macroscopic – Pertaining to something large enough to be seen without a microscope or other magnifying lens.

macular – Pertaining to or resembling a macule.

macule – A small spot or patch that is different in color than the surrounding skin. Macules are not raised above or depressed below the skin surface.

maculopapular – Pertaining to a skin lesion that is both raised above the skin surface (papule) and discolored (macule).

mail order pharmacy – A licensed pharmacy that uses the mail or other carrier (e.g., overnight carrier or parcel service) to deliver prescriptions to patients. In most cases, mail order pharmacies contract with health insurers and fill prescriptions at discounted rates for members of those plans.

maintenance dose – The amount of medication needed to provide a consistent amount of drug in the blood or other tissues.

maintenance drug – A prescription medication intended to treat a chronic medical condition. In many cases, maintenance drugs may also be used to treat acute medical problems. For example, the anti-inflammatory drug ibuprofen may be used for long-term treatment of arthritis. It may also be used to treat the short-term pain of a sprained joint.

maintenance therapy – Treatment intended to control a condition for the long-term benefit of the patient. In some cases, initial treatment of a disorder may require multiple drugs or aggressive doses to establish control of symptoms. Once control has been established, the drugs and doses necessary to continue to control the disease are considered to be maintenance therapy.

malabsorption – The inability to transport from the intestine to the bloodstream sufficient amounts of one or more nutrients. Malabsorption is usually due to a disease of the intestinal tract.

malacia – A softening of a structure. For example, osteomalacia is a softening of bone due to lack of calcium and vitamin D.

malaise – A general feeling of discomfort or illness. Malaise is often a symptom of infection, particularly the common cold or influenza.

malformation – An abnormality in the structure of an organ or organism. Malformations that occur in a fetus and are apparent at or after birth are often called birth defects.

malfunction – Improper working of an organ or piece of equipment.

malignant – In reference to cancer, the ability of the tumor to spread and invade other areas.

Also, progressive and resistant to treatment. For example, malignant hypertension is a condition characterized by a rapidly increasing blood pressure that resists control by medication or other treatments.

malignant melanoma – *See melanoma.*

malnutrition – A physical state where the inability or unwillingness to eat properly or the inaccessibility of vital nutrients leads to deterioration of body tissues. Malnutrition may also refer to medical conditions that are caused by overeating, and thus nutritional imbalances.

malpractice – Negligence or misconduct on the part of a health care professional that causes or leads to harm to a patient.

malpractice insurance – Insurance policy held by a health care professional to protect the policyholder against financial loss from judgements or settlements for proven or alleged malpractice. Malpractice insurance usually also covers the costs of legal representation.

mammary – Pertaining to the breasts.

mammo- – Prefix designating the breasts.

mammogram – The picture produced by mammography.

mammography – A procedure by which x-rays are passed through the breast and recorded on a photographic film (mammogram). Mammography is used for the detection and diagnosis of breast disease, particularly fibrocystic breast disease and breast cancer. Mammography is capable of locating cysts and tumors before they can be found any other way.

managed care – *See managed health care.*

M

managed care organization (MCO) – A health plan that uses princi-ples of managed health care to provide health services while also controlling costs. MCOs use a variety of incentives to providers as well as administrative controls to achieve these goals. While managed care organizations initially started in the 1970s they did not become a dominant factor in health care until the 1990s when they demonstrated that they could control the alarming escalation of health care costs. Since then, their meth-ods of controlling costs have initiated considerable controversy and political debate.

Health maintenance organizations (HMOs) and preferred provider organizations (PPOs) are examples of managed care organizations.

managed health care – A system of health care delivery that inter-venes to regulate the utilization and cost of services and meas-ures performance. The goal of managed health care is to provide access to high-quality, cost-effective health care.

Also, a system of insurance that pays for these services.

mania – A mental illness whose symptoms include loss of contact with reality, excessive physical and mental energy, rapid speech, abnormal stream of thoughts, poor concentration, and grandios-ity.

manic-depressive – Pertaining to bipolar affective disorder.

Also, a person who has bipolar affective disorder.

manic-depressive illness – *See bipolar affective disorder.*

manifestation – A sign or symptom of a disorder or an alteration of normal function.

marasmus – A condition of extreme malnutrition caused by long-term dietary deficiency of protein and calories. Marasmus occurs most commonly in children and is characterized by wasting of muscle and subcutaneous tissue.

margin – The border or edge of a structure or lesion.

marginal – Pertaining to a margin.

marrow – The soft tissue that fills the inside of bones. Bone marrow is the site of production of red blood cells, platelets, and most white blood cells.

masculinization – The process of forming the physical features of an adult male. Masculinization occurs during puberty of males as the result of testosterone production. It can also occur in females who are treated with testosterone-like drugs or who produce abnormally large amounts of testosterone themselves. Signs of masculinization include growth of body hair under the arms and on the face, skeletal muscle development, and deepening of the voice.

mask – A sign of a dermatological condition whereby the face is discolored.

masking – Hiding or concealment. For example, a drug that reduces fever can hide or conceal (mask) an early sign of infection.

mass – A lump or aggregation of cells or other material. Detection of a mass can be a sign of cancer.

Also, a putty-like mixture of active drug with excipients that can be rolled into a cylinder, measured, cut, and rolled into pills.

mast- – Prefix designating the breast.

mast cell – A large cell found in connective tissue that contains a wide variety of biochemicals, including histamine. Mast cells are involved in inflammation secondary to injuries and infections and are sometimes implicated in allergic reactions.

mastectomy – The surgical removal of a breast. A simple mastectomy involves removal of only breast tissue. With a radical mastectomy, the breast, some of the pectoral muscle in the chest, and the lymph nodes under the arm are all removed. Rehabilitation from a radical mastectomy is much more difficult than that following a simple mastectomy.

mastication – The act of chewing.

mastitis – Inflammation of a breast, usually due to infection. Mastitis may occur during breastfeeding or as the result of a chronic infection such as tuberculosis.

M

masto- – Prefix designating the breast.

mastopathy – A general term designating any disease of the breast.

matching – The deliberate process of dividing participants in a study into two or more groups so that a comparison can be made between like populations. For example, a study may be age-matched so that range of ages within each group is similar to that of every other group.

materia medica – Now obsolete, a term used in the first half of the twentieth century and earlier. Materia medica includes the study of the origins of drugs, extraction of drugs from natural sources (pharmacognosy), drug actions (pharmacology), as well as the physical aspects of prescription preparation.

maximum allowable cost (MAC) list – A listing of the highest price a third party payer is willing to reimburse a pharmacy for a prescription filled with a generic drug. MAC lists are usually lengthy, including prices for hundreds of drugs, dosage forms, and strengths. MAC lists are adopted by managed care organizations and Medicare and distributed to participating pharmacies.

maximum allowable cost (MAC) program – A system for reimbursing pharmacies for dispensing prescriptions filled with generic drugs. Since the costs for any specific generically-available drug can vary widely from one manufacturer to another, payer groups such as insurance companies and Medicaid often determine the price they are willing to pay. This price is usually based on the cost of one of the least expensive, identical products available or on the average cost of two or three such products. For example, a payer will "MAC" the price of a 20 mg tablet of the diuretic furosemide based on the price charged by one of the least expensive manufacturers.

maximum benefit – The upper limit an insurer will pay for claims over a specific period of time. For example, an insurance policy may stipulate a maximum benefit of $500 per quarter for prescription drugs.

M.B. – Abbreviation for bachelor of medicine, a medical degree commonly conferred in the United Kingdom. Equivalent to a doctor of medicine (M.D.) degree in the United States.

mcg – Abbreviation for microgram.

MCO – *See managed care organization.*

M.D. – Abbreviation for doctor of medicine. The medical degree commonly conferred in the United States.

MDI – *See metered-dose inhaler.*

measles – A viral infection that causes high fever, inflammation of respiratory mucous membranes, cough, and a widely dispersed red rash. Measles, also called rubeola, can be prevented by immunization during childhood. *See also rubella.*

mechanism of action – The specific means by which a drug achieves its effect. For example, penicillin's mechanism of action is to substitute itself for an amino acid certain bacteria incorporate into their cell walls. Substituting penicillin in place of the amino acid creates a weak point in the wall, and the cell wall ruptures when the bacterium grows.

media – Plural of medium.

Medicaid – A program funded by the federal government and the states that pays for health services delivered to enrolled indigent persons. Medicaid covers medical and pharmacy expenses.

medical director – A physician employed by a hospital, insurance company, or other corporation to advise management concerning medical issues. In some cases, particularly in hospitals and clinics, a medical director may supervise the clinical care given by other physicians. In an insurance company, the medical director usually has the final determination on payment or denial of payment for unusual claims and for approving policies relating to medical care.

medical insurance – A contract agreeing to pay the costs of specified medical and related expenses. Medical insurance may be purchased by individuals or by employers as part of the employee benefit package.

medical necessity – The need to provide a medical service or treatment for the health of a patient in accordance with local or national standards of practice. In questionable cases, an insurer

M

may deny payment for services rendered or deny authorization prior to the delivery of service. Physicians may be required to submit a statement of medical necessity to the insurance company. Unusual cases are normally reviewed for medical necessity by a staff member, often a nurse. Cases may be further reviewed by an insurance company physician prior to a final determination. Examples of cases that may be denied for lack of medical necessity include cosmetic surgery and treatment of fungal infections of toenails.

medical record – The clinical record relating to a patient's care. A medical record may be written on paper or stored in an electronic medium. Typically, a medical record contains demographic information, insurance information, laboratory test values, and health care workers' notations regarding the patient's specific problems, diagnosis, treatments given, and changes in status.

medicament – A medication.

Medicare – A federally funded health insurance program managed by the Health Care Financing Administration (HCFA) that provides coverage for individuals over 65 years of age and others in selected categories. Medicare's parts A and B cover hospitalization, outpatient care, and a few other specific services. With the exception of medications administered in a hospital and some intravenous medications given by a home health care provider, Medicare does not currently cover prescription or nonprescription medicines.

Medicare supplement – Insurance through a private carrier that covers some of the medical expenses that Medicare does not. Some Medicare supplement policies also cover prescription medications, although the coverage is often limited. Also called Medigap.

medicate – The act of taking a medicine or giving a dose to someone else.

Also, the treatment of a disorder with a medicine.

medication – A legal drug. The term usually connotes that the drug has a proven benefit.

medicinal – Relating to something that has the properties of a medicine.

medicine – A drug. Normally used in the context of a legal drug that has proven therapeutic value.

Also the body of science that deals with health and the diagnosis and treatment of disease.

medico- – Prefix designating medical.

medicolegal – Pertaining to issues that involve the legal aspects of the practice of medicine. This includes laws and regulations that relate to medicine as well as medical malpractice.

Medigap – *See Medicare supplement.*

medium – A substance that facilitates the action of something else. For example, a culture medium is a nutritive solution or gel that supports the growth of microorganisms in a laboratory for the purpose of identification of the cause of an infection. A contrast medium is a special dye or other substance injected or infused into tissue prior to x-ray examination. Contrast media block or alter x-rays so that abnormalities in the area of interest appear on the x-ray film.

mega- – Prefix designating large.

megakaryocyte – A large cell normally found in the bone marrow and rarely in circulating blood that serves as a precursor cell for platelets.

megal- – Prefix designating large.

megalo- – Prefix designating large.

megaloblastic anemia – A low red blood cell count associated with abnormally large red blood cells. The most common causes of megaloblastic anemia are pernicious anemia due to vitamin B_{12} deficiency, and megaloblastic anemia caused by folic acid deficiency.

-megaly – Suffix designating large. For example, splenomegaly is an enlargement of the spleen.

M

melan- – Prefix designating a black or dark color.

melano- – Prefix designating a black or dark color.

melanoma – A skin cancer derived from cells that are capable of forming the pigment melanin. Melanomas may form on any part of the body and are most commonly associated with exposure to sun or ultraviolet radiation from tanning booths. Often patients discover a mole with irregular borders that spread outward from its original location. Sometimes referred to as malignant melanoma, this condition is an extremely dangerous form of cancer that requires immediate, aggressive treatment. Once advanced, melanoma is nearly always fatal and can invade the lymph nodes, liver, lungs, and brain.

melena – Passage of dark, tar-like stool. Melena is caused by the interaction of digestive acids and enzymes on blood. The source of the blood is usually a bleeding ulcer or some other form of gastrointestinal bleeding. Melena is a sign of a serious condition that needs immediate medical attention.

melenemesis – Vomiting of dark-colored material. Often an indication of bleeding in the upper gastrointestinal tract.

member – A person covered by a health insurance plan and who is entitled to services under that plan.

Also known as an enrollee, eligible, eligible dependent, or covered life.

membrane – A material that covers the surface of a cell, organ, or tissue, divides a space, or lines a cavity. For example, a mucous membrane covers and protects the inside of the mouth, nose, throat, and other structures.

membranous – Resembling a membrane.

memory – The mental process that receives information, processes that information, and then stores it for later retrieval. Short-term memory relates to the ability to recall events that happened recently. Long-term memory is considered the permanent storage of information.

menarche – The first occurrence of a menstrual period. Menarche normally occurs between the ages of 9 and 17.

Meniere's disease – A chronic condition of the inner ear characterized by dizziness, nausea, vomiting, ringing in the ears, and progressive hearing loss. Meniere's disease is usually treated with bed rest and antihistamines. Surgery may be needed in some cases.

meninges – Plural form of meninx.

meningitis – An inflammation of one or more of the membranes (meninges) that cover the brain and spinal cord. Meningitis may be caused by viral or bacterial infection. Signs and symptoms of meningitis include severe headache, stiffness of the neck, vomiting, and high fever. Most cases of meningitis are viral, self-limited, and pass with minimal treatment. Some forms of bacterial meningitis, however, are extremely dangerous and require aggressive treatment of the patient and also preventive treatment of those recently exposed to the patient.

meningococcus – *Neisseria meningitidis*, the bacterium that causes the most dangerous type of bacterial meningitis.

meninx – One of the three membranes that cover the brain and spinal cord.

meno- – Prefix designating menses.

menopause – The permanent end of menstruation and menstrual cycles. Menstrual cycles typically end between the ages of 45 and 60 when the ovaries stop producing the hormone estrogen.

menorrhagia – Abnormally heavy or prolonged menstruation. Repeated episodes of menorrhagia may be due to hormonal problems, uterine disease, or cancer. Menorrhagia may lead to iron deficiency anemia.

menses – The periodic loss of blood from the female reproductive tract that signals the beginning of the menstrual cycle.

menstrual – Pertaining to menses or menstruation.

menstrual cycle – The repeating chain of events within the female reproductive system that leads to menses. The human menstru-

M

al cycle averages 28 days in length and is comprised of four phases: proliferative, secretory, premenstrual, and menstrual.

Proliferative phase: The uterine lining reestablishes itself and normalizes. The endometrium becomes thicker and establishes its blood supply. This phase lasts until one of the ovaries releases an egg, about 14 days before the beginning of menses.

Secretory phase: The endometrium increases in thickness and glands secrete glycogen. The corpus luteum in the ovaries secretes progesterone. The endometrium becomes engorged with blood in preparation for implantation of a fertilized egg. The secretory phase lasts 10 to 14 days.

Premenstrual phase: If fertilization and implantation have not taken place, the arteries supplying the endometrium constrict, reducing blood flow to the area. The premenstrual phase lasts about two days.

Menstrual phase: Dead tissue breaks away in patches from the wall of the uterus accompanied by bleeding. The menstrual phase usually lasts four to five days.

Because it is easy to observe, the first day of menses is considered to be the first day of the menstrual cycle.

menstruation – The shedding of the cells lining the interior of the uterus and the bleeding associated with it.

menstruum – Menstrual fluid.

mental – Pertaining to thought processes.

Also, pertaining to the chin.

mental health – The emotional and behavioral state of mind that allows a person to adjust to the stresses of life in a normal and socially acceptable fashion.

mental illness – A general term used to describe irrational emotional reactions to life situations. Symptoms of mental illness may include hallucinations, delusions, nervousness, and depression. Mental illness may be caused by toxicity induced by drugs or environmental chemicals, genetic predisposition, or social fac-

M

tors. Types of mental illnesses include anxiety, depression, schizophrenia, bipolar affective disorder, substance abuse, and many others. All generally recognized mental illnesses are listed in and described in the *Diagnostic and Statistical Manual of Mental Disorders* (DSM) published by the American Psychiatric Association.

mentation – The process of thinking.

mEq – Abbreviation for milliequivalent.

mercurial – Pertaining to mercury.

mercurial diuretic – A class of medications that increase urine production. Mercurial diuretics are now obsolete with the development of less toxic diuretics that are also more effective and easier to administer.

metabolic – Pertaining to metabolism.

metabolic rate – The speed with which a metabolic reaction occurs.

metabolism – The chemical changes that take place inside living cells. As a result of metabolism, an organism may grow, maintain body functions, release or store energy, produce and eliminate waste, digest nutrients, or destroy toxins.

Living organisms can also metabolize drugs. The purpose of these reactions is typically to alter the chemical nature of a drug so that it is easier for the organism to eliminate the drug from the system. Although there are many exceptions, drug metabolism usually terminates the pharmacological activity of the drug.

metabolite – The chemical product that results from metabolism. When a drug is metabolized, its metabolite(s) may be either active or inactive. An active metabolite is a product of drug metabolism that still possesses pharmacological activity. An inactive metabolite is one that has lost its pharmacological activity as the result of the metabolic reaction.

metal – A chemical element capable of carrying a positive charge. A heavy metal is a polyvalent, positively charged element. Heavy metals such as lead, iron, mercury, and cadmium can be extremely toxic if ingested in excessive amounts.

M

metastasis – The spread of a disease from one part of the body to another. Typically used in the context of a spreading cancer. In cancer, cells from the original (primary) tumor break away from that tumor and are carried in the blood to almost all parts of the body. Cells that are deposited in tissues that provide a hospitable environment are capable of seeding that area and growing a new tumor. This way, the primary cancer can produce secondary tumors in locations far from the original site.

Cancers usually follow a typical metastatic pattern. For example, breast cancer metastasizes to the lymph nodes, bone, brain, and liver. Colon cancer typically metastasizes to the liver and lungs. Malignant melanoma spreads to the lymph nodes, liver, lungs, and brain.

Cancer growing in metastatic sites retains the characteristics of the original cancer. For example, when breast cancer spreads to the bone, brain, and liver, it does not become cancer of the bone, cancer of the brain, or cancer of the liver. Instead, it is more properly thought of as breast cancer that is growing in the bone, brain, and liver.

metastasize – The process of invading the body by means of metastasis.

metastatic – Pertaining to metastasis.

meter (m) – A unit of measure in the metric system of weights and measures, sometimes referred to as the European system. A meter is equal to 39.37 inches in the English system of weights and measures.

metered-dose inhaler (MDI) – A device that delivers a measured amount of medication via aerosol spray. MDIs are used to administer precise doses of medication to treat asthma and other respiratory diseases.

methyl – Pertaining to methane.

Also, the chemical radical represented by the formula -CH_3.

methylation – The chemical process of adding a methyl radical to a compound. Some metabolic processes involve adding one or more methyl groups (methylation) or removing them (demethylation).

M

metr- – Prefix designating the uterus.

metra- – Prefix designating the uterus.

metro- – Prefix designating the uterus.

metropathic – Pertaining to a disease of the uterus.

metropathy – A general term that refers to any disease of the uterus.

metroperitonitis – Inflammation of the outer surface of the uterus.

metrorrhagia – Uterine bleeding that occurs independent of the normal menstrual period. Metrorrhagia may be caused by hormonal imbalances, cancers such as cervical cancer, or other uterine disease.

metrostaxis – Continuous loss of small amounts of blood from the uterus. If not corrected, metrostaxis can lead to iron deficiency anemia.

mg – Abbreviation for milligram.

MI – *See myocardial infarction.*

MIC – *See minimum inhibitory concentration.*

micr- – Prefix used to designate one-millionth.

Also, a prefix designating an extremely small quantity.

micro- – Prefix used to designate one-millionth.

Also, a prefix designating an extremely small quantity.

microbe – *See microorganism.*

microbial – Pertaining to a microorganism.

microbiologist – A person who specializes in the study of microorganisms. A microbiologist may or may not be a physician.

microbiology – The study of the life processes of microscopic and submicroscopic organisms. These organisms include bacteria, fungi, viruses, spirochetes, and rickettsiae.

Microbiology is one of the basic sciences that provides the foundation for medicine.

M

microchemistry – A specialized branch of chemistry that analyzes extremely small specimens.

microcirculation – The portion of the circulatory system that is comprised of the smallest blood vessels. The microcirculation includes arterioles, capillaries, and venules.

microdose – An extremely small dose of medication.

microgram (mcg) – A measurement in the metric system that is comprised of one-millionth of a gram.

microorganism – A life form that cannot be seen without a microscope. Microorganisms include bacteria, fungi, algae, protozoa, viruses, spirochetes, and rickettsiae.

microscope – An optic instrument that uses a lens or series of lenses to visualize substances that cannot be seen with the naked eye. Microscopes are essential tools in the diagnosis of infectious diseases, blood diseases, and the pathologic examination of biopsy tissue.

microscopic – Pertaining to a size that can only be seen with the use of a microscope.

Also, pertaining to a microscope.

microsurgery – A surgical operation performed with the assistance of a specially designed microscope. Some types of vascular and eye surgery are performed in this manner.

mid- – Prefix designating middle.

migraine headache – A type of pain in the head that is normally limited to one side or one specific spot in the head and is associated with dizziness, vomiting, and intolerance to light and noise. In some cases, a migraine headache may be preceded by an aura, where visual disturbances such as seeing unusual colors or blurred vision may warn the sufferer of an impending attack. A migraine headache may last for hours or days and may be incapacitating. In susceptible persons, headaches may be brought on by loud noise, bright light, an allergic reaction, emotional stress, alcohol use, tobacco smoke, or certain foods.

milk – A nutrient-rich substance produced by the mammary glands of females for the purpose of feeding their young.

In pharmacy, a milk is a suspension of an insoluble drug in a water vehicle that gives the appearance of milk when shaken; for example, milk of magnesia.

milliequivalent – One-thousandth of an equivalent, the mass of a chemical ion that will combine with one gram of hydrogen or eight grams of oxygen. An equivalent weight may be determined by dividing the atomic weight of an element by its valence. Concentrations of electrolytes (e.g., sodium, potassium, etc.) in the body are measured in milliequivalents.

milliliter (ml, mL) – One-thousandth of a liter.

millimeter (mm) – One-thousandth of a meter.

mineralocorticoid – A type of hormone produced in the adrenal gland that causes sodium and water retention in the kidneys. Mineralocorticoids are important factors in the control of hydration in the body. Deficiency of mineralocorticoids leads to diabetes insipidus, a condition characterized by excessive loss of urine and dehydration. Aldosterone is the principal mineralocorticoid.

mineral supplement – A source of inorganic nutrients beyond that received in the diet. Elements frequently used in this way include iron, calcium, magnesium, and zinc. Mineral supplements may be provided in the form of a single-ingredient product (e.g., ferrous sulfate, calcium carbonate), in combinations with other minerals, or combined with vitamins.

minim – 1/60th of a fluiddram in the apothecary system of weights and measures. A minim is roughly equivalent in size to a drop of water.

minimum inhibitory concentration (MIC) – The lowest concentration of an antibiotic that stops the growth of a strain of bacteria in the laboratory. The MIC gives an indication of how effective a specific antibiotic is likely to be for a specific infection. In general, it is preferable to treat an infection with an antibiotic that has a low MIC.

M

miotic – Pertaining to constriction of the pupils.

Also, an agent that constricts the pupils. Miotics are often used to treat glaucoma.

miscarriage – Loss of a fetus before the 20th week of pregnancy. In most cases miscarriage results because of fetal malformation that is incompatible with life outside of the womb. Over 10% of pregnancies end with miscarriage. Also known as spontaneous abortion.

miscible – Pertaining to the ability of two fluids to be mixed together without separating upon standing. For example, water and alcohol are miscible while water and oil are not.

misdiagnosis – An error in identifying an illness. Causes of misdiagnosis may include faulty laboratory results, misinterpretation of laboratory or physical findings, failure of the patient to accurately report symptoms, or malpractice.

mite – A small, sometimes microscopic, parasite that lives on or under the surface of the skin. In most cases mites cause no clinical problem. However, some mites such as those found on dogs, cats, and in house dust may trigger allergic or asthmatic reactions in susceptible persons. Some mites (e.g., chiggers, scabies) cause intense itching.

mixture – A substance containing two or more ingredients that do not chemically combine, do not necessarily occur in fixed proportions, do not lose their individual characteristics, and can be separated from each other if necessary. For example, the various powders that are combined together in a capsule (active drug, filler, stabilizer, etc.) have all of these characteristics.

ml – Abbreviation for milliliter.

mL – Abbreviation for milliliter.

mm – Abbreviation for millimeter.

mobilization – The process of shifting stored chemicals from one area or tissue of the body to another. For example, fat may be mobilized into the blood to provide energy when blood glucose levels are low.

mold – A fungus without stems or roots that lives on the surface of decaying matter or nonorganic materials.

molecule – The smallest part of a substance that can exist in the free state and still retain its characteristics. Molecules may consist of a single atom (e.g., iron) or a combination of atoms (e.g., H_2O— water). Molecules can also be extraordinarily complex, containing thousands of atoms (e.g., DNA).

mon- – Prefix designating one or single.

mono- – Prefix designating one or single.

monoamine oxidase inhibitor – A class of antidepressants usually reserved for treatment-resistant cases of depression. The usefulness of these drugs is limited by their ability to cause serious reactions when taken along with a wide variety of other medications and foods.

monoclonal antibody – Protein derived from a single cell or homogeneous group of cells. Monoclonal antibodies can be developed to prevent rejection after transplantation surgery or to attack specific types of cancer cells.

monocyte – A large white blood cell that normally represents 3% to 7% of the circulating white blood cells. Monocytes are capable of ingesting viruses, bacteria, and other foreign material in the blood or tissues. Monocytes may transform into macrophages.

monocytopenia – An abnormally low percentage of monocytes in blood.

monocytosis – An abnormally elevated percentage of monocytes in blood.

mononucleosis – An abnormally high number of monocytes in blood. Most commonly used in the context of infectious mononucleosis, a viral infection that typically causes fever, sore throat, extreme fatigue, swollen lymph nodes, and enlargement of the spleen and liver. Infection usually provides lifelong immunity thereafter.

monoxide – Any chemical molecule that contains only one atom of oxygen. For example, carbon monoxide.

M

morbid – Pertaining to sickness or illness.

morbidity – A state of illness or disease. For example, it could be said that the bacterium *Streptococcus pyogenes* causes a high rate of morbidity (illness). Contrasted to mortality.

morbidity rate – The proportion or percentage of a population that develops illness when exposed to a noxious factor. Factors may include viruses, bacteria, or environmental toxins.

morning-after pill – A type of contraception that consists of a single, large dose of estrogen or estrogen-progestin combination given to a woman within 72 hours of intercourse. Morning-after contraception is usually reserved for emergency use after a rape, incest, or other unprotected intercourse. It is not intended for routine contraception.

mortal – Pertaining to death or causing death.

mortality – Death or the state of being subject to dying.

mortality rate – The proportion of a population that dies over a specific period of time or as a result of exposure to a noxious factor. Factors may include infections with viruses or bacteria, side effects to drugs, or exposure to various toxins.

mortar – A bowl commonly used in pharmacy, chemistry, and cooking in which substances are ground into smaller particles. In pharmacy, mortars are also used to mix one powder with another, dissolve a powder into a liquid, or make emulsions. The instrument that is used to do the grinding or mixing is a pestle.

mouth – The opening through which a person takes in food and drink. Also, the opening to an organ or cavity.

mouthwash – A liquid that is normally swished around the inside of the mouth to improve oral hygiene. Mouthwashes may contain ingredients to improve breath or kill some of the bacteria that contribute to dental disease.

M.P.H. – Abbreviation for the degree of master of public health.

M.R.C.P – Abbreviation for Member of the Royal College of Physicians of England.

M.R.C.S. – Abbreviation for Member of the Royal College of Surgeons of England.

M.R.C.V.S. – Abbreviation for Member of the Royal College of Veterinary Surgeons of England.

MS – *See multiple sclerosis.*

muco- – Prefix designating mucus.

mucolytic – A drug or other agent capable of dissolving or liquefying mucus. Dilute solutions of salt in water are both soothing to inflamed tissue and mucolytic. Because of these properties salt water nose sprays and throat gargles are sometimes used to treat nasal congestion during a cold or sore throat.

mucosa – *See mucous membrane.*

mucosal – Pertaining to mucus or a mucous membrane.

mucous – Pertaining to mucus.

mucous membrane – A moist, mucus-secreting tissue that lines cavities and channels that are exposed to air. Mucous membranes have a rich supply of blood and become pale when anemia is present. Mucous membranes cover and protect the inside of the mouth, nose, throat, genitals, and other structures.

mucus – The clear, slippery secretion of a mucous membrane. Mucus traps bacteria, pollen, and other particles and protects the mucous tissue from dehydration.

multi- – Prefix designating many.

multigravida – A woman who has been pregnant more than once.

multi-infarct dementia – A type of mental deterioration caused by a succession of strokes. Multi-infarct dementia and Alzheimer's disease are the two most common forms of dementia. Many people experience both forms concurrently. *Also see dementia.*

multipara – A woman who has given birth to more than one live infant.

multiple myeloma – A cancer of bone marrow that rapidly spreads through the marrow and invades the surrounding bone, includ-

M

ing the skull. Eventually the tumors destroy bone and lead to multiple bone fractures and pain.

multiple sclerosis – A progressive neurologic disease characterized by deterioration of the myelin sheath that normally covers the nerve fibers of the brain and spinal cord. Early signs are mild, easily mistaken for other illnesses, and include abnormal sensations in the face or limbs. As the disease progresses, signs and symptoms may include muscle incoordination, weakness, dizziness, problems with vision, paralysis, difficulty speaking, and difficulty urinating. Patients may have periods where symptoms remit, followed by relapse. In time, remissions become fewer and shorter.

multisource drug – A pharmaceutical that is available from more than one manufacturer. A generic drug.

mumps – A viral infection that typically causes fever, earache, and painful swelling of the parotid glands in the neck. Most cases of mumps can be prevented with immunization during childhood.

mural – Pertaining to the wall of any cavity. For example, a mural thrombus is a blood clot attached to the wall of the heart.

murmur – A consistent, repeating, abnormal sound usually heard only with the aid of a stethoscope. Normally used in the context of the heart, where a murmur may be indicative of a disruption of blood flow through the chambers of the heart.

muscle – A tissue composed of fibers that are able to contract, thus causing movement of another body part or tissue. Muscles are normally categorized as skeletal (or voluntary), smooth (or involuntary), or cardiac.

Skeletal muscles are attached at one or both ends to bone and are responsible for all voluntary or willful movements that involve the skeleton and other structures (e.g., the eyes). These include the movements involved in walking, chewing, standing, and sitting.

Smooth muscles control internal organs and tissues. For example, they control the contraction and dilation of blood vessels, thus controlling blood pressure. They are involuntary muscles in

M

the sense that persons cannot consciously control their contractions. Instead, they are regulated by internally produced chemicals that cause them to contract or relax according to the body's needs at the time.

Cardiac muscle is found only in the heart. The rhythmic contractions of this muscle force blood through the lungs and into the general circulation.

muscle relaxant – A drug that reduces the contraction of muscle. Some are given intravenously during surgery to reduce tissue damage during incision. Others are used orally to reduce pain and muscle spasm following trauma. Still others are used to treat muscle spasms that occur as a result of chronic neurologic conditions such as multiple sclerosis.

mustard plaster – A paste made with mustard powder and spread onto a cloth which is then applied to the skin. The mustard irritates the skin and may cause symptomatic relief of muscle strain.

In previous times, mustard plasters were commonly used for a wide variety of illnesses. It was thought that the plaster drew illness out of the body. Now, it is more common to use a counterirritant cream or liniment to treat muscle or joint pain.

mutagen – An agent that causes genetic change in an organism. Mutagens may be drugs or environmental toxins such as chemicals or radiation.

mutagenic – Capable of causing mutation.

mutation – A sudden change in the nature of a gene as opposed to a gradual genetic change that develops over the course of generations. In some cases, mutations are innocuous, but in other cases may cause devastating medical problems. Mutations may be passed to future generations of progeny.

mute – A person who is unable or unwilling to speak, or the condition of being unable or unwilling to speak.

myalgia – A general term for a pain in a muscle. Myalgias are usually dull, aching pains associated with other illnesses, particularly infections.

M

myasthenia – Weakness in one or more muscles.

myasthenia gravis – A chronic, progressive muscular disease characterized by weakness and fatigue in the skeletal muscles. Symptoms typically start in the face and throat and eventually spread to the rest of the body.

Mycobacterium – Genus name of a group of microorganisms that cause diseases such as tuberculosis, Hansen's disease (leprosy), and pneumonia in persons with poorly functioning immune systems.

Mycobacterium avium complex (MAC) – An opportunistic infection that occurs in immunosuppressed persons, particularly those with AIDS. Signs and symptoms of MAC include pneumonia, fever, and weight loss.

mycologist – A biologist who specializes in mycology. A mycologist may or may not be a physician.

mycology – The study of the characteristics of fungi and the diseases they cause.

mydriasis – Dilation of the pupil of the eye.

mydriatic – A medication that dilates the pupil of the eye. Mydriatics are commonly used during eye examinations to permit examination of the retina. A common side effect of mydriatic medications is temporarily blurred vision.

myel- – Prefix designating bone marrow, the spinal cord, or the fiber that covers nerve fibers.

myelin – A substance that covers most nerve fibers. Myelin is composed of various fats, proteins, and cholesterol.

myelitis – Inflammation of either the spinal cord or the bone marrow. For example, osteomyelitis is an inflammation, usually due to bacterial infection, of the bone marrow and surrounding bone.

myelo- – Prefix designating bone marrow, the spinal cord, or the fiber that covers nerve fibers.

myeloma – A tumor that develops in the blood cell-forming tissue of bone marrow. *Also see multiple myeloma.*

M

myelopathy – Any disease of the spinal cord or bone marrow.

myeloproliferative – Pertaining to unusual growth or generation of bone marrow tissue. Leukemia is an example of a myeloproliferative disease.

myelosuppression – Inhibition of the blood-cell forming elements in bone marrow. Myelosuppression may lead to low red blood cell, white blood cell, and/or platelet levels. Myelosuppression is commonly caused by cancer chemotherapy and radiation.

myelotoxic – Pertaining to an agent that is harmful to bone marrow. Radiation and many cancer chemotherapy drugs are myelotoxic.

myo- – Prefix designating muscle.

myocardial – Pertaining to the heart muscle.

myocardial hypertrophy – Enlargement of the heart muscle. Myocardial hypertrophy is often an indication of heart failure.

myocardial infarction (MI) – Sudden death of a segment of the heart muscle caused by an abrupt interruption of blood flow to part of the heart. A heart attack.

Myocardial infarction is most often caused by a blood clot that occludes a coronary artery. The occlusion cuts off blood flow and oxygen supply to an area of the heart. As a consequence, that section of the heart dies if thrombolytic medications are not started within a few hours. Myocardial infarctions can range from relatively small and causing few long-term effects, or they can be massive, causing immediate death.

myocarditis – Inflammation of the heart muscle. Myocarditis may be caused by infection, an immune reaction, or a toxin.

myocardium – The heart muscle.

myoclonus – Spasm or twitching of a single muscle or group of muscles.

myometrium – The muscle within the wall of the uterus.

myoneural – Pertaining to both nerves and muscles.

M

myoneural junction – The point at which a nerve fiber has contact with a muscle fiber. The nerve fiber periodically secretes chemicals that cause the muscle to contract.

myopathy – Any disease or abnormality of a muscle.

myopia – Nearsighted vision. The inability to clearly see objects at a distance. Myopia is caused by the inability of the eye to properly focus light on the retina.

myositis – Inflammation of a muscle. Myositis may be caused by parasitic infestations, infection, or injury.

myring- – Prefix pertaining to the tympanic membrane, the eardrum.

myringitis – Inflammation of the tympanic membrane, the eardrum.

myringo- – Prefix pertaining to the tympanic membrane, the eardrum.

myxedema – A potentially fatal condition caused by severe hypothyroidism. Myxedema is characterized by swelling of the hands, face, feet, and the area around the eyes. It may also cause body cavities to fill with fluid, muscle weakness, hair loss, and slowed thought processes. It most often occurs after thyroid surgery or loss of function of the thyroid gland. Myxedema can be prevented and treated with thyroid hormone supplements.

N – Chemical symbol for nitrogen.

Na – Chemical symbol for sodium.

nadir – The lowest point. Often used in the context of cancer chemotherapy, where the nadir is the lowest level the normal blood cells reach following a course of chemotherapy. During the nadir, a patient is at greatest risk of hemorrhage or infection. Opposite of zenith.

nano- – Prefix designating one-billionth (10^{-9}).

nanogram (ng) – One billionth of a gram.

narco- – Prefix designating stupor.

narcolepsy – A neurologic disorder that causes individuals to fall asleep without warning. Episodes may occur several times a day and may last from a few minutes to hours. Although treated with stimulant drugs, the results are often disappointing.

narcosis – A state of unconsciousness induced by a drug or chemical agent other than an anesthetic. Narcosis may be drug induced or may be caused by metabolic toxicity caused by kidney or liver failure.

narcotic – A pain-relieving drug derived from opium or a drug chemically and pharmacologically similar to such opium-derived drugs. Narcotics are noted for their ability to relieve pain and cause sedation. In addition to their pain-relieving properties, narcotic drugs are sometimes used to treat cough, diarrhea, and some respiratory problems. Narcotics are also noted for their ability to produce dependence in susceptible persons.

In common usage, all drugs of abuse are sometimes erroneously referred to as narcotics.

nares – Plural of naris.

naris – A nostril.

nasal – Pertaining to the nose.

nascent – In chemistry, any substance released from a chemical compound that is more reactive in its uncombined state. For example, hydrogen peroxide is an effective antiseptic because it

N

releases nascent oxygen. These newly liberated oxygen molecules seek to immediately combine with other molecules. Often the molecules they find are those in bacterial cell membranes. The reaction of oxygen with these cell membranes weakens the membranes and kills the bacteria.

naso- – Prefix designating the nose.

nasogastric – Pertaining to both the nose and the stomach.

nasogastric intubation – A process of introducing a tube through the nose and threading it down the digestive tract and into the stomach. The purpose of a nasogastric tube is to either suction material out of the stomach (e.g., poisons, blood, secretions, etc.) or to instill materials (e.g., food, fluids, medicine) into the stomach.

nasopharyngeal – Pertaining to both the nose and the throat.

nasopharyngitis – An inflammation of the mucous membranes of both the nose and the throat.

National Committee on Quality Assurance (NCQA) – The national accrediting body for managed care organizations. A nonprofit organization, NCQA establishes standards for performance and reviews records of managed care plans to determine the degree of compliance with those standards. Depending upon the results of this review, a plan may be denied accreditation, awarded full accreditation, or given a lesser level of accreditation. NCQA is not required for licensing a health plan; however, many corporations that buy health insurance consider NCQA accreditation as a factor in choosing an insurance company.

national drug code (NDC) – The American coding system for prescription drugs whereby each drug is individually identified down to its package size. The NDC employs an eleven-digit design formatted thus: XXXXX-YYYY-ZZ. In this scheme, the first set of five digits represents the drug's manufacturer or distributor (e.g., 00069 signifies Pfizer, 00173 is GlaxoWellcome, 00002 is Lilly). The second set of four digits represents the name and strength of the drug, and the last set of two digits indicates the package size. Only the first set of digits is standardized. All the other numbers are assigned by the drug companies themselves.

N

The NDC is commonly used to identify the exact drug dispensed to a patient. It is easier and more accurate for a pharmacy to electronically transmit an NDC number to a payer than to try to describe the drug in other terms.

***National Formulary* (NF)** – A publication detailing the standards for the preparation of various pharmaceuticals. Beginning with its first edition in 1888, the NF was originally intended to standardize the way pharmacists compounded prescriptions. The publication later became the property of the American Pharmaceutical Association. As part of the Pure Food and Drug Act of 1906, the NF was recognized by the federal government as an official standard. In time, the NF evolved into a guideline for the manufacture of pharmaceutical products. The *National Formulary* is now incorporated into the *United States Pharmacopeia* (USP).

National Institutes of Health (NIH) – A branch of the United States Public Health Service that performs clinical and basic science research on a wide variety of medical problems. In addition, the NIH funds research at centers around the country and monitors the progress of the studies they fund. NIH is composed of several federally sponsored institutes, such as the National Cancer Institute (NCI); the National Heart, Lung, and Blood Institute (NHLBI); the National Institute of Mental Health (NIMH); and others. NIH is located in Bethesda, Maryland.

natriuresis – Excretion of sodium in the urine. Natriuresis is a property of most diuretics.

natriuretic – A substance, such as a diuretic, that causes loss of sodium into the urine.

natural active immunity – Resistance to an infectious disease that occurs as the result of contracting the disease and then developing antibodies to it.

natural birth control – A form of contraception that does not employ hormone manipulation or barrier contraception. Instead, couples estimate the time of ovulation and abstain from sexual intercourse during those times. Examples of natural birth control include the rhythm and Billing's methods.

N

natural passive immunity – Resistance to an infection that occurs as the result of antibodies passed to a fetus during pregnancy. Natural passive immunity usually lasts only a few months after birth. After that, children must develop their own antibodies either through exposure to diseases or by vaccination.

natural remedy – A drug derived from a biological source such as a plant or animal. Some individuals mistakenly equate "natural" with nontoxic. Their reasoning is that a chemical produced in nature cannot do harm. In fact, natural remedies can and do cause side effects in some people and are less well studied than those marketed as commercial prescription or nonprescription drugs. *Also see herbal remedy.*

naturopathy – A type of health practice where only naturally derived treatments are used. These include herbal drugs, massage, diet, exercise, yoga, etc.

nausea – The feeling of sickness in the stomach that makes one feel that vomiting may follow.

nauseant – An agent that causes feelings of nausea.

nauseated – Having feelings of nausea.

nauseous – Pertaining to an agent that causes feelings of nausea. Commonly incorrectly used in place of nauseated.

NCQA – *See National Committee on Quality Assurance.*

NDA – *See new drug application.*

NDC – *See national drug code.*

nebulize – To cause a liquid to break into fine particles.

nebulizer – A machine that converts liquids into a fine spray. Nebulizers are commonly used to mix liquid medications with water for the purpose of treating respiratory conditions such as asthma. Typically, a mask is placed on the patient's face and the patient breathes the mist of water and medicine.

neck – The part of the body between the head and the shoulders. Also, any similarly shaped structure.

N

necklace – A rash that encircles the neck, similar in appearance to a piece of jewelry.

necr- – Prefix designating death.

necro- – Prefix designating death.

necropsy – A surgical examination of a body after death to determine cause of death and presence of any undiagnosed diseased states. An autopsy.

necrosis – Localized death of a group of cells in a tissue or organ.

necrotic – Pertaining to necrosis.

needle – A hollow metal instrument intended to puncture the skin and underlying tissue for the purpose of injecting material into the area or aspirating material out of the area. A needle is normally attached to a syringe; however, it may also be attached to a catheter (e.g., intravenous catheter) or other device.

negative – Indication as part of a physical examination or a laboratory test that a finding is normal or not present. For example, a negative pregnancy test indicates that the subject is not pregnant. *Also see false negative.*

negotiated discount – A method of payment from a health insurance program to a health care provider (e.g., pharmacy, physician, hospital) whereby the provider agrees to accept a fee lower than usual in return for being allowed to participate in the health plan. Participation in the health plan usually brings the provider a larger volume of patients.

Neisseria – A genus of gram-negative bacteria. *Neisseria* may cause gonorrhea (*Neisseria gonorrhoeae*) or bacterial meningitis (*Neisseria meningitidis*).

neo- – Prefix designating new.

neonatal – Pertaining to the first 28 days of life.

neonatal intensive care unit (NICU) – A hospital floor specializing in treating critically ill newborn babies. Many of these babies are born prematurely, with serious birth defects, or addicted to drugs.

N

neonate – A baby for the first 28 days of life.

neonatologist – A pediatric physician who specializes in the care of newborn babies.

neonatology – The subspecialty of pediatrics that deals with the diagnosis and treatment of medical conditions in babies during the neonatal period.

neoplasm – An abnormal growth of new tissue that forms itself into a tumor. Neoplasms may be either benign or malignant.

neoplastic – Pertaining to a neoplasm.

nephr- – Prefix designating kidney.

nephrectomy – Surgical removal of one or both kidneys.

nephritic – Pertaining to nephritis.

nephritis – Inflammation of the kidneys. Usually one particular part of the kidney is involved and the specific condition takes its name from that structure. For example, interstitial nephritis is an inflammation of the connective tissue in the kidney. Glomerulonephritis is an inflammation of the glomerulus, the portion of the kidney that filters fluid from blood. Pyelonephritis is an infection of the innermost structures of the kidney.

nephro- – Prefix designating kidney.

nephrologist – A physician who specializes in disorders of the kidneys.

nephrology – The specialty of internal medicine that deals with the diagnosis and nonsurgical treatment of kidney diseases.

nephron – The functional unit of the kidney. The nephron filters fluid and waste products out of the blood and concentrates them to form urine. The newly formed urine travels by means of the ureters to the urinary bladder, where it is stored until it can be expelled. A normal kidney contains over a million nephrons.

nephropathy – Any disease of the kidneys.

nephrotomy – Surgical incision into a kidney. Contrasted to nephrectomy, the removal of a kidney.

N

nephrotoxic – Pertaining to a nephrotoxin.

nephrotoxin – A drug or chemical agent that kills or disables kidney cells.

nerve – A bundle of message-carrying fibers that connect the brain and the spinal cord to other parts of the body. Nerves can be afferent (carrying messages from the brain and spinal cord to other parts of the body) or efferent (carrying messages to the body from the brain).

nervous – Pertaining to feelings of anxiety.

nervous breakdown – A nonspecific colloquial term that can apply to any type of acute psychiatric disturbance.

net income per member per month – A means of calculating profit for an insurance company where monthly expenses are subtracted from monthly revenues and the difference is divided by the number of lives covered that month.

network – A group of health care providers (e.g., pharmacies, physicians, hospitals, etc.) who contract with a health insurer to offer a wide range of medical services. Networks may be "open," meaning that health plan members may see providers outside of the network but may then be responsible for additional charges. Networks may be "closed," meaning that health plan members will not receive any insurance benefits for services received from any health care practitioners they see outside of the health plan's contracted network.

neur- – Prefix designating a nerve or nervous system.

neural – Pertaining to the nerves or nerve cells.

neuralgia – Pain that follows the course of a nerve. Neuralgia is usually intense and throbbing.

neurasthenia – A feeling of exhaustion that often follows an episode of depression.

neuri- – Prefix designating a nerve or nervous system.

neuritis – Inflammation of a nerve. Symptoms of neuritis may include neuralgia, anesthesia, paralysis, decreased reflexes, or wasting

N

of an associated muscle. Causes may include trauma, infection, toxins, vitamin deficiency, or diabetes mellitus.

neuro- – Prefix designating a nerve or nervous system.

neuroblastoma – A malignant cancer that affects immature nerve cells. Neuroblastoma occurs most commonly in infants and children.

neurodynia – *See neuralgia.*

neuroendocrine – Pertaining to the functions that the nervous and endocrine systems have in common. In many cases hormones are released into the blood after their parent glands receive a signal from the central nervous system.

neurohormone – A chemical produced by and stored in nerve cells. When released, these chemicals (neurohormones) elicit a response from the target organ. For example, some nerve cells produce and store acetylcholine. When this neurohormone is released into a skeletal muscle, it causes contraction of that muscle.

neuroleptic – A drug used to control symptoms of psychosis. Also known as an antipsychotic or major tranquilizer.

neurologist – A physician who specializes in neurology.

neurology – The specialty within medicine that deals with the diagnosis and treatment of diseases of the brain and nerve tissue.

neuroma – A tumor composed of nerve cells or originating from nerve cells. A neuroma may or may not be malignant.

neuromuscular – Pertaining to the relationship between nerves and muscles.

neuromyopathy – A muscle disorder caused by a diseased condition of the muscle's nerve supply (e.g., multiple sclerosis).

neuron – A nerve cell, the basic structural element of the nervous system.

neuronal – Pertaining to a neuron.

neuropathy – Any disease of the nerves.

N

neuropharmacology – The specialty within pharmacology that deals with the effects of drugs on nerves and diseases affecting nerves.

neuropsychiatry – The branch of medicine that deals with the interrelationship of mental illness and the influences of nerve functions.

neurosis – An obsolete term that was used to describe a group of psychiatric illnesses that all had anxiety as their basis. These conditions are now called anxiety disorders.

neurosurgeon – A physician who practices neurosurgery.

neurosurgery – The specialty within medicine that deals with surgical operations on the brain, spinal cord, and nerve tissue.

neurosyphilis – The manifestations of syphilis on the nervous system. Signs and symptoms of neurosyphilis include loss of reflexes, loss of feeling in parts of the body, and dementia. Neurosyphilis does not usually occur until late in the course of the illness.

neurotic – An obsolete term describing a person who has an anxiety disorder. *See neurosis.*

neurotoxin – An agent that is harmful to nerve tissue.

neurotransmitter – A biochemical that is formed in and released from a neuron in order to stimulate or inhibit the actions of another cell. Examples of neurotransmitters include serotonin, dopamine, acetylcholine, norepinephrine, and epinephrine.

neutr- – Prefix designating neutral.

neutro- – Prefix designating neutral.

neutropenia – Abnormally low number of neutrophils in the blood. Neutropenia makes a person more susceptible to infection. Causes include acute leukemia, overwhelming infection, and rheumatoid arthritis.

neutrophil – A white blood cell that is capable of ingesting bacteria and foreign materials in blood. The concentration of neutrophils in blood rises during infections. Neutrophils normally account for 55% to 65% of white blood cells in the blood.

N

neutrophilia – A condition of increased neutrophils in blood.

neutrophilic – Pertaining to one or more neutrophils.

new chemical entity – A new molecule that has not been previously tested for pharmacologic activity in humans.

new drug application (NDA) – A formal submission to the United States Food and Drug Administration (FDA) asking for approval to market a new drug product. Approval is granted only after the FDA is satisfied that the drug has been sufficiently tested in animals and humans and that it has been shown to be safe and effective for its intended use.

new molecular entity – A term used by the United States Food and Drug Administration (FDA) to describe a newly developed drug.

NF – *See National Formulary.*

ng – Abbreviation for nanogram.

NICU – *See neonatal intensive care unit.*

NIDDM – *See noninsulin-dependent diabetes mellitus.*

NIH – *See National Institutes of Health.*

nit – The egg of a louse. Lice typically attach their nits to hair shafts in the affected areas of the body. When treating a lice infestation, the nits must also be killed and removed to effect a cure.

nitrates – A class of drugs that cause dilation of blood vessels with a corresponding decrease in the heart's demand for oxygen. Nitrates are used to treat angina pectoris and congestive heart failure. Nitroglycerin is an example of a nitrate drug.

nitrogen – A relatively inert gas that is sometimes used in pharmaceutical packaging to displace air from a container so that the medication does not deteriorate prior to use.

nitrogenous – Pertaining to nitrogen. For example, nitrogenous wastes are the by-products of protein metabolism that contain nitrogen.

Nocardia – A species of gram-positive bacteria. Some species are capable of causing nocardiosis.

N

nocardiosis – An infection usually caused by *Nocardia asteroides* that causes pneumonia and may cause abscesses in the brain and subcutaneous tissues around the body. Nocardiosis is sometimes mistaken for tuberculosis because of the microscopic appearance of the organism and the similarity of symptoms.

noci- – Prefix designating pain or injury.

nociceptor – A type of nerve whose function is to detect injury and transmit that information to the brain in the form of a pain sensation.

nocturia – Excessive urination at night, especially when it disturbs sleep. Among the causes for nocturia are excessive fluid consumption prior to sleep, diabetes mellitus or insipidus, use of diuretics including caffeine, and urinary tract disease, especially infections and prostate problems.

noncellular – Pertaining to an organism such as a virus that does not have a cell structure.

noncompliance – The failure of a patient to follow medical directions. Noncompliance may be willful or unintentional (e.g., the patient forgot to take prescribed medicine). Examples of noncompliance include failure to keep appointments, failure to follow prescribed diets or exercise programs, and omission of doses of medication. Noncompliance also includes failure to take doses of medication as prescribed, resulting in overdosing or underdosing. In some cases, patients are noncompliant with their medications because they feel they cannot afford to take full doses. This leads to situations where these patients may derive no benefit at all from the medicine they do take.

noncontributory – In the context of insurance, a noncontributory plan is one where the plan members do not pay any premiums. All premiums are paid by the employer or some other party.

nongonococcal urethritis – An infection of the urethra that cannot be attributed to gonorrhea. Most cases are caused by *Chlamydia*.

noninsulin-dependent diabetes mellitus (NIDDM) – A form of diabetes mellitus where individuals are able to produce some of

N

their insulin needs. Also called type II diabetes mellitus. *Also see diabetes mellitus.*

noninvasive – Pertaining to a diagnostic or therapeutic procedure that does not require insertion of an instrument through the skin or into an orifice. Examples include taking a blood pressure reading or swallowing a tablet of medicine.

nonmember hospital – A hospital that is not part of an insurance plan's network. *Also see network.*

nonpar – *See nonparticipating provider.*

nonparticipating provider (nonpar) – A health care provider who has not agreed to join the network of providers within a health insurance plan. Depending upon the insurance policy, plan members who receive services from nonparticipating providers may be reimbursed for only a portion of their expenses or may receive no reimbursement at all.

nonpathogenic – Pertaining to something that does not cause disease. For example, bacteria that normally live on the skin or in the intestines but do not cause clinical illness are said to be nonpathogenic.

nonprescription drug – A drug that does not require a prescription. In some cases, nonprescription drugs contain the same ingredients as prescription drugs, but often in lower concentrations. Nonprescription drugs may be purchased in pharmacies, grocery stores, convenience stores, department stores, and other retail outlets. Also called over-the-counter drugs.

nonproductive cough – A sudden ejection of air from the lungs and through the mouth that does not expel (produce) mucus or fluid from the throat or lungs.

nonproprietary name – *See generic name.*

nonsedating – Pertaining to a drug or other agent that does not cause drowsiness.

nonsteroidal anti-inflammatory drug (NSAID) – A class of drugs that reduces inflammation, relieves pain, and lowers fever. NSAIDs are not chemically related to corticosteroids and have different

N

side effects than corticosteroids. Uses for NSAIDs include arthritis, headache, muscle ache, menstrual cramps, pain following injury, and many other conditions. Examples of NSAIDs include ibuprofen and naproxen.

normal value – A test reading or result that is within the range of values exhibited by the majority of people. Deviation beyond the normal range may indicate the presence of a disease.

normo- – Prefix designating normal or usual.

normochromic – Pertaining to the typical color of something. Most often used in the context of red blood cells where normochromia usually indicates the presence of the usual amount of hemoglobin.

normocytic – Pertaining to normal sized cells. Most often used in the context of red blood cells.

normoglycemia – Normal level of glucose in the blood.

noso- – Prefix designating disease.

nosocomial – Pertaining to a disease contracted in a hospital. Nosocomial infections, also called hospital-acquired infections, may occur because of cross-contamination with another patient or for unknown cause. Nosocomial infections are often difficult to treat because the causative organisms may be resistant to a wide variety of antibiotics.

nosology – The science of the description and classification of diseases.

nostril – The opening to the nasal cavity.

nostrum – A remedy, typically one that is represented to have special powers or ability to treat disease. The term connotes a degree of deception or quackery.

noxious – Harmful or damaging to tissue.

NSAID – *See nonsteroidal anti-inflammatory drug.*

nuclear – Pertaining to a nucleus.

N

nuclear medicine – A subspecialty of radiology that concentrates on diagnosis of disease through the use of radioactive isotopes.

nuclear medicine specialist – A physician who is certified to practice nuclear medicine. Nuclear medicine specialists administer chemicals that are tagged with a radioactive isotope (radiopharmaceuticals). Once in the body, the physician uses a specially designed camera to determine where the chemical-isotope complex collected. Depending upon the type of test administered, the procedure may reveal information about metabolism, circulation, tumors, fractures, or other conditions. The nuclear medicine physician is able to provide valuable diagnostic information to the patient's attending physician.

nuclear pharmacy – A pharmacy that is specially licensed to work with radioactive materials. Nuclear pharmacies tag radioactive elements to other drugs or chemicals for use in nuclear medicine. Previously called radiopharmacy.

nucleus – A structure at the center. In a cell, the nucleus is located in the cell's center, regulates many of the functions of the cell, and stores most of the cell's DNA.

Also, the center of an atom where the protons and neutrons are located.

nuclide – The nucleus of any atom. If it is radioactive, it is often referred to as a radionuclide. *Also see isotope.*

numbness – Loss or lack of sensation in an area.

nurse – A person who is specially trained, usually in a college or university setting, to care for the physical and emotional needs of patients, to prevent disease, and to promote good health practices.

Nurses may practice in a wide variety of settings and specialties. They may work in hospitals, clinics, physicians' offices, schools, or corporations. Nursing specialties include dermatology, public health, anesthesia, obstetrics, psychiatry, and surgery. Many of the nursing specialties require certification or a master's degree. *Also see licensed practical nurse, registered nurse.*

Also, to breastfeed.

N

nurse practitioner – A registered nurse with advanced academic and clinical training that encompasses the physical and psychosocial health of patients. Nurse practitioner programs usually award a master's degree upon completion. Nurse practitioners work under the supervision of a physician and carry out assessments, diagnosis, and treatment functions. Areas where nurse practitioners may specialize include family practice, mental health counseling, women's health, and pediatrics.

nursing home – A licensed facility that provides long-term residential care for patients with disabling illnesses who do not need to stay in a hospital but cannot be cared for at home. Nursing homes provide medical, nursing, and custodial care to their residents.

nutraceutical – There is no general agreement on the definition of this term. Some consider a nutraceutical to be an herbal remedy or plant constituent formulated into a pharmaceutical dosage form such as a tablet or capsule (e.g., vitamin C tablets, broccoli capsules). Others consider nutraceuticals to be foods that may be used to treat or prevent disease (e.g., vitamin-fortified milk, bread, etc.). Still others consider nutraceuticals to be only commercially-produced food supplement products (e.g., Ensure, Sustical, etc.).

nutrient – A food or other substance (e.g., vitamin, mineral, amino acid) that provides part of the elements necessary for nourishment.

nutrition – All the processes involved in ingesting and utilizing foods for the maintenance of the organism.

nutritionist – A person who specializes in the study of nutrition. While some nutritionists possess graduate degrees from highly respected programs, nutritionists are not licensed and vary widely in knowledge and competence. Without required licensing or certification, anyone can claim to be a nutritionist.

nystagmus – Uncontrollable rhythmic movement of the eyes. Nystagmus is often a side effect of drugs that affect the central nervous system.

O

O – Chemical symbol for oxygen.

Oath of Hippocrates – *See* Hippocratic Oath.

OB – Abbreviation for obstetrics or obstetrician.

OB/GYN – Abbreviation for obstetrics and gynecology. *See obstetrician and gynecologist.*

obese – Pertaining to someone who is excessively overweight.

obesity – The state of being overweight. Obesity is normally considered to be an actual bodyweight greater than 30% of normal. At one time normal bodyweight values were determined solely by a combination of height and body frame size (small, medium, large). While this method is still used as a general screening method, a much better indicator is measurement of total body fat.

OBS – *See organic brain syndrome.*

observation unit – A floor or collection of rooms in a hospital that are reserved for patients who need to be medically monitored for up to 23 hours and 59 minutes. Within that amount of time the patient must either be discharged or admitted to another hospital unit. Observation time, also called a 23-hour admission, is usually billed at a different rate than the daily hospital rate.

obsessive-compulsive disorder (OCD) – An anxiety syndrome characterized by repetitive thoughts (obsessions) along with ritualistic actions (compulsions). OCD is usually treated with psychotherapy and antidepressants.

obstetrical services – The care given to a woman in relation to pregnancy and childbirth. Obstetrical services ideally start as soon as the woman suspects she is pregnant and continues for a few weeks after the delivery.

obstetrician (OB) – A physician who specializes in obstetrics.

obstetrician and gynecologist (OB/GYN) – A physician who specializes in both obstetrics and gynecology.

obstetrics (OB) – The specialty of medicine that deals with the health of women during pregnancy, delivery of their babies, and their health in the six weeks that follow delivery.

O

occlusion – A closure or blockage.

occlusive dressing – A bandage that prevents air or moisture from reaching a wound.

occult – Hidden. Not apparent. For example, occult blood is blood that comes from a source that cannot be immediately determined, such as a peptic ulcer.

occupational therapist (OTR) – A person with a specialized baccalaureate or master's degree and who must also pass a certification examination administered by the American Occupational Therapy Association. Most states also require occupational therapists to be licensed.

occupational therapy – According to the American Occupational Therapy Association, occupational therapy is "the use of purposeful activity with individuals who are limited by physical injury or illness, psychosocial dysfunction, developmental or learning disabilities, poverty and cultural differences, or the aging process to maximize independence, prevent disability, and maintain health. The practice encompasses evaluation, treatment, and consultation." In short, occupational therapy helps individuals who have permanent or temporary disabilities adjust to the physical demands of daily living, including work-related and normal household activities.

OCD – *See obsessive-compulsive disorder.*

ocular – Pertaining to the eye or the eyepiece of an instrument such as a microscope.

oculo- – Prefix designating the eye.

oculogyric – Pertaining to the rotation of the eye.

oculogyric crisis – A spasm in the muscles that control eye movements causing the eyes to rotate involuntarily. Most commonly, the eye rotation is upward or to the side and may last from minutes to hours. Oculogyric crisis is most commonly seen in Parkinson's disease or as a side effect of antipsychotic medications. While the condition does not of itself cause permanent damage, the panic and visual disturbance it causes may cause a patient to fall or be otherwise injured.

O

O.D. – Abbreviation for doctor of optometry, the professional degree of optometrists. *See optometrist.*

od or o.d. – Abbreviation for the Latin *omni die*, or every day. An abbreviation commonly used on prescriptions to indicate that the drug should be taken once daily, every day.

Also an abbreviation for the Latin *oculus dexter*, meaning right eye. An abbreviation commonly used on prescriptions to indicate that the prescribed medicine is to be applied to the right eye.

OD – *See overdose.*

official – Pertaining to a drug or chemical that is listed in a pharmacopoeia and, consequently, meets certain standards.

off-label – A use for a drug that is beyond that officially approved by the United States Food and Drug Administration (FDA). Although physicians may legally prescribe drugs for off-label uses, some managed care plans do not cover drugs prescribed for nonFDA-approved uses.

Also see indication.

-oid – Suffix designating a resemblance to the root word. For example, fibroid is like a fiber.

oil – A lipid that feels greasy to the touch, is in liquid form at room temperature, does not mix with water, and may or may not be soluble in alcohol but is soluble in ether. Oils may be derived from animal, vegetable, or mineral (e.g., petroleum) sources.

ointment – A semisolid, greasy pharmaceutical product intended for external application. Because of their occlusive nature, ointments hold water beneath the skin and are most useful for treating dermatologic conditions that include dry skin as part of the problem. Medications that may be administered in ointment form include anti-inflammatory drugs, topical anesthetics, and antibiotics.

o.l. – Abbreviation used on prescriptions for the Latin *oculus laevus*, left eye.

-ol – Suffix indicating an alcohol, such as ethanol, methanol.

olfactory – Pertaining to the sense of smell.

O

olig- – Prefix designating little or few.

oligo- – Prefix designating little or few.

oligomenorrhea – Abnormally light menstrual periods.

oligospermia – A lower than normal concentration of sperm in semen.

oliguria – Abnormally small amount of urine produced, particularly if fluid consumption significantly exceeds urine output. Oliguria is often a sign of kidney disease, obstruction of the urinary tract, or dehydration.

-ology – Suffix designating a study of the root word. For example, pharmacology is the study of the effects of drugs. Dermatology is the study of the health and diseases of the skin.

-oma – Suffix designating a tumor or cancer. For example, lymphoma is a cancer of the lymphatic system.

oncho- – Prefix designating a tumor or mass.

onco- – Prefix designating a tumor or mass.

oncogene – A gene found in some viruses that may initiate transformation from normal to cancer in a host cell.

oncologist – A physician who specializes in the diagnosis and treatment of cancer. Such physicians may be medical oncologists (treat cancer primarily with medications), surgical oncologists (treat cancer primarily with surgery), or radiation oncologists (treat cancer primarily with radiation treatments). Depending upon the specific type of cancer, the disease may be treated by one of these specialists or by a team of them.

oncology – The medical specialty that deals with tumors and cancers.

oncolysis – Destruction of tissue in a tumor.

oncolytic – An agent that kills cancer cells. A cancer chemotherapy drug.

-one – Suffix designating a ketone, such as acetone.

on-line adjudication – A process whereby claims are entered into a computer at the place where service is provided (e.g., in a phar-

O

macy). The provider receives immediate approval or denial of coverage via computer. For example, when an HMO patient has a prescription filled at a network pharmacy, the pharmacist enters the patient's identification into the computer as well as information about the prescription itself. If the patient is eligible for service and if the medication is covered by the plan in the dose prescribed, the on-line adjudication system sends a message to the pharmacist that the plan will pay for the prescription. Many on-line adjudication systems also check for drug interactions, overdoses, underdoses, excessive refills, and other problems.

on-off phenomenon – The sudden changes that may occur in a patient taking levodopa for Parkinson's disease. Patients may fluctuate between improved mobility (on) to sudden stiffness and tremor (off). The fluctuations may occur rapidly and are not related to the time the last dose of levodopa was taken.

onych- – Prefix designating a fingernail or toenail.

onycho- – Prefix designating a fingernail or toenail.

onychomycosis – A fungal infection of the nails. Most cases of onychomycosis are benign and are only of cosmetic concern. Because the site of the infection is difficult to reach with topical antifungal drugs, treatment is usually given orally and may last for months before the infection is cured. Many managed care plans do not cover these treatments.

onychopathy – Any disease of the nails.

oo- – Prefix designating an egg or ovary.

oogenesis – The physiologic process that results in production of an egg.

oophor- – Prefix designating an egg or ovary.

oophorectomy – The surgical removal of one or both ovaries. If both ovaries are removed, the procedure causes immediate infertility and menopause. The most common reason for performing an oophorectomy is treatment of ovarian cancer or suppression of growth of an estrogen-dependent cancer.

O

oophoritis – An inflammation of one or both ovaries. This usually occurs along with an inflammation or infection of one or both fallopian tubes.

open access – A provision in some managed care plans that allows members to see specialists without a referral from a primary care physician. Open access is usually not allowed in the more tightly controlled plans.

open-angle glaucoma – The most common form of glaucoma, a condition of increased fluid pressure inside the eye. Open-angle glaucoma is usually present in both eyes and is caused by the inability of aqueous humor, the fluid in the front chamber of the eye, to drain properly. Open-angle glaucoma may be treated with a wide variety of oral medicines and eye drops.

open enrollment – A designated time, usually once a year, when employees in a company-sponsored health plan have an opportunity to change insurance plans without penalty and usually without providing evidence of insurability. Also the time when employees who previously declined insurance coverage may choose to enroll.

open formulary – A list of drugs a health plan prefers that physicians prescribe; however, coverage is not limited to these drugs. Contrasted with a closed formulary, where coverage is limited to drugs on the list.

open panel HMO – A contractual arrangement between a managed care plan and private physicians and other health care providers that allows plan members free movement between providers in the plan's network and those outside of the network. Typically the open panel providers must agree to the same reimbursement terms as the network providers.

operable – Pertaining to a condition that may be treated with surgery. For example, an operable tumor is one that lies in an area that can be reached and removed by means of surgery.

operation – A surgical procedure.

ophthalmia – An inflammation of the eye.

ophthalmic – Pertaining to the eye.

O

ophthalmic preparation – A pharmaceutical intended for use in the eye; for example, eye drops, eye ointments. Ophthalmic preparations must be sterile to prevent eye infections and should be isotonic to minimize burning. Medications in ophthalmic preparations include antibiotics, antivirals, decongestants, artificial tears, and topical anesthetics. Depending upon their active ingredients, ophthalmic preparations may be sold over-the-counter or may require a prescription.

ophthalmo- – Prefix designating the eye.

ophthalmologist – A physician who specializes in ophthalmology.

ophthalmology – The medical specialty that deals with the health and diseases of the eye as well as vision problems. Ophthalmologic treatments include corrective lenses (eyeglasses and contact lenses), drugs (e.g., for glaucoma), and surgery (e.g., repair of traumatic injuries, laser treatment for vision problems).

ophthalmopathy – Any disease of the eye.

ophthalmoplegia – Paralysis of one or more of the muscles that control the movements of the eye. Ophthalmoplegia is usually caused by disease that affects the function of the nerves that control these muscles.

ophthalmoplegic – Pertaining to ophthalmoplegia.

ophthalmoscope – An instrument consisting of a light and magnifying lenses that is used to examine the interior of the eye.

-opia – Suffix designating vision; for example, myopia (nearsightedness), presbyopia (age-related difficulty seeing things that are close to the eye).

opiate – Any chemical substance that is derived from the opium poppy. The term is most commonly applied to opiate narcotics (e.g., morphine, codeine) but also includes nonnarcotic drugs, such as the vasodilator papaverine, that are also found in opium.

opioid – Any drug that has narcotic analgesic properties similar to morphine but is not found in opium, e.g., meperidine (Demerol).

O

opioid receptor – A specialized molecule on the surface of a nerve cell that is stimulated by the presence of an opioid drug. When stimulated by an opioid, the receptor signals the nerve cell to send a message to the brain that causes the typical pharmacological response to a narcotic (e.g., pain relief, drowsiness, respiratory depression).

opioid receptor antagonist – An agent that prevents opioids from coming into contact with opioid receptors. These drugs are commonly used in the treatment of narcotic overdoses. They reverse the effects of narcotic poisoning.

opium – The milky substance produced in the seedpods of the *Papaver somniferum* (opium poppy) plant. At least 20 pharmacologically active substances have been isolated from opium. The most therapeutically useful of these are the analgesics morphine and codeine and the vasodilator papaverine.

opportunistic infection – A type of infection that rarely occurs in persons in good health when body defenses are intact. Examples include *Pneumocystis carinii* pneumonia in persons with AIDS or leukemia and staphylococcal skin infections in diabetics.

optic – Pertaining to the eye or vision.

optical – Pertaining to the eye or vision.

optician – An individual who fills prescriptions for eyeglasses and contact lenses and fits them to the patient.

optico- – Prefix designating optics.

optics – The science of light and its properties.

optional benefits – Insurance coverage that may be purchased in addition to the standard offering. Depending upon the standard plan, optional benefits may include coverage for prescription drugs, dental, mental health, or obstetrical care.

opto- – Prefix designating optics.

optometrist (O.D.) – A graduate of a doctor of optometry program who assesses vision problems, screens for diseases of the eye, and prescribes corrective lenses or eye exercises for vision prob-

O

lems. Optometrists must pass an examination and be licensed by the state before they can practice.

OPV – *See oral poliovirus vaccine.*

oral – Pertaining to the mouth.

oral contraceptive – A tablet taken by mouth intended to prevent conception. Oral contraceptives contain either a progesterone-like hormone called a progestin alone or in combination with an estrogen. Oral contraceptives work inhibiting ovulation, inhibiting implantation of fertilized eggs, by thickening cervical mucus to make it more difficult for sperm to enter the uterus, or a combination of these effects.

oral poliovirus vaccine (OPV) – A form of immunization against polio that involves swallowing a series of solutions of live, attenuated polioviruses.

oral route of administration – The process of giving medication by mouth. When medications are swallowed, they pass into the stomach and intestinal tract. Once there, they may be absorbed into the bloodstream or continue on through the intestines to exert their effects there.

Orange Book – A monograph compiled by the United States Food and Drug Administration (FDA) officially titled *Approved Drug Products with Therapeutic Equivalence Evaluations.* Commonly called the Orange Book because of the color of its cover. The Orange Book lists every strength of every generic drug approved for distribution in the United States. Each product is rated for its therapeutic equivalence to the innovator drug. State pharmacy boards and managed care organizations use this as a reference to determine which generic products are suitable for substitution for innovator drugs.

orbit – The eye socket.

orbital – Pertaining to bones of the eye socket.

orchi- – Prefix designating the testes.

orchiatrophy – Shrinking of the testes. Orchiatrophy is a potential side effect of abuse of anabolic steroids.

O

orchidic – Pertaining to the testes.

orchido- – Prefix designating the testes.

orchio- – Prefix designating the testes.

orchitis – Inflammation of the testes.

organ – A structure of the body, usually composed of several types of tissue, that performs a specific function. For example, the thyroid gland secretes thyroid hormone, the brain processes information and controls the function of other organs, the heart pumps blood, etc.

organic – Pertaining to a substance formed by living matter.

Also, pertaining to an organ.

organic brain syndrome (OBS) – Psychological or behavioral symptoms caused by disease or damage to brain tissue. Causes of OBS may include brain tumors, strokes, Alzheimer's disease, and trauma.

organic chemistry – The study of the chemical properties of molecules that contain at least one carbon atom.

organic compound – A chemical that contains at least one carbon atom.

organism – Any individual animal or plant having diverse organs and parts that function together as a whole to maintain life and its activities.

organo- – Prefix designating an organ or living (organic) material.

organogenesis – The formation and differentiation of organs during development. Drugs taken by a mother during pregnancy are usually most dangerous if taken during the period of organogenesis. Drug-influenced metabolic changes at this time can lead to devastating physical birth defects.

organophosphate – A class of drugs and chemicals that temporarily or permanently disable nerve function. Some organophosphates are used to treat resistant cases of glaucoma. More commonly, they are used as insecticides. Military nerve gases are another type of organophosphate.

O

oro- – Prefix designating the mouth.

orofacial – Pertaining to both the mouth and the face.

orolingual – Pertaining to both the mouth and tongue.

oronasal – Pertaining to both the mouth and nose.

oropharynx – Pertaining to both the mouth and throat.

orphan drug – An agent used for the diagnosis, treatment, or prevention of a rare disease or condition. According to the Orphan Drug Act of 1983, a rare disease is one that occurs in less than 200,000 people in the United States or one that occurs in more than 200,000 people but for which there is no reasonable expectation that a manufacturer would be able to recover its costs of developing the drug. The Orphan Drug Act provides financial incentives to manufacturers who develop such drugs.

orth- – Prefix designating straight or normal.

ortho- – Prefix designating straight or normal.

orthopedic surgeon – See orthopedist.

orthopedics – The specialty of medicine that deals with diseases of or trauma to the bones, joints, and the structures (e.g., muscles, tendons, ligaments) that support them. Also spelled orthopaedics.

orthopedist – A physician who specializes in orthopedics. Also spelled orthopaedist.

orthopnea – A condition where a person must stand or sit upright or inclined in order to breathe comfortably. Persons with this condition have difficulty breathing when lying flat. Orthopnea is common in congestive heart failure.

orthostatic – Pertaining to a standing or upright position or posture.

orthostatic hypotension – A condition where standing up from a lying or sitting position causes a precipitous drop in blood pressure that can cause dizziness or even fainting. Orthostatic hypotension is most commonly caused by the drugs that are used to treat hypertension.

o.s. – Abbreviation often used on prescriptions for the Latin *oculus sinister*, meaning left eye.

-ose – Suffix indicating a carbohydrate; for example, sucrose (table sugar) and lactose (milk sugar).

-osis – Suffix usually indicating a disease, action, or result; for example, diagnosis (determination of the character of a disease) and prognosis (the probable course of a disease).

osmosis – The process of fluid passing through a membrane from the side of lower concentration of solute to the side of higher concentration. The materials dissolved in the fluid are unable to pass through the membrane.

osseo- – Prefix designating bone.

ossi- – Prefix designating bone.

ossification – The process of bone formation.

ost- – Prefix designating bone.

oste- – Prefix designating bone.

osteitis – Inflammation of bone tissue.

osteo- – Prefix designating bone.

osteoarthritis – A slowly developing condition characterized by deterioration of cartilage in joints and overgrowth of bone tissue. Osteoarthritis most commonly affects the weight-bearing joints in the knees and hips, but can also affect the spine, fingers, and any other area where two bones meet. Osteoarthritis is characterized by pain and stiffness. The condition usually appears first during middle-age and worsens with time. Osteoarthritis is the most common form of arthritis. Also called degenerative joint disease or DJD.

osteodynia – Pain emanating from a bone.

osteomalacia – Softening of bone tissue due to loss of calcium. Sometimes called adult rickets. Osteomalacia is caused by either a dietary deficiency of calcium, phosphorus, and vitamin D or by an inability to absorb sufficient amounts of these nutrients from the digestive tract. Signs and symptoms of osteoma-

O

lacia include bone fractures, weakness, bone pain, and weight loss. Treatment usually consists of supplementing the diet with the deficient nutrients.

osteomyelitis – Inflammation, almost always due to bacterial infection, of a bone and the marrow within it. Infection is most commonly introduced as the result of surgery, trauma, infection that reaches the bloodstream, or invasion from a nearby infection, such as an infected diabetic skin ulcer. Treatment usually includes several weeks of intravenous antibiotic therapy.

osteopath – A physician trained in osteopathic medicine.

osteopathic medicine – Originally, a concept that disease results from misalignments of bone and muscle in the body and that correction of those misalignments could effect cure.

Now, osteopathy encompasses all of the usual forms of medical diagnosis and treatment, including drugs, nutrition, surgery, radiology, etc. Doctors of osteopathy (D.O.) are trained in the same areas of medicine as doctors of medicine (M.D.); however, osteopaths still emphasize the effect of the musculoskeletal system in the role of disease and treatment. Osteopaths take the same state licensing examinations as doctors of medicine (M.D.) and are entitled to practice in the same specialties as M.D.s (e.g., psychiatry, internal medicine, obstetrics-gynecology, etc.)

osteopathic physician – *See osteopath.*

osteopathy – *See osteopathic medicine.*

Also, any disease of bone.

osteoporosis – An abnormal decrease in the density of bone. Osteoporosis causes bone shafts to thin and become more susceptible to fracture.

Osteoporosis is much more common in women than men, eventually affecting about 30% of women. Osteoporosis usually starts to develop in susceptible women after menopause and is due to the inability of bone to regenerate itself. Osteoporosis is also more likely to occur in individuals, men or women, who are sedentary, immobilized, or taking long-term corticosteroids for chronic conditions.

O

Preventive treatments normally consist of calcium supplements, estrogen, and prescribed exercise. Some medications such as the bisphosphonates may stop the progression of the condition or even reverse it to some degree.

osteoporotic – Pertaining to any condition characterized by increased porosity of bone.

osteosarcoma – A malignant cancer of bone.

ostomy – A surgical opening that creates a channel from either the urinary tract or the gastrointestinal tract for the purpose of providing either a drain for body wastes or a means to introduce fluids and nutrition. Ostomies are usually performed because an obstruction or other problem prevents nutrients or wastes from being passed through the gastrointestinal tract in the usual way.

otalgia – Pain in the ear. Earache.

OTC – *See over-the-counter drug.*

otic – Pertaining to the ear. For example, otic drops are ear drops.

otitis – Inflammation of the ear. Inflammatory conditions or infections in the ear are usually further described by their location. For example, otitis externa is an inflammation or infection of the external ear canal. Otitis media is an inflammation or infection of the middle ear, the area inside the tympanic membrane (eardrum). Otitis interna is an inflammation or infection of the inner ear, the deepest part of the ear, also known as the labyrinth.

oto- – Prefix designating the ear.

otodynia – Pain in the ear. Earache.

otolaryngologist – A physician who specializes in otolaryngology. Otolaryngologists are often referred to as ear, nose, and throat (or ENT) specialists.

otolaryngology – The branch of medicine that deals with the diagnosis and treatment of diseases of the ears and throat. Otolaryngology usually also includes disorders of the upper respiratory tract, particularly the nose, air passages, and sinuses.

O

-otomy – Suffix designating a surgical procedure.

otopathy – Any disease of the ear.

otopharyngeal – Pertaining to both the middle ear and the throat.

ototoxic – Pertaining to an agent that is noxious to the ear. For example, the aminoglycoside antibiotics are considered to be ototoxic because under some circumstances, they are able to damage ear structures that are responsible for hearing and balance.

ototoxicity – The property of being noxious to the ear.

OTR – Abbreviation for occupational therapist, registered.

o.u. – Abbreviation often used on prescriptions for the Latin *oculus uterque*, meaning both eyes.

ounce (oz) – A weight in the English system of weights and measures that equals one-sixteenth of a pound or 28.349 grams.

Also a measure in the English system of weights and measures that equals one-sixteenth of a pint or 29.6 milliliters.

-ous – A suffix that indicates a chemical element whose salt forms are of a lower valence. For example, ferrous (iron) salts have a lower valence than ferric salts.

outcome indicators – Definitive signs occurring during the course of a disease or recovery from it that can be measured and analyzed. For example, the number of asthma attacks, hospital admissions, emergency room visits, heart attacks, strokes, etc.

outcomes – The results achieved through a specific health care intervention. Outcomes may include objective measures such as death rates, days of hospitalization, or incidence of conditions such as strokes, heart attacks, asthma attacks, or emergency room visits. Outcomes may also include subjective measures such as quality of life, stress reduction, and others.

For example, the desired outcomes of treatment of heart failure with ACE inhibitors is longer life with fewer symptoms. One desired outcome of an influenza vaccination program is reduced hospitalizations due to complications of influenza. A less clinical but also desirable outcome is improved satisfaction with treatment by physicians, pharmacies, hospitals, insurers, etc.

outcomes management – A continuous quality improvement approach intended to improve the end result of encounters between patients and their health care providers. Outcomes management typically attempts to modify practices in response to data analysis. Outcomes management often includes the development of clinical protocols or practice guidelines.

outcomes measurement – The formal process of collecting and analyzing data relating to the results (outcome) of encounters between patients and health care providers.

outcomes research – Formal studies intended to measure the effects of a given type of intervention (drug, surgery, etc.) on health or costs. Outcomes research is difficult to perform because many factors other than the one under study can contribute to or subtract from the effectiveness of the study factor.

outlier – A patient or provider whose costs of care far exceed the norm for the applicable disease state.

out-of-area – Health care received by a person outside of the geographic area normally covered by a health plan.

out-of-area benefits – Provision in a managed care insurance policy that describes the benefits available to members who need service outside of the geographic area normally covered by the plan.

out-of-network – Providers who have not contracted to participate with a given managed care organization.

out-of-network benefits – Provision in a managed care insurance policy that describes the benefits available to members who seek service outside of the group of contracted providers. In some cases, there may be no coverage at all. In other cases, coverage may be limited or may include higher deductibles.

out-of-pocket costs – The portion of payments for health services that must be paid by the enrollee, including copayments, coinsurance, and deductibles.

out-of-pocket maximum – Provision in a health insurance contract that states the greatest amount of money an insured member will be expected to pay for services over a specified period of time, usually one year. Once this limit is reached, insurance pays

100% of covered benefits. The out-of-pocket maximum includes deductibles and coinsurance.

outpatient – An individual being treated or evaluated in a setting other than a hospital (e.g., physician's office, clinic).

outpatient facility – A structure that provides service to patients who are not hospitalized. Outpatient facilities include clinics, doctors' offices, and departments within a hospital that are intended to be used by outpatients, including physical therapy, radiology, pharmacy, etc.

output – Product or work that is produced or expelled. Normally used in the context of either cardiac output (the amount of blood ejected by the heart over a measured amount of time) or urinary output (the amount of urine produced by the kidneys in a measured period of time).

ova – Plural of ovum.

ovari- – Prefix designating an ovary.

ovarian – Pertaining to an ovary.

ovario- – Prefix designating an ovary.

ovary – One of a pair of female reproductive organs that are responsible for producing eggs and releasing them for potential fertilization. The ovaries also produce and secrete female hormones. The ovaries are located on either side of the uterus.

overdose (OD) – A quantity of a medication or street drug taken or administered in an excessive amount. Overdoses may cause serious signs or symptoms of toxicity or even death.

override – A decision made by an individual that supersedes the normal process. For example, a pharmacist may override a drug interaction warning if he has properly counseled that patient. An HMO physician may override a claim denial upon successful appeal of the denial.

over-the-counter (OTC) drug – A drug that does not require a prescription. In some cases, nonprescription drugs contain the same ingredients as prescription drugs, but in lower concentra-

O

tions. Nonprescription drugs may be purchased in pharmacies, grocery stores, convenience stores, department stores, and other retail outlets.

ovi- – Prefix designating an egg or ovary.

ovicidal – Pertaining to an agent that kills eggs.

oviduct – See *fallopian tube*.

ovo- – Prefix designating an egg or ovary.

ovulation – The release of an egg from an ovary. Ovulation usually occurs during or near the fourteenth day of the menstrual cycle.

ovum – The female germ cell. The ovum carries half of the genetic code needed by an organism. Upon fertilization, a sperm cell provides the other half of the code. Thus the organism's genetic code is comprised of equal parts of the mother's and father's genes.

oxygenation – The addition of oxygen. For example, the primary function of the lungs is to oxygenate the blood.

oxytocic – An agent that causes the uterus to contract so that childbirth may progress more quickly.

oz – See *ounce*.

P – Chemical symbol for the element phosphorus.

P&T committee – *See pharmacy and therapeutics committee.*

PA – *See physician assistant.*

pacemaker – An artificial device that regulates the rhythm of the heart. A cardiac pacemaker may be either internal or external. An internal pacemaker is surgically implanted in the chest and works when the surgeon attaches electrodes directly to the heart. An external pacemaker is temporarily applied to the chest wall over the heart and works by sending electrical pulses through the chest. External pacemakers are typically used in emergency situations.

Also, the sinoatrial node, the portion of the heart that initiates the electrical pulses that result in heart contractions.

pack – A dressing or bandage. Packs may be dry or wet (dry pack, wet pack), hot or cold (hot pack, cold pack).

package insert – *See label.*

pain – An unpleasant feeling usually associated with a tissue injury or illness that triggers noxious nervous transmission to the brain. Pain may be described as mild, moderate or severe, acute or chronic, dull or sharp, burning or piercing, localized or generalized.

paint – A liquid pharmaceutical product that is applied over a large area by means of a swab or brush. Normally used to treat large skin lesions.

palliative treatment – A remedy that improves patient comfort but does not treat the underlying condition. For example, a narcotic may ease the pain of a cancer patient but does not change the course of the disease.

pallor – An unnatural paleness of the skin.

palm – The flat part of the hand between the wrist and the fingers, opposite the back of the hand.

palmar – Pertaining to the palm of the hand.

palpate – To examine by using the hands to touch and feel.

palpation – To examine by touch, feeling for normal or abnormal organs, masses, or movement.

palpitation – Forceful or fluttering heartbeat felt by the patient. Palpitations are usually faster or more forceful than normal heartbeats. Palpitations may be associated with either normal or abnormal heart rhythms.

palsy – Permanent or temporary paralysis or loss of sensations.

pan- – Prefix designating all or whole.

panacea – A single agent capable of treating all illnesses. A cure-all.

panalgesia – Pain that affects the entire body.

pancreas – A gland in the gastrointestinal tract that measures about five inches long and is positioned next to the duodenum. The pancreas secretes digestive enzymes into the duodenum. The pancreas also produces and secretes the endocrine hormones insulin and glucagon into the blood.

pancreat- – Prefix designating the pancreas.

pancreatic – Pertaining to the pancreas.

pancreatic enzyme – Any of the digestive agents produced by the pancreas and secreted into the duodenum. Pancreatic enzymes aid in digestion of food. The most important of these enzymes are trypsin, chymotrypsin, steapsin, and amylopsin.

pancreatitis – Inflammation of the pancreas. Pancreatitis may be acute or chronic. Chronic alcohol abuse is a common cause.

pancreo- – Prefix designating the pancreas.

pancytopenia – Abnormal reduction in the number of all circulating blood cells.

pandemic – The occurrence of a disease in a widely dispersed population, such as an entire country or the world.

pang – A sudden, sharp pain.

panic – Intense feeling of anxiety or dread for no apparent reason.

pant- – Prefix designating all or whole.

P

panto- – Prefix designating all or whole.

papilledema – Fluid collection in the optic disk, the area where the optic nerve attaches to the retina of the eye. Papilledema is often a sign of advanced hypertension.

pap smear – A test commonly used to screen for cancer of the cervix. Specimen cells are obtained by swabbing the uterine cervix during a pelvic examination. Microscopic examination of the specimen determines the presence or absence of abnormal cells. The test is named for George Papanicolaou, the physician who developed the technique.

papular – Pertaining to one or more papules.

papule – A small, raised lesion on the skin. *Also see macule, maculopapular.*

PAR – *See participating provider.*

para – The number of pregnancies that have resulted in a birth. For example, a woman who has brought one pregnancy to term is described as para I, two pregnacies, para II. Multiple births (e.g., twins, triplets, etc.) are counted as a single birth.

para- – Prefix designating a pair or next to.

paralysis – Loss of voluntary movement in a part of the body. Paralysis may be caused by disease, trauma, or mental illness.

paramedic – A nonphysician who is specially trained and certified to provide emergency medical care. Paramedics maintain radio contact with physicians for advice and treatment instructions.

paranasal – Pertaining to the area next to the nose.

paranoia – An irrational feeling that someone or something intends to do harm. The perceived threat may be centered on a specific person (e.g., spouse, employer), on an institution (e.g., hospital, military), or may be widespread (e.g., society in general). The perceived threat may be physical (e.g., assault) or nonphysical (e.g., criticism). Paranoia may occur as the result of chronic mental illness (e.g., schizophrenia), acute stress, or drug toxicity (e.g., substance abuse).

P

paranoid – Pertaining to paranoia.

paraplegia – Paralysis of the lower portion of the body. Paraplegics are able to maintain use of their arms but not their legs.

paraplegic – Pertaining to paraplegia.

parasite – An organism that lives on or within another living organism and extracts its nutrition from the host organism to the detriment of the host. Examples include lice and tapeworms.

parasitic – Pertaining to a parasite.

parasympathetic – The portion of the autonomic nervous system that opposes the effects of the sympathetic branch of the same nervous system. Some of the effects of the parasympathetic nervous system include slowing heart rate, reducing blood pressure, and increasing digestive activity. Also called the cholinergic nervous system. *Also see autonomic nervous system.*

parasympatholytic – An agent that decreases the actions of the parasympathetic nervous system.

parasympathomimetic – An agent that increases the actions of the parasympathetic nervous system.

parathyroid gland – One of four small glands attached to the thyroid gland. The primary function of the parathyroid glands is to secrete parathyroid hormone, which is responsible for absorption of calcium and its distribution in bone and blood.

parenteral – Pertaining to some means of administration other than the digestive tract.

parenteral injection – A dosage form usually intended to be administered intravenously, subcutaneously, or intramuscularly.

parenteral nutrition – A combination of amino acids, dextrose, fats, vitamins, minerals, electrolytes, and water administered intravenously. Parenteral nutrition is capable of providing all the nutrients needed to sustain life. Parenteral nutrition is often used for patients with gastrointestinal diseases that preclude eating or limit nutrient absorption (e.g., intestinal surgery) and for conditions where patients are not able to eat enough to maintain a nutritional balance (e.g., cancer). Parenteral nutrition

P

may be short-term, lasting for only a few days, or long-term, lasting for months to years.

paresthesia – An abnormal, usually unpleasant, sensation such as numbness, tingling, or prickling.

Parkinson's disease – A chronic, progressive, degenerative condition of the central nervous system characterized by tremors and muscle stiffness. As the disease progresses it causes difficulty walking and speaking.

parkinsonian – Pertaining to Parkinson's disease.

parkinsonism – *See Parkinson's disease.*

paroxysm – A sudden onset of a disease or symptom of a disease. Also, a sudden spasm or a convulsion.

participating (PAR) pharmacy – A pharmacy that agrees with a health plan to be a participating provider. *Also see participating (PAR) provider.*

participating (PAR) physician – A physician who agrees with a health plan to be a participating provider. *Also see participating (PAR) provider.*

participating (PAR) provider – An individual or institution that supplies health care services to consumers and who contracts with a managed care organization to provide those services to the organization's members. Participating providers may include physicians, pharmacists, hospitals, clinics, dentists, physical therapists, psychologists, etc.

particulate matter – In pharmacy, the granular or flocculent material found in a pharmaceutical preparation that should be free of any such matter. Particulate matter is primarily a concern when it appears in an intravenous solution. Particles may indicate the presence of microbial contamination or a chemical incompatibility between two or more of the solution's ingredients.

parturition – The process of childbirth.

paste – A semisolid pharmaceutical preparation intended for external use. Some pastes contain a medication while others are used for hygiene (e.g., toothpaste).

P

pastil – A lozenge intended to dissolve in the mouth. The medication in a pastil is intended to treat the mucosal lining of the mouth and throat.

pastille – *See pastil.*

patent – A legal grant of exclusivity to produce a product. Patents are granted by the United States Patent Office and stay in effect for 17 years after approval. In the case of drugs, this 17 years marks the time the patent holder can produce and market a drug without competition from generic manufacturers. During this time the manufacturer tries to recoup research and development costs plus make a profit.

patent medicine – A nonprescription drug whose ingredients are protected by patent. *Also see patent.*

path- – Prefix designating disease.

patho- – Prefix designating disease.

pathogen – A microorganism that is capable of producing disease. For example, most bacteria are considered either to be able to cause disease (pathogenic) or incapable of producing disease (nonpathogenic). In some cases, a microorganism may be pathogenic in one species (e.g., dogs) but not in another (e.g., humans).

pathogenesis – The origin of disease, specifically the biochemical process whereby the disease began and progressed.

pathogenic – Disease-producing.

pathognomic – Pertaining to a characteristic sign or symptom of a disease that is seen in no other condition. A pathognomic sign establishes a conclusive diagnosis for that condition. An example is Kopliks' spots, the characteristic rash inside the mouth that is only seen with measles infection.

pathologic fracture – A broken bone that is the result of a disease process. Pathologic fractures occur without any apparent trauma to the involved bone. For example, they result from a cancer that invades bone and weakens the bone to the extent that it breaks spontaneously.

P

pathologist – A physician who specializes in the diagnosis of disease and in providing facilities for other physicians to establish accurate diagnoses. A pathologist may examine or chemically test specimens from body fluids, biopsy, surgery, or autopsy. Pathologists also supervise clinical laboratories.

pathology – The specialty of medicine that involves all aspects of disease, most particularly the microscopic and biochemical changes that occur during the disease process.

pathway – A sequence of chemical reactions. Often used in the context of a metabolic pathway, the chemical chain of events that affects an agent from the time it enters the organism until it is eliminated.

-pathy – Suffix designating disease; for example, neuropathy.

patient – A person who is receiving the services of a health care practitioner.

patient chart – *See medical record.*

payer – Any individual or organization that is ultimately responsible for health care bills. Payers may include insurance companies, trade unions, employers, trusts, or foundations.

payor – *See payer.*

PBM – *See pharmacy benefit management company.*

p.c. – Abbreviation commonly used on prescriptions for the Latin *post cibum*, meaning after a meal.

PCP – *See primary care physician.*

ped- – Prefix designating child or foot.

pedal – Pertaining to the feet.

pedi- – Prefix designating child or foot.

pediatric – Pertaining to pediatrics.

pediatrician – A physician who specializes in the health of children. Depending upon local custom, pediatricians may treat children from birth up through ages 12 to 18.

pediatrics – The medical specialty concerned with the diagnosis and treatment of disease and the general health of children from birth through adolescence.

pediculosis – A lice infestation. Lice primarily affect hairy areas of the body, including the top of the head, eyebrows, eyelids, underarms, chest, and pubic area.

pedo- – Prefix designating child or foot.

peer review – A process where one or more physicians examine the appropriateness of the professional activities of other physicians. Peer review may examine diagnostic procedures, postsurgical complications, drug prescribing patterns, length of hospitalizations, and other factors. In a hospital, peer review may result in continuation or denial of privileges. In a managed care organization, peer review may result in continuation or discontinuation of a contract with a provider.

pellagra – A nutritional deficit that leads to diarrhea and skin ulcers. Pellagra is caused by a deficiency of niacin and tryptophan. Pellagra is most often caused by the inability to absorb niacin and tryptophan, poor diet, or chronic alcoholism.

pelvic inflammatory disease (PID) – An infection of the uterine lining that may spread into the fallopian tubes. Signs and symptoms include foul-smelling vaginal discharge and abdominal pain. The most common causes of PID are gonorrhea and chlamydia.

pemphigus – A serious skin condition characterized by the eruption of large, fluid-filled blisters that easily rupture, leaving raw skin. People afflicted with pemphigus often feel weak and are at risk of skin infections. Untreated pemphigus is usually fatal. Treatment consists of corticosteroids and any necessary supportive treatment (e.g., fluids, antibiotics). The cause of pemphigus is unknown.

-penia – Suffix designating a lack or deficiency. For example, neutropenia is a deficiency of neutrophils.

penicillin – A class of antibiotics derived in whole or in part from the mold *Penicillium notatum*. Penicillin G was the first purified antibiotic to be used clinically. Chemical derivatives of penicillin G are widely used in medicine.

penis – The male primary sex organ. Within the penis, the urethra delivers semen during copulation and also provides passage for urine during elimination.

pep pill – Colloquial term for a stimulant.

pepsin – The primary digestive enzyme in the stomach. The stomach secretes pepsinogen and hydrochloric acid when food enters. Hydrochloric acid converts pepsinogen to pepsin and churns these chemicals with the food to begin the process of digestion.

peptic – Pertaining to digestion or pepsin.

peptic ulcer – An erosion of the lining of either the stomach or the duodenum. More specifically, an ulcer in the stomach is called a gastric ulcer while one in the duodenum is called a duodenal ulcer. Duodenal ulcers account for about 90% of peptic ulcers. Although some individuals never experience significant discomfort, peptic ulcer typically causes a burning pain that may be temporarily relieved with food or antacids. Treatment usually consists of a combination of antacids and drugs that reduce acid secretion. Antibiotics may also be used if *Helicobacter pylori* (*see* *Helicobacter pylori*), a bacterium often found in association with peptic ulcer, is present. Since effective treatments for this organism have been discovered, patients improve faster and experience fewer relapses.

peptide – A chemical compound comprised of two or more amino acids.

per- – Prefix designating through or by.

per member per month (PMPM) – A mathematical expression commonly used by health insurers to determine the average monthly cost of a program for each member served by an insurance benefit. PMPM allows health plans to track their basic costs as the number of members fluctuates from one time period to another. PMPM is determined by dividing the cost of a program over a specific period of time by the number of participants in that program and dividing again by the number of months in

P

that time period. For example, if claims paid for a prescription drug program for a fiscal year quarter total $3,075,000 for 100,000 eligible members, the PMPM of this program can be determined by dividing the claims cost ($3,075,000) by the number of eligible members (100,000 members) and by the number of months covered (3 months). The PMPM for this program would be $10.25.

percolation – A process where drugs or other chemicals are extracted from their natural sources (e.g., leaves, roots, animal tissue) by passing a solute through a column of the source.

percutaneous – Pertaining to the passage of a substance through intact skin. Medicines in skin patches (e.g., estrogen, nicotine, etc.) reach the bloodstream by means of percutaneous absorption.

perforation – A hole or puncture. A perforated duodenal ulcer, for example, is an ulcer that has eroded all the way through the wall of the stomach or intestine.

perfusion – The passage of blood or other fluid into an organ or tissue.

peri- – Prefix designating around or about.

perianal – The area surrounding the anus.

pericarditis – Inflammation of the pericardium.

pericardium – The membrane that surrounds the heart. The space between the membrane and the heart is filled with a small amount of fluid for lubrication. The pericardium attaches to the blood vessels entering the heart and to the abdominal diaphragm. Its purpose is to hold the heart in its proper place.

perigastric – Pertaining to the area surrounding the stomach.

perigastritis – Inflammation of the outer lining of the stomach.

periglottis – The mucous membrane lining the tongue.

perinatal – The period of time ranging from 28 weeks of pregnancy to one week after birth.

P

perinatologist – A physician who specializes in perinatology.

perinatology – The subspecialty of obstetrics that deals with the diagnosis and treatment of medical problems of fetuses during the last few weeks of pregnancy.

perineal – Pertaining to the perineum.

perineum – The area between the legs that extends from the coccyx (tailbone) to the pubis. The perineum includes the anus and the genitals.

period – *See menstrual period.*

periodic – Pertaining to an event that happens at regular intervals.

perioperative – Pertaining to the period of time just before, during, and just after a surgical operation.

perioral – Pertaining to the area around the mouth.

periorbial – Pertaining to the area around the eye sockets.

periosteum – The membrane that covers the surface of bones everywhere except in the joints. The periosteum supports blood vessels and nerves that supply the bones.

peripheral – Pertaining to a position or location away from the center. For example, peripheral blood vessels are those that supply blood to the areas away from the heart and lungs.

peripheral resistance – The resistance of arteries to blood flow. The degree of peripheral resistance is determined by the diameter of blood vessels and the force of contraction exerted by vascular smooth muscle. Peripheral resistance is one factor that accounts for blood pressure.

peripheral vascular disease – Any abnormal condition of the blood vessels outside of the heart.

peristalsis – The rhythmic movement of the intestinal tract that propels nutrients and wastes along its course. Peristalsis is responsible for nutrients being digested properly and reaching their sites of absorption and for delivering solid wastes to the rectum and anus.

peristaltic – Pertaining to peristalsis.

peritoneal – Pertaining to the peritoneum.

peritoneum – The membrane that covers the inside of the abdominal cavity and the organs within the abdomen.

peritonitis – Inflammation of the peritoneum. Infections in the peritoneum spread quickly, are usually difficult to treat, and are extremely dangerous.

perkinism – A form of quackery that involves treatment with magnets and magic.

permeable – Capable of allowing fluids to pass through. Often used in the context of a permeable membrane, a barrier that allows passage of a fluid and materials dissolved in it.

pernicious – Pertaining to a condition that is usually fatal without adequate treatment.

pernicious anemia – A disorder of red blood cells that causes them to develop into an enlarged, misshapen form. Pernicious anemia is caused by the inability to absorb vitamin B_{12} from the diet.

peroral – By mouth.

peroxide – A molecule that has two linked oxygen atoms. Peroxides are chemically unstable and easily release one of the highly reactive oxygen molecules. The most commonly used example is hydrogen peroxide, an antiseptic.

peroxy- – Prefix designating a peroxide.

pestle – A grinding or mixing tool often used in the preparation of a compounded prescription. Normally used along with a mortar.

petechia – A minute hemorrhage about the size of a pinhead. Such hemorrhages usually indicate a lack of blood platelets or a dysfunction of platelets.

petechiae – Plural form of petechia.

petechial – Pertaining to petechiae.

P

petit mal epilepsy – A seizure disorder characterized by loss of consciousness, sometimes with muscle twitching. Petit mal epilepsy most commonly affects children.

petrolatum – A semisolid oily substance derived from petroleum and frequently used as a base in ointments. The best known trademarked form of petrolatum is Vaseline.

pg – Abbreviation for picogram.

pH – A chemical expression that indicates the degree of acidity or alkalinity of a solution. A solution with a pH 7 is considered neutral while solutions with values lower than 7 are considered acids and those with values higher than 7 are bases. The pH of human blood ranges from 7.35 to 7.45.

-phage – Suffix designating something that eats. For example, a macrophage is a large cell that engulfs and digests invading bacteria.

phago- – Prefix designating something that eats.

phagocyte – A cell that has the ability to ingest and digest bacteria, protozoa, and other cells and cellular debris. Phagocytes are an important part of the body's defense against infection.

phagocytosis – The process of eating and digesting foreign cells and cellular debris.

phall- – Prefix designating the penis.

phalli- – Prefix designating the penis.

phallic – Pertaining to the penis.

phallo- – Prefix designating the penis.

phallodynia – Pain in the penis.

phallorrhea – Any abnormal discharge from the penis. Phallorrhea is often an indication of infection, particularly a sexually transmitted disease.

pharmaceutic – *See pharmaceutical.*

P

pharmaceutical – Pertaining to drugs, pharmacy, or the sciences that form the basis of pharmacy.

Also, a commercially prepared or compounded medication.

pharmaceutical care – A strategy of involving pharmacists in the responsible provision of drug therapy for the purpose of achieving desirable treatment outcomes. In so doing, the pharmacist becomes an active participant in planning treatments, educating patients, communicating with physicians, and monitoring changes in patients' conditions.

Pharmaceutical Research and Manufacturers of America – The industrial association of approximately 100 companies that engage in the development and manufacture of new drugs. Formerly called the Pharmaceutical Manufacturers' Association.

pharmaceutics – The science that relates to the manufacture or extemporaneous compounding of drug dosage forms.

pharmacist – A graduate of a college of pharmacy. Prior to practicing, pharmacists must also pass a state-administered licensing examination. Currently, the pharmacy curriculum is a minimum of five years and culminates in a bachelor of science degree. By 2004 all new pharmacists must graduate from a six-year doctor of pharmacy (Pharm.D.) program.

pharmaco- – Prefix designating drugs.

pharmacodynamics – The study of the interaction of drugs with their sites of action. Pharmacodynamics examines the way drugs bind with their receptors, the concentration required to elicit a response, and the time required for each of these events.

pharmacoeconomics – The science concerned with assessing costs of drug therapy versus the likely results of those treatments.

pharmacognosist – An individual who is trained in pharmacognosy. A pharmacognosist may or may not be a pharmacist or physician.

pharmacognosy – The pharmaceutical science that deals with the identification of natural substances (e.g., herbs, animal tissue) that have medicinal value. Pharmacognosy also involves the identification and extraction of the medicinally active components.

P

pharmacokinetic – Pertaining to pharmacokinetics.

pharmacokinetics – The pharmaceutical science that deals with the absorption, distribution, metabolism, and elimination of drugs and the amount of time each of these requires. In many cases, pharmacokinetics can explain the reasons why different people react differently to a drug.

pharmacologic – *See pharmacological.*

pharmacological – Pertaining to pharmacology.

Also used to describe a dose of a hormone or nutrient far in excess of the normal amount. The term denotes that the natural substance is being used for drug effect rather than for its usual purpose. Higher doses may have different physiological effects and more side effects than usual. For example, the high doses of vitamin C some people take to treat or prevent common colds are pharmacological doses.

pharmacologist – An individual who is trained in pharmacology. A pharmacologist may or may not be a pharmacist or physician.

pharmacology – The study of how drugs affect living organisms.

pharmacopoeia – A reference book that contains the official standards for drug preparation and manufacture. In the United States, these standards are listed in the *United States Pharmacopoeia* (USP) and the *National Formulary* (NF).

pharmacotherapy – The use of drugs to treat disease.

pharmacy – The art and science that relates to the preparation and standardization of drugs. Pharmacy may include the cultivation and harvest of medicinal plants, extraction of drugs from plants, synthesis of chemicals with medicinal properties, chemical analysis of drugs, and examination of the effects of drugs on living systems. Pharmacists may compound prescriptions into dosage forms (e.g., tablets, capsules, ointments, solutions) appropriate for patient use. They also advise patients on the proper use of medicines.

Also, a drugstore where prescriptions are prepared and dispensed.

P

pharmacy and therapeutics (P&T) committee – In managed care, a panel, usually composed of physicians, pharmacists, and sometimes other health care practitioners, that advises management on issues that relate to the pharmacy benefit and the general use of medications within the plan. The P&T committee often makes the final determination regarding which drugs are included on the plan's formulary.

In a hospital, the P&T committee is comprised primarily of physicians and is a committee of the medical staff. The P&T committee determines which drugs are to be included in the hospital's formulary, approves policies relating to the function of the pharmacy department, and sets policies regarding the use of drugs within the hospital and its clinics.

pharmacy benefit management company (PBM) – Originally, a private organization that processed prescription drug claims for managed care organizations and other health care payers. PBMs have evolved to the point where they organize pharmacy networks, negotiate discounts with their network pharmacies, contract with pharmaceutical manufacturers for preferred pricing, and implement cost-control programs for their payer clients.

pharmacy claim – A request to an insurer for reimbursement for a professional service rendered. In most cases, pharmacy claims are for prescriptions dispensed. In some cases they may be for patient education or counseling services.

pharmacy services administrative organization (PSAO) – A network of pharmacies that seeks to contract with managed care organizations, employer groups, or pharmacy benefit management companies.

Pharm.D. – Abbreviation for doctor of pharmacy.

pharyng- – Prefix designating the throat.

pharyngeal – Pertaining to the throat.

pharyngitis – Inflammation of the mucous membranes that line the throat. Sore throat.

pharyngo- – Prefix designating the throat.

P

pharyngospasm – A sudden contraction of the muscles of the throat.

pharynx – The throat.

Ph.D. – Abbreviation for doctor of philosophy. A Ph.D. degree may be granted in almost any discipline and is usually considered to be the ultimate degree in its field.

phenothiazine – A class of drugs used primarily for the treatment of psychosis. Some of these drugs are used in pain control and treatment of nausea and vomiting.

Ph.G. – Abbreviation for graduate in pharmacy, a designation that dates back to the time before a bachelor of science degree was required in pharmacy.

-phil – Suffix designating a love of or affinity for. For example, a chemical is said to be hydrophilic if it is easily dissolved in water.

-phile – Suffix designating a love of or affinity for. For example, a chemical is said to be a hydrophile if it is easily dissolved in water.

-philia – Suffix designating a love of or affinity for. For example, a chemical is said to be hydrophilic if it is easily dissolved in water.

-philic – Suffix designating a love of or affinity for. For example, a chemical is said to be hydrophilic if it is easily dissolved in water.

phleb- – Prefix designating a vein.

phlebitis – An inflammation of a vein. Phlebitis may result from irritation caused by an intravenous catheter. Phlebitis is often accompanied by a blood clot (thrombophlebitis), a dangerous situation that can lead to a stroke or pulmonary embolus.

phlebo- – Prefix designating a vein.

phlebotomy – Entry into a vein with the intention of extracting blood for a laboratory test or blood donation.

phlegm – Thick or excessive mucus in the respiratory tract. Phlegm often accompanies asthma or a respiratory infection.

P

phobia – An unreasonable and persistent fear of a specific person, place, activity, or situation.

-phobia – Suffix designating an unreasonable and persistent fear; for example, microphobia (fear of bacteria), acrophobia (fear of heights), agoraphobia (fear of open places).

phobic – Pertaining to phobia.

phocomelia – A birth defect of the arms and/or legs that causes the hands or feet to attach close to the body so that they give the appearance of flippers. Phocomelia may occur in a child whose mother has taken thalidomide during pregnancy.

phot- – Prefix designating light.

photo- – Prefix designating light.

photodermatitis – Any inflammation of the skin caused by exposure to ultraviolet radiation. Photodermatitis includes increased sun sensitivity caused by drugs and allergic reaction to excessive sunlight.

photophobia – Unusual intolerance or sensitivity to light, especially light in the eyes.

photosensitization – Extreme reaction to light, particularly ultraviolet radiation from the sun. Photosensitization can be caused by a wide variety of drugs and typically causes severe sunburn after even brief exposure to sunlight.

phototoxic – Pertaining to a harmful exposure to light.

-phrenia – Suffix designating the diaphragm or the brain; for example, schizophrenia.

PHS – *See Public Health Service.*

physi- – Prefix designating physical.

physiatrist – A physician who specializes in evaluating and treating patients by means of physical therapy.

physical – Pertaining to the body as compared with the mind or emotions.

P

physical examination – An assessment of the body to determine its state of health. Physical examination involves observation of visible body tissues and structures, palpation of body structures, listening to body functions (e.g., heart, lung, and bowel sounds), and often X-ray examination and blood testing. In women, physical examination often includes breast and pelvic examinations. In men, it often includes prostate examination.

physical therapist – An individual trained in the evaluation and treatment of patients with physical disorders or limitations. Physical therapists have a minimum of a bachelor of science degree from an accredited physical therapy program and are licensed by the state.

physical therapy – The treatment of medical disorders by means of massage, manipulation, stretching, exercises, cold or heat applications, or a wide variety of other manual or manipulative treatments.

physician – A graduate of an accredited school of medicine who has passed the state licensure examination for medicine. A physician may hold either a doctor of medicine (M.D.) or doctor of osteopathy (D.O.) degree.

physician assistant (P.A.) – A person who works under the supervision of a physician and has been trained in physical examination, patient evaluation, and treatment of common medical problems. Physician assistants must graduate from a rigorous training program, pass a national certification examination, and participate in continuing education programs.

physician dispensing – A practice whereby a physician provides directly to the patient the medications he/she prescribes. Physician dispensing is a revenue-producing activity for the physician.

physio- – Prefix designating physical.

physiologic – See *physiological*.

physiological – Pertaining to normal body processes.

physiologist – A person trained in the science of physiology. A physiologist may or may not be a physician.

P

physiology – The science that deals with the normal physical and chemical processes of life. Physiology deals with how living organisms function. Physiology is one of the sciences that provides basic information for all of the health professions.

physiotherapist – See *physical therapist*.

physiotherapy – See *physical therapy*.

phyt- – Prefix designating plants.

phyto- – Prefix designating plants.

phytodermatitis – Any skin condition caused by exposure to plants (e.g., poison ivy rash).

phytoestrogen – A chemical agent derived from a plant that causes physiologic changes similar to the naturally occurring female hormone estrogen. Some of the herbal remedies that are used to treat symptoms of menopause contain phytoestrogens.

phytotoxin – A poison or poisonous substance derived from a plant.

pico- – Prefix designating one-trillionth (10^{-12}).

picogram (pg) – One-trillionth of a gram. Radioimmunoassay tests are able to detect amounts of substances this small.

PID – See *pelvic inflammatory disease*.

pigment – Any substance that gives color. For example, the iris of the eye, red blood cells, and skin all contain pigments that give them their characteristic colors.

pigmentation – The coloring of an organ or tissue. Pigmentation most commonly applies to the skin. Some diseases cause abnormal skin pigmentation.

pile – A single hemorrhoid. Also see *hemorrhoid*.

pill – A medicine initially compounded or manufactured as a putty. Measured portions of the putty are rolled into spheres that may or may not be coated. Pills are intended for oral administration.

Tablets are produced by an entirely different process and are often mistakenly referred to as pills. Birth control pills, for example, are actually tablets.

pill-rolling – A motion with the fingertips that resembles that of a pharmacist forming a pill. Pill-rolling motion is a common sign of neurologic disease, particularly Parkinson's disease.

pimple – A pus-filled skin lesion characteristic of acne. *Also see comedo.*

pinkeye – An acute, contagious infection of the eye. *Also see conjunctivitis.*

pint – A fluid measure in the English system of weights and measures. A pint contains 16 fluid ounces or 473.166 milliliters.

pinworm – A parasitic worm that infests the intestines and rectum.

pitting edema – An abnormal collection of fluid that, when pressed firmly, leaves an indentation. Pitting edema is most commonly found in the feet or ankles and indicates that water is not being properly eliminated. Pitting edema may be a sign of kidney or heart disease.

pituitary gland – A small endocrine organ attached to the base of the brain. The pituitary gland secretes a wide variety of hormones that either directly regulate body functions or cause secretion of other hormones that affect body functions.

placebo – An inert substance given to a patient instead of an active medicine. Placebos are often given to people who participate in studies intended to evaluate the effectiveness of a medicine. Studies of pain in postoperative patients have shown that over 30% of patients who receive a placebo report some relief of pain. *Also see control group, double-blind study.*

placenta – A structure within the uterus that transfers nutrients and oxygen from mother to fetus during pregnancy.

placental barrier – An impediment to the passage of drugs from a woman's bloodstream to her fetus. In reality, the placental barrier generally acts only as a filter, blocking passage only of drugs that have large molecules. Most drugs a woman takes during pregnancy reach her fetus as well. Some of these are capable of causing birth defects. *Also see barrier.*

plaque – A patch on the surface of the skin, a tooth, a mucous membrane, or the lining of an artery. Arterial plaques are caused by

P

lipid deposits and in susceptible individuals may lead to myocardial infarction, coronary artery disease, or stroke.

plasma – The fluid portion of blood that remains after all blood cells have been removed. Plasma consists of water and dissolved proteins and amino acids, glucose, fats and fatty acids, electrolytes, gases, and metabolic wastes.

plasma level – The concentration of a drug in blood plasma. Plasma levels are often used to determine if the dose of a drug is sufficient to produce a therapeutic effect and to prevent toxicity.

plateau – A flattened area of a graph. In pharmacy, plateau refers to the period of time where blood levels of a drug flatten out, i.e., the rate of drug absorption equals the rate of drug elimination.

platelet – A blood cell formed in bone marrow that initiates blood clotting. Platelets are essential for controlling bleeding episodes; however, platelets can also trigger inappropriate blood clots inside veins. These clots can lead to myocardial infarctions, strokes, or pulmonary emboli.

platelet inhibitor – A drug that reduces the clotting ability of blood platelets. Platelet inhibitors can reduce the risk of myocardial infarction and stroke in patients at risk of those conditions. Aspirin is the most commonly used platelet inhibitor.

-plegia – Suffix designating paralysis; for example, paraplegia.

pleura – The membrane that lines the outside of the lungs. The pleura contains a plasma-like fluid that reduces friction during respiration.

pleurisy – An inflammation of the pleural lining of the lungs. Pleurisy causes intense pain with breathing.

PMPM – *See per member per month.*

PMS – *See premenstrual syndrome.*

-pnea – Suffix designating breath or breathing; for example, hyperpnea, apnea.

pneumo- – Prefix designating the lungs or air.

pneumococcal – Pertaining to *Streptococcus pneumoniae*, the bacterium that causes most cases of pneumonia.

pneumococcemia – Presence of *Streptococcus pneumonia*e in the blood.

pneumococci – Plural form of pneumococcus.

pneumococcus – *Streptococcus pneumoniae*, the bacterium that causes most cases of pneumonia.

pneumoconiosis – Any lung disease caused by chronically breathing dust or other particles. Black lung disease of coal miners is one form of pneumoconiosis.

P*neumocystis carinii* – An opportunistic protozoa that primary infects immunosuppressed persons. The organism can cause a difficult-to-treat form of pneumonia in infants, the elderly, and cancer patients. It most commonly affects persons with AIDS. Signs include fever, cough, and rapid heart rate. Diagnosis is difficult, usually involving examination of cells obtained from the linings of the bronchi.

pneumon- – Prefix designating the lungs or air.

pneumonia – Inflammation of the lung characterized by fluid filling the alveoli and bronchioles. Pneumonia may be caused by inhaling irritating chemicals or by infection with bacteria, viruses, fungi, protozoa, or rickettsiae. Over 50 causes of pneumonia are known, but the most common cause is bacterial infection with the pneumococcus *Streptococcus pneumoniae*.

pneumonic – Pertaining to the lungs.

pneumono- – Prefix designating the lungs or air.

p.o. – Abbreviation often used on prescriptions for the Latin *per os*, meaning by mouth.

pod- – Prefix designating the foot or the likeness of a foot.

podiatric – Pertaining to podiatry.

podiatrist – A health care practitioner trained in the diagnosis and treatment of disorders of the feet and ankles. Treatments may include physical therapy, drug therapy, and surgery. After successfully completing a course of study at a college of podiatry,

P

podiatrists are granted a doctor of podiatric medicine degree (D.P.M.). Podiatrists must be licensed by the state before they can practice.

podiatry – The health care specialty that deals with the health of the feet and ankles.

poditis – Any inflammation of the foot.

podo- – Prefix designating the foot or the likeness of a foot.

-poiesis – Suffix designating production or formation; for example, hematopoiesis, production of blood cells.

poikilothermia – A condition where body temperature increases or decreases to match environmental temperature.

poison – A substance that causes illness or death when ingested or absorbed, even if administered in small amounts. Poisons may come from synthetic sources (e.g., nerve gas) or from natural sources such as plants (e.g., cyanide, strychnine).

poisonous – Pertaining to the characteristics of a poison.

polio – *See poliomyelitis.*

poliomyelitis – A potentially fatal viral infection that causes inflammation of the spinal cord, often with resulting permanent paralysis. Signs and symptoms of acute poliomyelitis include fever, sore throat, headache, vomiting, and stiffness in the neck and back. Most cases of poliomyelitis can be prevented with vaccination.

pollen – The male sex cells formed in flowering plants, trees, and grasses. Airborne pollens may trigger allergic reactions in susceptible persons.

pollinosis – Allergic rhinitis (hay fever) caused by allergic reactions to inhaled pollen.

poly – Abbreviated form of polymorphonuclear leukocyte, a neutrophil.

poly- – Prefix designating multiple.

polyarthritis – Inflammation of more than one joint at the same time.

P

polycythemia vera – An abnormal increase in production of blood cells. Polycythemia vera is a serious condition that can be controlled by removing blood and by chemotherapy that reduces the activity of bone marrow cells.

polydipsia – Excessive thirst. Polydipsia is often a symptom of undiagnosed or poorly controlled diabetes mellitus.

polymyalgia – Pain in more than one muscle group.

polyneuritis – Painful inflammation in more than one nerve, and usually in a large number of nerves.

polyphagia – Excessive food intake. Polyphagia is often a symptom of undiagnosed or poorly controlled diabetes mellitus.

polypharmacy – The practice of prescribing multiple medicines to a single patient simultaneously. In general, it is better to use as few medicines as possible. Polypharmacy increases the patient's costs of treatment as well as increasing the chances for side effects and drug interactions.

polysaccharide – A carbohydrate composed of three or more sugar molecules. A complex carbohydrate.

polyuria – Excessive elimination of urine. Polyuria is often a symptom of undiagnosed or poorly controlled diabetes mellitus.

population – A statistical and epidemiologic term that designates all the objects or people in a class or study group.

positive – Indication as part of a physical examination or a laboratory test that a finding is present. For example, a positive pregnancy test indicates that the subject is indeed pregnant.

Also see false positive.

posology – The specialty within pharmacology that deals with determining proper doses of drugs.

post- – Prefix designating after or behind.

postfebrile – After a fever.

postictal – After a seizure or a stroke.

P

postmarketing surveillance – Research on drugs already on the market conducted by independent investigators and funded by drug manufacturers. The purpose of postmarketing surveillance is to gain further knowledge about new drugs that have been released on the market. Postmarketing surveillance provides further information about clinical uses of drugs and side effects and is required by the United States Food and Drug Administration (FDA).

postmenopausal – Pertaining to the time following the permanent cessation of menses.

postpartum – After childbirth.

postprandial – After a meal.

postural – Pertaining to the position of the body.

postural hypotension – A condition where standing up from a lying or sitting position causes a precipitous drop in blood pressure that can cause dizziness or even fainting. Postural hypotension is most commonly caused by the drugs that are used to treat hypertension.

potassium – An electrolyte found in blood, nerve tissue, and muscle fibers. Potassium is necessary for normal cardiac and muscle function.

potency – Strength or power, including that of a medicine. Depending upon context, potency may refer to the amount of active drug in a dosage form, particularly if the drug is close to its expiration date.

Potency may also refer to the pharmacologic activity of a drug based on its milligram strength. For example, the diuretic hydrochlorothiazide (HCTZ) is 10 times as potent as its relative chlorothiazide (CTZ). Thus, a 25 mg dose of HCTZ produces the same amount of urine as a 250 mg dose of CTZ.

potentiation – An interaction between two drugs that causes an effect greater than would have been expected from the additive properties of the drugs involved. For example, alcohol potentiates the sedating effects of the tranquilizer diazepam when the two drugs are ingested at the same time.

P

potion – A large dose of liquid medicine or poison.

pound – A weight in the English system of weights and measures that equals 16 ounces or 454 grams.

powder paper – In pharmacy, a square or rectangular paper folded into the shape of an envelope and filled with a dose of powdered medicine. The patient usually prepares a dose by opening one of the envelopes and mixing the contents with water or other suitable vehicle and consuming the mixture.

PPO – *See preferred provider organization.*

practice – The application of a health care profession. Such practice may include evaluation, diagnosis, treatment, and maintenance of health in patients.

practice guidelines – A set of instructions or protocols for physicians to follow in diagnosing and treating certain conditions. Practice guidelines may be highly flexible or tightly controlled. Managed care organizations often use practice guidelines to determine whether a patient's medical care complies with organizational policies and procedures. Practice guidelines may be developed by the managed care organization itself, by a government agency, by a professional association, or by a private company.

practitioner – A person who engages in the application of a health care profession. Practitioners include physicians, pharmacists, nurses, physical therapists, dentists, and many others.

pre- – Prefix designating before or in front of.

precancerous – Pertaining to a lesion that has the potential to become cancerous.

precipitation – The formation of a solid in what was formerly a solution. In some cases precipitation is a desired outcome because it is an indication of the formation of a desired drug or chemical. In other cases (e.g., intravenous solutions), precipitation is highly undesirable and can cause serious harm to a patient if it is administered.

preclinical – Before the onset of disease or before use in humans.

P

preclinical research – When new drugs are developed they are tested for safety and effectiveness in laboratory animals (preclinical testing) before being tried in humans. The results of preclinical testing indicate whether or not the proposed drug is likely to be effective for treating disease and what side effects to anticipate when used in humans.

precursor – That which comes before and is the source for something else.

preeclampsia – Development of serious hypertension along with fluid retention and loss of protein in the urine that develops in 5% to 7% of pregnancies after the fifth month. Symptoms resolve when the pregnancy ends.

preexisting condition – Any medical disorder diagnosed or treated within a specified period of time before a new health insurance policy takes effect. The preexisting conditions that most concern health insurers are chronic conditions and pregnancy. Depending upon the insurance contract, an insurer may provide full coverage for preexisting conditions, not cover them at all, or begin coverage after a specified period of time.

preferred provider – Physicians, hospitals, and other health care providers who contract to provide health services to persons covered by a particular health plan. Preferred providers usually offer substantial discounts to managed care organizations in return for patient referrals.

preferred provider organization (PPO) – A health plan that contracts with providers of medical care for significant discounts on service in return for patient referrals. PPOs select providers in a wide variety of specialties (e.g., primary care, cardiology, surgery, dermatology, etc.) to provide as many types of medical service within its own network as possible. While it is easier for a PPO member than an HMO member to see a specialist or an out-of-network provider, there are usually financial incentives (e.g., deductibles, copayments, etc.) for members to stay within the PPO network.

PPOs and health maintenance organizations (HMOs) are the two principle types of managed care organizations. However, PPOs

P

are usually less tightly controlled and their premiums are often higher.

pregnancy – The condition of carrying one or more embryos in the uterus from conception to birth.

preload – The pressure of blood entering the heart from the general circulation. In congestive heart failure, excessive preload over-fills the heart chambers and reduces the force of contraction. Reducing preload, usually with a nitrate drug like nitroglycerin, reduces filling pressure and allows the heart to pump more efficiently.

premature – Occurring before expected. For example, a premature baby is an infant who is born before the 37th week of pregnancy.

premenstrual – Pertaining to the time before menses.

premenstrual syndrome (PMS) – A condition that may occur several days before onset of menses. Symptoms are due to changing hormone levels and include irritability, weight gain, headache, breast discomfort, and mood changes. Symptoms subside when menstruation begins.

premium – The money paid to a health plan to provide insurance coverage. Premiums are usually paid monthly. In some cases an employer may pay 100% of premiums or it may pay part of the premium while employees pay the remainder. In the case of individual plans, the insured pays the entire premium.

prepubertal – Prior to sexual maturity.

prepubescent – Pertaining to the time immediately before sexual maturity.

presby- – Prefix designating advanced age.

presbyo- – Prefix designating advanced age.

presbyopia – Age-related difficulty clearly seeing or reading material at close range. Presbyopia usually occurs after age 40.

prescribe – To order the preparation and consumption of medicine.

prescriber – A health care practitioner who is legally allowed to write prescriptions. Depending upon the state and the circumstances,

P

prescribers may include physicians, pharmacists, nurses, physician assistants, dentists, podiatrists, psychologists, and optometrists.

prescription – A written order for the preparation of medication. A prescription includes at least the following: the name of the patient, the name and strength of the drug and the amount of medicine to be dispensed, the directions for use, and the name of the prescriber.

Also, the medicine so ordered.

prescription drug – A medication that can only be legally dispensed to a patient with a valid prescription. Most prescription drugs are so designated by the United States Food and Drug Administration (FDA); however, states can also designate specific drugs or devices as prescription items. Prescription drugs may only be dispensed by a pharmacist or by the prescriber.

prescription drug plan – The portion of a health insurance policy that provides coverage for prescription drugs. Depending upon the policy, drugs may be fully covered, fully covered after a copayment, covered in part (e.g., 80% coverage), or covered in whole or in part after a deductible.

preservative – A chemical added to foods or drugs to keep them from spoiling. Although a rare occurrence, preservatives in medicines can cause side effects.

pressor – An agent that raises blood pressure. Natural pressors include epinephrine and norepinephrine.

prevalence – The number of cases of a problem or disorder that exist within a geographic location at any point in time. For example, about 1% of the United States population, or approximately 2.5 million Americans, has schizophrenia.

Contrasted with incidence, which is the number of new cases of a disorder or problem that occur in a specified period of time.

preventive care – Any intervention intended to keep a disease from occurring or to keep a mild form of disease from progressing. Preventive care may include regular physical examinations, vaccinations, diet, exercise, smoking cessation, prenatal care, physical therapy, drug therapy, and many others.

P

primary care – The initial level of attention given to a patient. Primary care is usually the basic service given to a patient for a medical condition or as an early detection or preventive measure. Patients with more complicated problems may be referred to a specialist (secondary care).

primary care physician (PCP) – A physician who is trained to diagnose and treat a wide variety of illnesses. The primary care specialties are internal medicine, pediatrics, family practice, and general practice. Some health plans also consider obstetrics-gynecology to be a primary care specialty since gynecology may encompass the general medical care of women.

Most health maintenance organizations (HMOs) require members to select a primary care physician as their entry point into the health care system. Any referrals to specialists are made by the primary care physician.

primary hypertension – High blood pressure that occurs without known cause and accounts for over 90% of cases of high blood pressure. *Also see hypertension.*

primigravida – A woman who is in her first pregnancy.

primipara – A woman who has completed one pregnancy through to childbirth.

Prinzmetal's angina – Sharp pain in the chest or arm that occurs during rest. Unlike more common forms of angina pectoris, Prinzmetal's angina is caused by spasms of the coronary arteries unrelated to exertion.

prior auth – *See prior authorization.*

prior authorization (prior auth) – The process of gaining approval from an insurance company for a treatment or procedure before the service is rendered. For example, a health plan may only pay for some uses of a prescription drug but not for other uses. A physician may receive authorization to use a weight control drug for a patient who is dangerously overweight but not for a patient who only needs to lose a few pounds.

privileges – *See clinical privileges.*

P

p.r.n. – Abbreviation often used on prescriptions for the Latin *pro re nata*, meaning when necessary or as needed.

pro- – Prefix designating before or in front of.

procedure – A specific way of accomplishing a task.

Also, a surgical or diagnostic operation.

proct- – Prefix designating the rectum.

proctitis – Inflammation of the mucous membrane in the rectum and anus.

procto- – Prefix designating the rectum.

prodrome – The early signs or symptoms of a disease.

prodrug – A drug that is metabolically converted to its active form once it is in the body. For example, the antiparkinson prodrug levodopa must be metabolized to its active form, dopamine. The advantage of levodopa is that after an oral dose it is absorbed into brain tissue while dopamine is not. Once in the brain, levodopa is converted to dopamine.

productive cough – A cough that brings up fluid or mucus from the lungs.

profiling – An analytical method used by managed care organizations that summarizes a health care provider's practice patterns over a period of time. Profiling can indicate whether a provider is over- or underutilizing resources for patient care. Providers are typically sent copies of their profiles periodically for the purposes of cost containment and quality improvement.

progesterone – A hormone secreted primarily in women. Progesterone prepares the uterine lining for possible implantation of a fertilized egg during the second half of the menstrual cycle.

progestin – A synthetically produced drug that has progesterone-like properties.

progestogen – Any natural or synthetically produced agent that has progesterone-like properties.

P

prognosis – A prediction of the course and outcome of a disease. For example, the prognosis for a case of influenza in a healthy young adult is full recovery.

progress note – Comments made in a patient's chart that indicate the patient's medical state at the time the notation was made. Progress notes are typically written by a health care professional at the time of contact with the patient. Progress notes provide a history of the patient's past health and medical problems for comparison to present and future encounters.

progressive disease – A medical condition that continues to advance, causing increasing illness or disability; for example, Parkinson's disease.

prolactin – A hormone produced in the pituitary gland that stimulates breast growth and milk production. Both males and females are capable of producing prolactin.

proliferation – Growth and reproduction of cells. For example, the proliferative phase of the menstrual cycle is characterized by thickening of the uterine lining.

proliferative disease – A medical condition that features inappropriate replication of cells; for example, leukemia and lymphoma.

prophylactic – Pertaining to prophylaxis.

Also, a condom used to prevent pregnancy or sexually transmitted diseases.

prophylaxis – The prevention of a disease, usually accomplished by controlling the factors that cause the disease. For example, a single dose of an antibiotic is sometimes injected immediately prior to surgery to prevent postoperative infection.

proprietary name – A trademark assigned by a manufacturer and registered with the United States Patent Office. For example, Tylenol is the proprietary name of drug acetaminophen.

prospective drug evaluation – A review process where the appropriateness of a drug is reviewed before the prescription is dispensed from the pharmacy. When the pharmacist enters a prescription into the pharmacy computer system, a prospective

P

drug evaluation program scans for problems that may include drug interactions, inappropriate dose, time since last refill, compliance with health plan formulary, and other factors. Any problems are reported immediately to the pharmacist for resolution.

prostaglandin – A hormone-like substance originally detected in prostate fluid. Low concentrations of prostaglandins in blood affect a wide variety of bodily functions including pain transmissions, inflammation, gastrointestinal mucus secretions, and uterine contractions.

prostaglandin inhibitor – A drug that reduces the production of prostaglandins in the body. The most commonly used prostaglandin inhibitors are aspirin and the nonsteroidal anti-inflammatory drugs (NSAIDs).

prostate – A gland in males that lies at the base of the urinary bladder and surrounds the urethra. The prostate produces seminal fluid and constricts the urethra during an erection, thus preventing urination during intercourse.

prostatectomy – Surgical removal of all or part of the prostate. Prostatectomy may be performed to treat advanced prostatic hyperplasia or prostate cancer.

prostatic hyperplasia – Enlargement of the prostate. Signs and symptoms include difficulty passing urine, passing only small amounts of urine, and the need to urinate frequently. Prostatic hyperplasia is initially treated with drug therapy but advanced cases may require surgery. Prostatic hyperplasia is common in older men and is not related to prostate cancer.

prostatic hypertrophy – *See prostatic hyperplasia.*

prostatitis – Inflammation of the prostate, usually caused by infection.

prostration – Total exhaustion. Physical collapse. Often caused by exposure to heat (heat prostration) or emotional stress (nervous prostration).

protein – A complex molecule composed of multiple amino acids. Protein comprises about 75% of the mass of most cells once

P

water is removed. Protein is essential for the physical structure of cells and is a major source of energy. Concentrated dietary sources of protein include milk, eggs, red and white meat, fish, and soybeans.

proteinuria – Presence of protein in the urine. Usually an indication of kidney disease.

protocol – The procedures to be followed during an experiment, an examination, or a treatment. Protocols for research studies are usually extensive, written plans that detail selection of subjects for the study, the study design, and the methods for collection and analysis of data.

prototype – The first of its kind. In pharmacy, the first drug in a new class. For example, penicillin G was the prototype for all of the variations on penicillin that followed.

provider – Any individual or institution that supplies health care services to consumers, including physicians, pharmacists, hospitals, clinics, dentists, physical therapists, psychologists, laboratories, etc.

pruritic – Pertaining to pruritus.

pruritus – Itching.

PSAO – *See pharmacy services administrative organization.*

pseud- – Prefix designating false.

pseudo- – Prefix designating false.

pseudoanaphylaxis – A condition that has the same clinical manifestations as an anaphylactic reaction but is not caused by an allergic reaction. Pseudoanaphylaxis is just as dangerous as anaphylaxis and is treated in the same manner. The most common example of pseudoanaphylaxis is an asthmatic reaction to aspirin and related drugs. *Also see anaphylaxis.*

pseudomembranous colitis – An acute, potentially fatal inflammation of the intestine resulting in the formation and passage of intestinal membranes in the stool. Signs and symptoms include vomiting, bloody diarrhea, and abdominal pain. Pseudomembranous colitis is most commonly caused by antibiotic therapy that allows overgrowth of *Clostidium perfringens* in the large intestine.

pseudoparkinsonism – A condition resembling Parkinson's disease. Pseudoparkinsonism is a common side effect of some antipsychotic medications. Unlike Parkinson's disease, pseudoparkinsonism is not progressive and symptoms improve if the dose of the causative agent is reduced or the drug is discontinued.

psoralen-ultraviolet A (PUVA) – A treatment for psoriasis consisting of a dose of a medication (psoralen) that makes skin more sensitive to light, followed by exposure to high intensity ultraviolet (uv-a) radiation. The treatment is intended to make psoriasis lesions shrink.

psoriasis – A chronic skin condition characterized by raised red patches covered with white scale. Psoriasis most often appears on the elbows, knees, scalp, genitalia, and trunk. Patches of psoriasis may also appear at sites of trauma.

psoriatic – Pertaining to psoriasis.

psoriatic arthritis – The combination of psoriasis and joint pain that resembles rheumatoid arthritis. Psoriatic arthritis primarily affects the joints of the fingers and toes.

psych- – Prefix designating the mind.

psyche- – Prefix designating the mind.

psychedelic – Pertaining to a wide range of psychologic symptoms ranging from pleasure to terror, induced by the ingestion of drugs. Such drug ingestions are usually voluntary. Lysergic acid diethylamide (LSD) is an example of a drug capable of causing psychedelic effects.

psychiatric – Pertaining to psychiatry.

psychiatrist – A physician who specializes in the diagnosis and treatment of mental illness.

psychiatry – The specialty of medicine that deals with the diagnosis and treatment of mental illness.

psycho- – Prefix designating the mind.

P

psychoactive drug – *See psychotropic drug.*

psychologic – Pertaining to psychology.

psychological – *See psychologic.*

psychologist – An individual who is trained in psychology. Psychologists may specialize in clinical psychology, industrial psychology, animal psychology, experimental psychology, or any of a number of other areas.

A clinical psychologist is trained in evaluating, diagnosing, and treating mental and emotional conditions in humans. Clinical psychologists must possess a minimum of a master's degree in psychology, serve a supervised internship, and pass a state licensure examination.

psychology – The science that deals with normal and abnormal thought processes and their effects on behavior.

psychopharmaceutical – A drug used in the treatment of mental illness.

psychopharmacology – A subspecialty within pharmacology that deals with drugs that are used to treatment mental illness as well as drugs that cause psychiatric side effects.

psychoses – Plural of psychosis.

psychosis – A mental disorder characterized by loss of contact with reality. Psychosis may occur from no apparent physical cause (functional psychosis) or may be the result of physical illness or drug ingestion (organic psychosis). Symptoms of psychosis may include hallucinations, depression, agitation, anxiety, delusions, and social isolation. Psychosis may be short-term (e.g., drug ingestion) or may be chronic (e.g., schizophrenia). Even in cases of chronic mental illness, psychotic symptoms may remit with treatment.

psychosomatic illness – A disorder caused by the interaction of emotional stress with one or more organs of the body. For example, peptic ulcer may be induced by intense anxiety. A common misconception is that psychosomatic illnesses are not real. Successful treatment of psychosomatic illness usually involves

P

treatment of the physical ailment along with the underlying emotional cause.

psychotherapist – A counselor who is specially trained in psychotherapy techniques. Psychotherapists include physicians, psychologists, social workers, nurses, school counselors, and others.

psychotherapy – Treatment of emotional disorders by means of verbal and nonverbal techniques rather than by physical means (e.g., drugs, surgery). Psychotherapy usually involves a series of sessions where the therapist and patient discuss the patient's problems, causes of those problems, and ways to resolve the emotional issues involved. Psychotherapy may be done individually or in a group.

psychotic – Pertaining to psychosis.

psychotropic drug – A chemical substance that affects mood, behavior, or any other mental function. The term includes drugs used for treatment (e.g., antidepressants, tranquilizers) as well as drugs of abuse (e.g., cocaine, amphetamine).

PT – Abbreviation for physical therapy or physical therapist.

pt – Abbreviation for patient.

ptosis – *See blepharoptosis.*

puberty – The stage in life where an adolescent begins the physical process of sexual maturity. In girls, the first signs of puberty may appear as early as age 8 and puberty is usually completed by age 16. In boys, the first signs usually appear between ages 10 and 12 and puberty is completed by age 18.

Public Health Service (PHS) – A department of the United States Department of Health and Human Services (HHS) and led by the Surgeon General of the United States. The Public Health Service conducts medical research, administers hospitals and clinics, and controls epidemics and infectious diseases. As part of HHS, the PHS is associated with the Food and Drug Administration, National Library of Medicine, National Institutes of Health, and the Centers for Disease Control.

P

pulmo- – Prefix designating the lungs.

pulmon- – Prefix designating the lungs.

pulmonary – Pertaining to the lungs.

pulmonary circulation – The blood flow and blood vessels within the lungs and between the lungs and the heart.

pulmonary embolus – A blood clot or fat deposit formed in a peripheral blood vessel that breaks free from its site of formation and lodges in a blood vessel in the lung. Signs and symptoms include sudden chest pain and difficulty breathing. If treatment is not initiated in a few hours, the portion of the lung normally supplied by the blocked blood vessel may die. Severe cases of pulmonary embolus are often immediately fatal.

pulmonary hypertension – High blood pressure within the lungs, usually due to high resistance to blood flow. Pulmonary hypertension may precipitate congestive heart failure.

pulmonary medicine – The specialty of medicine that deals with diagnosis and treatment of diseases of the respiratory tract.

pulmono- – Prefix designating the lungs.

pulse – Rhythmic throbbing of an artery caused by contraction and relaxation of the muscles in the arterial wall. After a heart contraction ejects blood into the blood vessels, the rhythmic contractions of the arteries keeps blood moving through the body in a wave-like fashion. Arterial pulses increase or decrease in frequency as the heart rate increases or decreases.

pump – A device that causes liquids or gases to move. For example, an infusion pump is an electronic device that forces a precisely measured amount of intravenous fluid into a patient's vein over a predetermined amount of time.

pupil – The opening at the center of the iris of the eye. Light entering the pupil strikes the retina, causing the perception of an image.

purgative – A laxative.

purulent – Forming or containing pus.

P

pus – A fluid, usually yellow in color, that results from inflammation, most commonly due to bacterial infection. The main constituents of pus are water, protein, and white blood cells.

pustule – A small swelling or bump in the skin that contains pus.

PUVA – *See psoralen-ultraviolet* A.

pyel- – Prefix designating the pelvis of the kidney.

pyelo- – Prefix designating the pelvis of the kidney.

pyelonephritis – An inflammation, usually due to bacterial infection, of the kidney. In most cases, pyelonephritis results from a bladder infection that travels up one or both ureters to the kidneys. Untreated or inadequately treated pyelonephritis can lead to kidney failure.

pyemia – A bacterial infection of the blood that causes formation of abscesses in multiple sites around the body.

pylorus – The muscle at the juncture of the stomach and the duodenum that controls the flow of stomach contents into the small intestine. The pylorus is normally closed but opens to allow the stomach to push partially digested food into the duodenum.

pyo- – Prefix designating pus.

pyoderma – An infection of the skin that causes pus formation; for example, impetigo.

pyogenic – Pertaining to pus formation.

pyorrhea – A discharge of pus, particularly from a dental abscess.

pyr- – Prefix designating fire or heat.

pyretic – Pertaining to fever.

pyrexia – Fever.

pyro- – Prefix designating fire or heat.

pyrogen – An agent that produces fever. Pyrogens include proteins, toxins, bacteria, viruses, and fungi.

pyrogenic – Pertaining to the ability to cause fever.

P

pyuria – The presence of pus in the urine. Pyuria may be caused by kidney disease or a urinary tract infection.

Q

q. – Abbreviation often used on prescriptions for the Latin *quaque*, meaning every.

QA – *See quality assurance.*

q.d. – Abbreviation often used on prescriptions for the Latin *quaque die*, meaning every day.

q.h. – Abbreviation often used on prescriptions for the Latin *quaque hora*, meaning every hour.

QI – *See quality improvement.*

q.i.d. – Abbreviation often used on prescriptions for the Latin *quarter in die*, meaning four times a day.

q.s. – Abbreviation often used on prescriptions for the Latin *quantum sufficiat*, meaning a sufficient quantity.

quack – A person who pretends to have medical knowledge but actually treats patients or sells remedies to patients fraudulently.

quackery – The methods used by a quack.

quadrant – An anatomic area, most commonly the abdomen, that is divided into fourths. The quadrants of the abdomen are the right upper, right lower, left upper, and left lower quadrants. Physicians often use these terms to describe the location of signs and symptoms such as masses and pain.

quadriplegia – Paralysis of all four limbs. Most commonly caused by a traumatic injury.

quality assurance (QA) – A formal monitoring program that assesses the level of care being provided by health care professionals or institutions. The observed level of care is measured against an expected standard. QA is usually part of a quality improvement program.

quality improvement (QI) – A process that identifies problems, implements possible solutions, and then reexamines the situation to determine whether satisfactory improvement has occurred.

quality of life – A subjective evaluation of the impact a treatment has had on a patient's comfort, normal activities, and decision-mak-

Q

ing ability. For example, narcotic treatment for a patient with terminal cancer is intended to improve the quality of the patient's life by relieving pain and the disability it causes. An antihypertensive drug may decrease a specific patient's quality of life because, while reducing blood pressure, it also causes intense, physically limiting side effects.

quarantine – Detention of persons or animals suspected of having a contagious disease. Quarantine of persons is rare in developed countries. Instead, persons with infectious diseases may be placed in isolation where visitors must take appropriate precautions during visits and when leaving.

quicksilver – Colloquial term for the element mercury.

quinolones – *See fluoroquinolones.*

R

R&C – *See reasonable and customary.*

Ra – Chemical symbol for the element radium.

RA – *See rheumatoid arthritis.*

rabies – A viral infection of the central nervous system that initially causes fever, headache, decreased nerve sensations, and muscle pain. After several days, signs and symptoms include delirium, painful muscle contractions, seizures, coma, and usually death. Rabies is carried by warm-blooded animals including dogs, cats, raccoons, skunks, bats, and foxes. The virus is usually present in the saliva of a rabid animal and is transmitted by means of a bite. Rabies may be prevented by vaccination. Once symptoms appear, death is imminent unless intensive treatment is instituted.

racemic – Pertaining to a mixture of molecules that contains an equal number of separable molecules that rotate a beam of light to the left (levorotatory) and to the right (dextrorotatory). *See dextrorotatory, levorotatory.*

rachitic – Pertaining to rickets.

rad – A unit of measure that indicates the amount of radiation absorbed by a gram of tissue.

radiation – The waves of energy or charged atomic particles (e.g., protons, electrons) emitted by an atom. Ionizing radiation (e.g., alpha particles, beta particles, gamma rays) is capable of destabilizing cells. While this is often a useful property in treating cancer, excessive exposure to ionizing radiation can also cause cancer in the exposed areas.

radiation therapy – The use of radioactivity to treat disease. Radiation therapy is most commonly employed in treatment of cancer.

radical – In chemistry, a group of positively or negatively charged molecules or atoms that pass from one molecule to another. Radicals are not able to exist in a free state.

radio- – Prefix designating radiation.

R

radioactivity – The ability of certain elements to give off energy rays or charged particles. Some unstable isotopes have this property as well as all elements with an atomic number greater than 83.

radiograph – The picture produced when radiation, particularly x-rays, interacts with a photographic plate.

radioimmunoassay – A method for determining the concentration of a protein, such as an antigen or antibody, by tagging a radioactive isotope to a substance known to interact with the protein. The radiation activity of the complex is measured, revealing the concentration of the target protein. Radioimmunoassay is extremely sensitive, capable of measuring picograms (trillionths of a gram). Radioimmunoassay is sometimes used to detect minute concentrations of drugs in tissues or to determine how drugs interact with their receptors.

radioisotope – The radioactive form of an element. All elements with an atomic number greater than 83 are radioactive. However, most other elements (e.g., hydrogen, carbon) also have radioactive forms.

radiologist – A physician who specializes in radiology.

radiology – The medical specialty that deals with diagnosis and treatment of disease by means of radiation.

radionuclide – The nucleus of an atom that emits radiation and undergoes radioactive decay.

radiopaque – A substance that does not allow passage of x-rays. Radiopaque materials (e.g., barium enema) are used to help image structures in the body that ordinarily do not visualize well with x-rays. Radiopaque materials appear white on x-ray films.

radiopharmaceutical – A drug that is or has been made to be radioactive. Although a few radiopharmaceuticals are used to treat diseases (e.g., radioactive iodine), most are used as diagnostic agents.

radiopharmacy – *See nuclear pharmacy.*

radiotherapy – Treatment of disease (e.g., cancer) by means of radiation.

R

rale – Bubbling or crackling sound heard through a stethoscope during physical examination of the chest. Rales are caused by the movement of air through excessive mucus secretions or fluid in the bronchioles and alveoli. Rales are often present in lung infections and congestive heart failure.

randomized clinical trial – An evaluation of a treatment or diagnostic procedure using human subjects where the subjects have been placed in study groups by means of chance selection. Randomization prevents study coordinators from stacking a group with subjects that are more likely or less likely to respond to the study agent.

rapid eye movement (REM) – A period of sleep where the eyes move laterally or in circles. REM sleep is thought to occur in association with dreams. Drugs that impair REM sleep decrease the restfulness of the sleep period.

rational drug therapy – A decision process whereby the most appropriate drug is prescribed for a patient's condition. Rational drug therapy includes selecting a drug that is likely to be effective for the disease state, a form of the drug the patient or caregiver is able to reliably administer, a dose that is appropriate, consideration of potential drug interactions, and the patient's previous medical history.

rbc – *See red blood cell.*

RBC – *See red blood cell.*

R.C.P. – Abbreviation for Royal College of Physicians.

R.C.S. – Abbreviation for Royal College of Surgeons.

R.D. – Abbreviation for registered dietician.

RDA – *See recommended dietary allowance.*

reaction – An adverse response to a treatment; for example, allergic reaction, adverse drug reaction.

In chemistry, a change or transformation that takes place when two or more atoms or molecules interact with each other.

R

reagent – A chemical added to one or more other chemicals in order to produce a chemical reaction.

reasonable and customary (R&C) – The normal fee a health care provider charges for a specific service. Many managed care contracts require pharmacies and other providers to bill the plan the lower of either a discounted rate or the provider's usual charge. Also known as usual and customary.

rebate – An agreed upon amount of money a drug manufacturer pays back to a payer after the manufacturer's product has been used. In pharmacy, drug manufacturers often pay rebates to managed care plans that successfully help the manufacturer increase its products' market shares among plan participants.

rebound – A phenomenon whereby symptoms opposite to the effects of a drug appear as the effects of the drug diminish. For example, discontinuing a sleep medication after several nights' use commonly produces a rebound effect characterized by difficulty getting to sleep and fragmented sleep patterns. Normal sleep patterns return after a few nights off of the medication.

Rebound is a separate phenomenon from dependence or addiction and is not necessarily related.

recalcification – The replacement of lost or depleted calcium to a tissue, particularly bone tissue.

recall – A process for retrieving defective drugs once they have been shipped from the manufacturer. Reasons for drug recalls include mislabeling, packing the wrong drug or dose in a bottle, and adulteration of the drug product.

receptor – The site on a cell surface or within a cell that binds with specific intrinsic substances (e.g., hormones) or drugs. Drugs may either stimulate receptors or block them. For example, beta receptor agonists are drugs that mimic the effects of epinephrine on receptors and relieve symptoms of asthma. Beta receptor blockers are drugs that inhibit the effects of epinephrine on its receptors and are useful for treating hypertension.

recidivism – The tendency to return for treatment of recurrences of the same illness. The term is most commonly applied to rehospitalization for mental illness.

R

recombinant DNA – The insertion of deoxyribonucleic acid (DNA) taken from one organism into another. Also known as gene splicing. DNA transferred in this way continues to function as it did in its original host. Recombinant DNA technology allows scarce human hormones (e.g., insulin, growth hormone) to be grown in large quantities in microorganisms for future harvest and use to treat human disease.

recommended dietary allowance (RDA) – An estimate of the total quantity of a vitamin a normal, healthy person should consume from all sources (diet and/or supplement) in an average day. RDAs are established by the Food and Nutrition Board of the United States Department of Health and Human Services.

reconstitution – The process of adding water or other solvent to a powdered form of a medicine to make a solution or suspension. Reconstitution is commonly used to prepare for administration a medicine that has short stability in the liquid form.

recovery – The process of recuperating from an illness.

Also the recuperation from general anesthesia following surgery.

recovery room – The area in a hospital, usually adjacent to the operating suite, where patients receive postsurgical care and emerge from anesthesia.

recrudescence – Relapse of a disease or symptoms of a disease after a period of remission.

recruitment – The gathering of participants for a scientific study. Potential subjects must meet the parameters of the study, must be informed of the benefits and risks of participation, and must give their consent.

rect- – Prefix designating the rectum.

rectal – Pertaining to the rectum.

Also a route of drug administration intended for suppositories and enemas.

recto- – Prefix designating the rectum.

R

rectum – The structure, approximately 5 inches long, found between the end of the large intestine and the anus. The rectum holds feces until they are ready for defecation.

recuperation – Recovery from illness.

recurrence – Return of symptoms after a period of improvement.

red blood cell (rbc, RBC) – The most common cell in blood. Also known as erythrocyte. Red blood cells contain hemoglobin, a complex organic compound that binds oxygen from the lungs. As RBCs travel through the body, they exchange oxygen for carbon dioxide. Once back in the lungs, the erythrocytes exchange carbon dioxide for oxygen and repeat the cycle.

reentry – The restimulation of heart tissue by an impulse for the second time. Reentry occurs when the normal impulse pathway is blocked and the impulse returns along parts of its original route. Reentry often leads to arrhythmias.

referral – The process of sending a patient to a specific health care provider for evaluation or treatment.

reflex – The impulsive, involuntary movement of an organ or tissue in response to a stimulus. Reflexes depend upon an intact nerve pathway from the site of the stimulus, to the spinal cord, and back again. Diminished reflexes may indicate nerve or muscle disease.

reflux – Unintended backward flow of fluids or other materials. For an example, see gastroesophageal reflux.

regimen – A controlled therapeutic program. Regimens may include exercise, drugs, diet, or other treatments.

regional anesthesia – Loss of sensation in an area of the body induced by injecting a local anesthetic medication near a nerve that normally carries sensations from that part of the body to the brain. Regional anesthesia may be used in surgery, childbirth, or for other applications.

registered nurse (R.N) – An individual who has completed a prescribed course of study in an approved program. Studies include disease processes, therapeutic interventions, and supportive

R

care of patients. Registered nurses must have a minimum of two years of academic training in an approved program and must pass a state-administered examination.

regression – A state where progress made toward resolving a condition is lost as symptoms reappear or worsen.

Also, the state where a tumor or lesion shrinks in size.

regurgitation – A backward flow, particularly blood that flows backward in the heart because of a damaged valve.

rehab – *See rehabilitation.*

rehabilitation (rehab) – A therapeutic program intended to return a person to normal health after an injury or disease, particularly substance abuse.

rehydration – Restoration of fluids to a person suffering from dehydration. Depending upon the severity of the situation, rehydration may be accomplished with intravenous or oral fluids.

reinfection – An infection caused by the same organism that caused a previous infection. Reinfection is different than a relapsing infection. In relapse, the infection was never completely eliminated. Reinfection implies that a previous infection was cured but that microorganisms have been reintroduced to the body. Reinfection is common in urinary tract infections.

rejection – A response to a transplanted organ or tissue whereby the recipient's immune system recognizes the transplant as foreign to the body and tries to destroy it. Rejection can often be prevented with drugs that suppress the immune system.

relapse – Return of symptoms after a period of improvement. Relapse may occur in association with a wide variety of diseases including infections, substance abuse, and diabetes.

Also see reinfection.

REM – *See rapid eye movement.*

remedy – Any treatment for a disease. Most commonly used in the context of a medicine; for example, a home remedy or an herbal remedy.

R

remineralization – Replacement to the body of minerals lost because of disease or diet. Remineralization is accomplished by means of mineral supplements, not by dietary changes.

remission – Lessening in the severity of disease or even the complete disappearance of disease, particularly one that fluctuates in intensity. In cancer, a long remission may be an indication of cure.

remodeling – The process healthy bone tissue goes through where minerals from bone are continually lost to and reabsorbed from blood. Remodeling continually rebuilds healthy bone.

renal – Pertaining to one or both kidneys.

reni- – Prefix designating the kidney.

renin – An enzyme produced in the kidneys to facilitate the conversion of angiotensinogen to angiotensin I. Since angiotensin I and its metabolite angiotensin II cause blood vessels to constrict, renin plays a major role in controlling blood pressure.

reno- – Prefix designating the kidney.

reportable disease – Infections that physicians must report to their local health departments, who in turn report to the Centers for Disease Control. Examples of reportable diseases are hepatitis, AIDS, sexually transmitted diseases, and tuberculosis. The purpose of reporting these diseases is to monitor for epidemics and take appropriate containment actions to prevent widespread disease.

rescue – A therapeutic maneuver where a toxic dose of medication is intentionally administered to a patient, followed by an antidote. Leucovorin rescue is a technique commonly used in treating cancer. In this case, a high dose of the chemotherapy agent methotrexate is administered to a patient, followed by a series of doses of the folic acid metabolite leucovorin. Methotrexate poisons cells' ability to properly use folic acid. Administering doses of leucovorin rescues normal cells. However, some types of cancer cells are not able to absorb leucovorin and, consequently, die from folic acid deficiency.

R

resident – A graduate physician or other health care worker in a clinical training program. Physicians must complete at least one year of residency, formerly called internship, before they can be licensed. Most medical specialties require a minimum of three years of residency. Most pharmacy residencies are one- or two-year programs.

Residencies are usually hospital-based and include rotations in a wide variety of medical practice settings.

resistance – The ability of cells, particularly microorganisms and cancers, to adapt their metabolism or cellular structure to withstand the effects of drugs. Resistance of bacteria to antibiotics has become an enormous public health problem, caused primarily by the overuse of antibiotics.

respiration – The act of breathing whereby oxygen is inhaled and mixed with blood in the lungs while carbon dioxide is removed from blood and exhaled.

retching – The act of vomiting without expelling stomach contents. Retching usually occurs after a previous episode of vomiting has already emptied the stomach. Colloquially called dry heaves.

retention enema – An infusion of fluid into the rectum that is intended to be held in the rectum or small intestine for a prolonged period of time. Retention enemas usually contain either a medication that needs time to be absorbed or a diagnostic aid (e.g., barium enema).

reticulocyte – A newly formed red blood cell. Reticulocytes normally account for only 1% of circulating red blood cells.

reticulocytopenia – Decreased number or total absence of reticulocytes in the blood. Reticulocytopenia may be an indication of bone marrow disease.

reticulocytosis – Increased number of reticulocytes in the blood. Reticulocytosis occurs when the body is recovering from blood loss or anemia.

retina – The light-sensitive, multilayered structure in the back of the eye that converts light to electronic impulses and transmits these impulses to the brain via the optic nerve.

R

The retina is the only place in the body where blood vessels can be observed directly. Consequently, retinal examination is an important part of the evaluation of patients with diseases such as hypertension and diabetes mellitus that can damage blood vessels.

retinal – Pertaining to the retina.

retinitis – Inflammation of the retina. Symptoms of retinitis include photophobia, distortion of shapes, and diminished vision.

retinopathy – Any degeneration of the blood vessels supplying the retina of the eye that is not caused by inflammation.

retrograde amnesia – Loss of memory of past events. Retrograde amnesia can be caused by a drug reaction, drug abuse, or by neurologic disease.

retrospective drug evaluation – A review process where the appropriateness of drug therapy is reviewed sometime after the patient has started taking a medication. Retrospective programs are commonly used to analyze physicians' prescribing practices.

reversal – A change to the opposite direction. Reversals can be either beneficial or harmful. Reversal of a condition that is improving is undesirable; however, reversal of progression of disease is a sought-after outcome.

Also, a process where a pharmacist nullifies or reverses an electronic claim for a prescripion.

reversible – Not permanent. Capable of changing course. For example, dizziness is a reversible side effect of some medications.

Reye's syndrome – A metabolic disorder that affects primarily the central nervous system of children and adolescents. Reye's syndrome usually follows a viral infection and has been associated with the use of aspirin. Early signs are indistinguishable from minor illness and include vomiting and rash occurring approximately a week after onset of viral illness. Symptoms progress to confusion, disorientation, seizures, coma, and respiratory arrest. Depending upon severity, the mortality rate varies from 20% to 80%. There is no specific treatment for this condition.

R

rhabdomyolysis – Potentially fatal destruction of skeletal muscle. Rhabdomyolysis is a rare side effect of some drugs.

rheumatic fever – An inflammatory condition varying in severity and duration that may follow an infection by Streptococcus. The most common cause is an untreated or inadequately treated strep throat infection. Rheumatic fever is more common in children than in adults. Rheumatic fever may cause serious heart and/or kidney damage. Signs and symptoms include pain in joints, rash, chest pain, and heart palpitations.

rheumatic heart disease – Damage to the heart muscle and valves as a result of rheumatic fever. Signs and symptoms may include heart murmurs, abnormal pulse and heart rhythms, and potentially heart failure.

rheumatism – Colloquial term for rheumatoid arthritis or rheumatic fever.

rheumatoid arthritis (RA) – A chronic, painful inflammation of the joints that, while most commonly affecting the hands and feet, can involve multiple joints in the body. Rheumatoid arthritis is initiated when the body's immune system begins to attack connective tissue in the joints. RA causes swelling of affected joints, often with permanent disfiguration. RA most often affects women during middle age. The cause of RA is unknown.

rheumatologist – A physician who specializes in rheumatology.

rheumatology – The medical specialty that deals with diagnosis and treatment of arthritis and other forms of muscle and joint disease.

rhin- – Prefix designating the nose.

rhinitis – Inflammation of the mucous membrane of the nose. Signs and symptoms include itching, sneezing, congestion, and production of excess mucus. Allergic rhinitis (hay fever) is a common example.

rhino- – Prefix designating the nose.

rhinopharyngitis – An inflammation of the mucous membranes of both the nose and the throat.

R

rhinorrhea – Excess fluid discharge from the nose.

rhinoscope – An instrument designed to examine the interior of the nose.

rhonchi – Plural of rhonchus.

rhonchus – A whistling sound made during inhalation. Presence of rhonchi indicates an obstruction of airflow through the lungs.

ribonucleic acid (RNA) – An endogenous chemical that assists with the formation of cellular proteins. RNA is found in both the cytoplasm and nuclei of cells.

rickets – A condition caused by either dietary deficiency of vitamin D, calcium, and phosphorus or by the inability to absorb any or all of these nutrients from the diet. While the condition also affects the liver and spleen, most of its effects are on bone. Rickets causes softening of bone tissue with deformities that include knock-knees and bowed legs. Treatment is primarily restoration of deficient nutrients.

rickettsia – Small bacteria incapable of living free of a host. Rickettsiae are usually found in lice, fleas, ticks, and mites. Rickettsiae cause Rocky Mountain spotted fever and typhus.

rigor – Uncontrollable shivering caused by fever.
    Also rigidity in a muscle (e.g., rigor mortis).

ringworm – Any fungal infection of the skin or nails.

R.N. – Abbreviation for registered nurse.

RNA – *See ribonucleic acid.*

Rocky Mountain spotted fever – An infection caused by a tick-borne rickettsia. Originally, the condition was thought to occur only in the western areas of the United States. Now it is known that Rocky Mountain spotted fever can occur in any area where ticks are indigenous. Signs and symptoms include fever, chills, rash, headache, and muscle ache. The mortality rate without adequate antibiotic treatment is approximately 20%.

roentgen – A measure of ionizing radioactivity.

R

roundworm – An intestinal parasite of the class Nematoda.

route of administration – The pathway by which a drug is given to a patient. Depending upon the patient's condition and the characteristics of the drug, the route of administration may include oral, rectal, vaginal, topical, intravenous injection, intramuscular injection, subcutaneous injection, transcutaneous patch, inhalation, and many others.

R.Ph. – Abbreviation for registered pharmacist.

-rrhagia – Suffix designating a discharge (e.g., menorrhagia).

-rrhea – Suffix designating a flow (e.g., diarrhea).

rubefacient – An agent that causes reddening when applied to the skin. Rubefacients are often used as counterirritants. *Also see counterirritant.*

rubella – A viral infection that produces signs and symptoms of a mild upper respiratory infection, lymph node enlargement, and a fine red rash. Rubella is also known as German measles or the three-day measles because of its short duration. Rubella can be prevented by vaccination.

rubeola – *See measles.*

rubescent – Reddening or flushing of an area of skin.

Rx – Abbreviation often used on prescriptions for the Latin *recipe*, meaning take.

S

s – Abbreviation often used on prescriptions for the Latin *sine*, meaning without.

sacr- – Prefix designating the sacrum.

sacro- – Prefix designating the sacrum.

sacroiliac – Pertaining to the juncture of the sacrum and ilium bones in the pelvis.

sacroiliitis – An inflammation of the joint where the sacrum and the ilium meet.

sacrum – The large triangular bone in the back of the pelvis that joins with the hip bones. The sacrum forms the base of the spinal column.

safety – The property of being free from danger of injury. The United States Food and Drug Administration (FDA) applies a safety standard before approving any new drug for marketing. However, safety is relative to the class of drugs under consideration. For example, a new antihistamine would be expected to cause few side effects because other antihistamines currently on the market cause few problems. However, a new cancer treatment may be approved despite the fact that it causes a high incidence of serious side effects as long as it can be shown to have other advantages over similar drugs.

salicylate – A class of drugs derived from salicylic acid. Salicylates relieve pain and inflammation and reduce fever. Aspirin is the most commonly used salicylate.

saline – A solution of salt in water. Normal, also called physiologic, saline is a solution of 9 grams of sodium chloride per 100 milliliters of water.

saliva – The mixture of water and mucus produced by the salivary glands. Saliva also contains digestive enzymes and electrolytes. Saliva moistens food, aids in chewing and digestion, and suppresses the growth of bacteria in the mouth.

salivary – Pertaining to saliva.

salivary glands – The small organs that form saliva and secrete it into the mouth. Humans have three pairs of major salivary glands

S

that produce most of the saliva needed plus numerous small glands that supplement the actions of the major glands.

salping- – Prefix designating a tube, particularly the fallopian or eustachian tubes.

salpingitis – An inflammation or infection of a fallopian tube in the female abdomen or a eustachian tube that connects the throat to the middle ear.

salpingo- – Prefix designating a tube, particularly the fallopian or eustachian tubes.

salpingo-oophorectomy – The surgical removal of one or both ovaries and fallopian tubes.

salt – A chemical compound formed by the interaction of an acid with a base. While the term is most commonly used to describe sodium chloride, common table salt, it actually encompasses hundreds of chemicals.

salve – An obsolete term for an ointment.

sample – Free goods provided by drug manufacturers to physicians and other prescribers for distribution to patients. The intent of a sample is to allow a patient to take a few doses of a new medicine free of charge to determine the patient's response to the treatment. If the response is satisfactory, the physician usually writes a prescription for a larger amount of medicine.

sanita- – Prefix designating health.

sanitarium – An institution intended for the long-term treatment of a medical or psychiatric condition. In the past, mental health facilities and tuberculosis hospitals were often called sanitariums.

sanitary – Clean. Free of dirt. Encouraging health.

sanitation – Action taken to improve health or prevent disease. Includes disposal of excrement and trash.

sanity – Presence of good mental health.

SA node – *See sinoatrial node.*

S

saponification – The process of combining a fatty acid with a base to form a soap.

sarcoidosis – A disease that causes nodules to form in the lungs, liver, lymph nodes, skin, spleen, eyes, small bones of the hands and feet, and other organs. The nodules usually disappear over time but leave scar tissue on the affected areas.

sarcoma – A highly malignant tumor that begins in connective tissue such as that in muscle or bone. The specific type of tumor is usually named after the tissue of origin. For example, osteogenic sarcoma originates in bone.

saturate – To cause a substance to combine to the full extent of its ability. For example, to dissolve the maximum amount of a substance in a fluid or to fill up all of a compound's chemical binding sites.

saturated fatty acid – A fatty acid that has all of its carbon atoms bound to hydrogen. *See fatty acid.*

sc – Abbreviation for subcutaneous. Typically used to describe a site of drug injection.

scabies – A dermatologic condition caused by a mite that burrows into the skin, causing intense itching. Female mites lay their eggs beneath the skin surface, causing the infestation to continue. Scabies may be found anywhere on the trunk or extremities. The condition is highly contagious and requires treatment with specially formulated insecticides.

scall – An inflammation of the scalp that produces a crusty lesion.

scalp – The skin on the head. The area normally covered by hair.

scan – The visual display created by introduction of a source of radiation into an organ of the body. The visual display indicates features of the organ's function. For example, a brain scan can indicate the precise location of restricted blood flow. A bone scan can indicate minute fractures that do not appear on typical x-rays. Scanning procedures often involve injection of a radio-pharmaceutical that collects in a specific organ or tissue. Radiation from that location is captured in a scintillation detector that produces a picture for diagnostic interpretation.

S

scar – The tough skin that replaces that damaged by injury. Initially scar tissue is red in color. Later, it turns white and glistening. Scar tissue has no blood vessels.

scheduled drug – One of the five groupings for drugs that have abuse potential. *Also see controlled substance.*

schedule of benefits – The portion of an insurance policy that explains which items are covered, to what extent they are covered, and which items are not covered.

schizoid – A personality disorder characterized by social isolation, difficulty in forming interpersonal relationships, and extreme shyness.

schizophrenia – A mental illness characterized by distortion of reality, disorganized thought patterns, social withdrawal, hallucinations, and poor judgement. Schizophrenia is one of the most devastating forms of mental illness. Schizophrenia occurs in approximately 1% of the population.

scientific method – A systematic approach to conducting research and confirming results. The scientific method includes clearly stating the problem to be resolved or investigated, developing a hypothesis, employing an appropriate protocol or experimental procedure, collecting data, analyzing results, and formulating conclusions. Researchers usually publish their findings and invite others to perform similar experiments to confirm or refute their conclusions.

scintillation – The discharge of energy caused by the disintegration of radioactive elements.

scintillation detector – An instrument that collects and measures radioactive discharges. Scintillation detectors are used to read radioactivity during a nuclear medicine scan.

sclera – The white of the eye. The white covering over the eye that maintains the eye's size and shape. The sclera also contains blood vessels that supply the eye.

sclerae – Plural form of sclera.

scleral – Pertaining to the sclera.

S

scleroderma – An immune system disorder that causes skin to become tight, tough, and hyperpigmented. The disease may progress to involve the kidneys, lungs, heart, and digestive tract. The condition is normally treated with drugs that suppress the immune system and with physical therapy to improve mobility.

scleroid – Pertaining to a tissue that has a hard or tough texture.

-scope – Suffix designating an instrument used for viewing (e.g., microscope, endoscope).

scorbutic – Pertaining to scurvy.

scratch test – A procedure intended to identify substances that cause allergic reactions in a specific person. The procedure involves making a small scratch on the patient's skin, then placing a drop of antigen-containing solution on the scratch. An inflammatory reaction at the site of the test indicates that the patient may be allergic to the antigen applied to that site. Patients may be tested with dozens of antigens at a single sitting.

screening test – A test applied, often to a large number of people, to detect the possibility of disease; for example, skin tests for exposure to tuberculosis. Screening tests are usually not diagnostic of a disease. Rather, they are intended to identify people who are at significant risk of disease so that further testing can be done on those individuals.

scrotal – Pertaining to the scrotum.

scrotum – The pouch of skin comprising the part of the male external genitalia that contains the testes.

scurvy – A nutritional disease characterized by bleeding from the gums and skin, anemia, pain in the legs and joints, loosening of teeth, and muscle pain. Scurvy is caused by a diet devoid of vitamin C.

seasonal allergic rhinitis – An allergy-mediated inflammatory reaction in the upper respiratory tract that occurs in individuals at specific times of the year. Also known as hay fever. *Also see allergic rhinitis.*

S

seborrhea – A skin condition characterized by overproduction of the oil glands of the skin. Oily skin. Seborrhea may also occur in some chronic diseases, e.g., Parkinson's disease.

seborrheic – Pertaining to seborrhea.

seborrheic dermatitis – A common skin condition characterized by itchy, reddened, oily patches of skin. The lesions often shed large dandruff-like scales. Seborrheic dermatitis is often mistakenly called seborrhea.

sebum – Naturally produced skin oil. Sebum is formed by sebaceous glands in the skin. Its main function is to retain the water content of the skin. Sebum helps to prevent dry skin conditions.

secondary care – Medical care delivered by specialists as opposed to primary care physicians. In most managed care settings, secondary care is arranged upon the referral of a primary care physician.

secondary hypertension – Elevated blood pressure due to a known cause, usually kidney disease.

Also see hypertension.

sedation – A state of calmness or sleep. Sedation is often achieved by means of a drug.

sedative – Any agent that produces calm or sleep. Sedative drugs may be given by mouth or by injection.

seizure – An epileptic attack. A forceful series of uncontrolled muscle contractions that may affect the arms, legs, trunk, and/or head. The patient may lose consciousness and have no memory of the seizure.

selective serotonin reuptake inhibitor (SSRI) – A class of antidepressants that primarily affect the storage of the neurotransmitter serotonin in the brain. The first SSRI marketed was fluoxetine (Prozac).

self-insurance – A health insurance plan funded entirely by an employer. In most cases, self-insured plans employ the services of an insurance company to process and administer claims. The employer then pays the insurer the cost of the claim plus an

S

administrative fee. Although there is risk of one or more employees incurring an expensive illness, self-insured plans usually save money over traditional health care insurance policies. In some cases, an employer purchases a separate policy to protect itself from catastrophic claims.

self-medication – A process where a patient determines his own drug treatment. In most cases, self-medication involves selecting an over-the-counter drug; however, some patients practice self-medication with old prescription medicines or with a friend's or family member's prescription medication. Self-medication with prescription medicines can have disastrous outcomes.

semen – The thick, yellowish-white, sperm-containing fluid males ejaculate during intercourse. Males normally ejaculate 2 to 5 milliliters of semen during an orgasm.

semi- – Prefix designating half.

seminal – Pertaining to semen or seed.

semipermeable – Pertaining to the property of a membrane that allows water or solvents to pass through freely but restricts or prevents passage of materials dissolved in the fluid.

semisynthetic – Pertaining to a chemical, a portion of which came from nature. The term is used to describe a drug whose principle chemical structure is isolated from nature, usually from a plant source, and then is chemically altered to enhance the drug's activity or reduce its side effects. For example, the antibiotics ampicillin and amoxicillin are semisynthetic derivatives of naturally-occurring penicillin.

senescence – The state of aging or growing old.

senile – Pertaining to old age. Commonly used in the sense of deterioration of physical or mental faculties.

senility – Mental or physical deterioration due to old age.

sensation – The perception of a physical stimulus to a part of the body. Sensations are perceived by nerves and transmitted to the brain. In the case of permanent or temporary neurological damage or injury, sensations may occur without physical cause. For

S

example, individuals in drug detoxification programs often complain of the sensation of insects crawling on their skin when there are no insects present.

sense – The mechanism for perceiving external stimuli. The five senses are sight, hearing, taste, touch, and smell.

sensible – Capable of being perceived or measured.

sensitivity – Susceptibility to a drug or other agent.

sensitivity test – A laboratory assessment of the ability of a variety of antibiotics to inhibit the growth of a microorganism. Sensitivity tests are routinely performed to determine the most effective antibiotic for an infection in a specific patient.

sensitization – The process of making a person allergic to a substance. For example, repeated exposures to penicillin increase the likelihood of future allergic reactions to the drug.

sepsis – The presence of pathogenic bacteria in tissue. Signs of sepsis usually include fever and inflammation of the infected area.

septic- – Prefix designating sepsis.

septicemia – An infection of the blood. Septicemia may be caused by direct injection of bacteria into blood as with a contaminated needle or, more commonly, by an infection anywhere in the body that spreads into the blood. Septicemia is a serious problem that can cause shock, coma, and death if not treated aggressively with appropriate antibiotic therapy.

septicemic – Pertaining to septicemia.

septico- – Prefix designating sepsis.

septic shock – A precipitous drop in blood pressure due to overwhelming infection. Treatment includes aggressive treatment of the infection as well as intravenous fluids to support blood pressure.

sequela – A condition or situation that follows from something else. For example, the natural sequela of untreated leukemia is death.

sequelae – Plural of sequela.

S

serendipity – An accidental discovery made while looking for something else. For example, while physicians were using it to treat arthritis, ibuprofen (Motrin) was serendipitously found to be effective for relieving menstrual cramps.

sero- – Prefix designating serum.

seroconversion – The sudden appearance of antibodies in serum following exposure to microorganisms or following immunization.

serology – The branch of science concerned with the protein components of serum. Serology includes testing for changes in antibodies that may indicate the presence of infection.

seronegative – The absence of a specific antibody. A patient may be seronegative because she has not been exposed to the suspected infection, has been exposed but is not capable of forming antibodies to it, or has lost the ability to make antibodies to resist this organism.

seropositive – The presence of a specific antibody. Depending upon the test, a seropositive result may indicate exposure to a specific microorganism or the presence of an immune disorder such as rheumatoid arthritis.

serous – Pertaining to a body fluid that has the appearance or consistency of serum.

serum – The clear, sticky portion of blood that remains after removal of all cells and clots. Serum differs from plasma in that plasma still contains clotting factors.

Also, any clear fluid that exudes from a skin lesion.

Serum is often used as a synonym for antitoxin.

service area – The geographic area served by a health plan. Health plans must submit their proposed geographic boundaries to the state department of insurance and receive approval before they can implement services in any new areas.

sexually transmitted disease (STD) – Any of several contagious diseases passed from an infected person to another person as a consequence of sexual intercourse. STDs include gonorrhea, syphilis, chlamydia, AIDS, genital herpes, genital warts, and crab lice.

S

shedding – The presence of live viruses in body fluids or secretions. The common cold is most contagious when viruses are shed in nasal mucus.

shingles – *See herpes zoster.*

shock – A condition where insufficient blood is returned to the heart to sustain normal circulation. Shock may occur due to loss of body fluids or a profound drop in blood pressure. Shock is a serious condition that requires immediate treatment because organs and tissues do not receive adequate oxygenation. Causes of shock may include hemorrhage, dehydration, allergic reaction, myocardial infarction, and infection.

shunt – To redirect blood flow from one blood vessel to another or around an obstruction; or a device that shunts blood. A shunt may be inserted into a patient's arm to facilitate connection to a hemodialysis (artificial kidney) machine.

sialorrhea – Excess salivation with or without drooling.

sickle cell anemia – A genetically based disease of red blood cells characterized by abnormal hemoglobin and the tendency to form themselves into a sickle shape. The red blood cells in sickle cell anemia are diminished in number and fragile. Because of their abnormal shape, sickled cells can obstruct capillaries and cause extreme pain.

sickling – The propensity for red blood cells to change themselves into a curved form in patients with sickle cell anemia.

side effect – An outcome other than that intended. Most commonly used in the context of drug therapy where a side effect is an unwanted consequence of the drug in use. Common side effects include nausea, vomiting, and diarrhea. Some side effects are of little clinical consequence while others may be fatal.

siderosis – A high, usually toxic, level of iron in circulating blood. Causes of siderosis include frequent blood transfusions and prolonged ingestion of iron supplements in persons who do not need them.

Also, a lung disease caused by chronic inhalation of dust particles.

S

Sig – Abbreviation for the Latin *signa*, meaning mark or label. The Sig is the portion of a prescription where the prescriber writes the directions for use.

sign – An objective, observable, often measurable manifestation of disease. Signs can be observed by someone other than the patient. Examples of signs include skin rash, blood pressure readings, and laboratory test results. A*lso see symptom.*

simple – A plant with medicinal properties.

single-source drug – A drug that is available from only one manufacturer. Single-source drugs are protected by patents, and generic drug manufacturers cannot manufacture these drugs until their patents expire.

sinoatrial (SA) node – The portion of the atrium in the right side of the heart that initiates the electrical impulses that cause the heart to contract. The sinoatrial node fires more often during exercise and at a slower rate during rest. Disorders of the SA node lead to irregular heart rates. In some cases these problems can be treated with medications. Some persistent problems with the SA node may require an artificial pacemaker.

sinus – A hollow space in a bone (e.g., paranasal sinuses).

sinusitis – An inflammation, usually due to infection, of the mucous membranes lining the paranasal sinuses. Sinusitis can cause fever, congestion, and severe pain.

sinusoid – Pertaining to or resembling a sinus.

site – A place or location. For example, an injection site is the place where an injection is administered. A receptor site is the position on or within a cell where a drug or biochemical attaches and triggers its action.

Sjögren's syndrome – A collection of signs and symptoms that include dryness of the mucous membranes of the eyes, nose, and mouth, purplish spots on the face, and enlargement of glands in the neck. Sjögren's syndrome is more common in postmenopausal women and persons with rheumatoid arthritis.

S

skeleton – The 206 bones of the body that provide shape, structure, and protection for the body and its internal organs.

skilled nursing care – Residential medical care provided under the supervision of at least one registered nurse.

skilled nursing facility (SNF) – A residential health care institution that provides convalescence and rehabilitation services for long-term care or for transition from a hospital environment to a patient's home. In the past SNFs were referred to as nursing homes.

skin – The membrane that covers the exterior of the body. The skin is the largest organ in the body and consists primarily of two layers, the epidermis and the corium. Each of these has several components.

sleep – A natural, recurring condition of rest for the body and mind during which the eyes close and there is little or no conscious thought. Sleep may occur in up to four layers of depth, termed stages one through four. Sleep may also be characterized as REM (rapid eye movement) sleep or nonREM (nonrapid eye movement) sleep. Dreams usually occur during REM sleep.

slough – To shed dead cells or tissue.

small calorie (c, cal) – The amount of heat necessary to raise one gram of water one degree Celsius. The unit of measure people refer to in terms of nutritional calories is actually a large calorie or kilocalorie.

Also see kilocalorie.

small intestine – The lengthy, tube-like lower portion of the digestive tract that runs from the stomach to the large intestine. The small intestine is intended primarily for food digestion and nutrient absorption. The small intestine is composed of the duodenum, jejunum, and ileum.

smear – A small amount of material, usually cellular material, spread on a surface for examination. Examples of smears include blood smears, pap smears, and bacterial smears. These smears are spread on a glass slide and prepared for microscopic examination.

S

smooth muscle – *See muscle.*

sneeze – Sudden expulsion of air from the nose and mouth. Sneezes are commonly initiated by irritation to the nose, allergic reactions, and upper respiratory infections.

SNF – *See skilled nursing facility.*

snore – A sound-producing vibration of the palate during sleep. Snoring does not respond to any drug therapy; however, drugs with sedating effects can make the condition worse.

SNS – *See sympathetic nervous system.*

snuff – A medicated powder breathed in through the nose.

Also, a tobacco product that is inhaled into the nose or placed in the mouth.

soap – A molecule of a metallic element, particularly sodium or potassium, combined with a long-chain fatty acid. The resulting compound can be used with water to clean or wash.

SOAP note – A method of organizing the progress notes section in medical records. SOAP is an acronym for subjective, objective, assessment, and plan.

social worker – An individual trained to help patients access available resources to assist them in their care. Resources may include health care settings such as skilled nursing facilities, hospice, or home care. Social workers also assist patients with financial aspects of their care, including insurance reimbursement, Medicare, and Medicaid.

In addition, psychiatric social workers are trained to conduct psychotherapy with the mentally ill.

socialized medicine – The total control of health care delivery systems and reimbursements for services by a government agency.

sodium – An element with atomic number 11. Sodium is essential for the function of all cells in the body. Excessive sodium leads to water retention and can worsen disorders such as hypertension and heart failure.

sol – *See solution.*

S

soln – *See solution.*

solubility – The amount of a substance that can dissolve in a fluid under specific conditions such as temperature and barometric pressure.

soluble – Capable of passing into solution.

solute – A substance that is dissolved in a fluid.

solution (sol, soln) – The dispersion of a substance in another, usually a fluid, to form a homogeneous mixture.

solvent – A material, usually a fluid, that can dissolve another substance. Common solvents include water, alcohol, and acetone.

somat- – Prefix designating the body.

somatic – Pertaining to the body or structures of the body as opposed to the mind or the imagination.

somatico- – Prefix designating the body.

somato- – Prefix designating the body.

somatotherapy – Treatment directed at physical rather than psychological disorders.

somatotropic – Pertaining to an agent that stimulates body growth (e.g., growth hormone).

somnambulism – A sleep disorder that causes a person to walk, and sometimes even talk to others, while still asleep. Sleepwalking.

somnolence – Prolonged drowsiness that may last hours to days.

somnolent – Sleepy. About to fall asleep.

soporific – A drug or other agent that causes sleep.

sore – An open lesion in the skin or mucous membrane.
Also, pertaining to an area that is painful or tender.

spacer – A cylindrical device added to a metered dose inhaler. The purpose of the spacer is to assist patients, particularly children, who have trouble properly inhaling aerosol medication for asthma and other respiratory diseases. One end of the spacer is

S

attached to the mouthpiece of the aerosol canister and the other end goes into the patient's mouth. Upon activation of the canister, a dose of medication swirls around the spacer and the patient inhales the aerosol until it is all consumed.

spasm – An uncontrollable muscle contraction. Affected muscles may include those in the limbs, hollow organs such as the uterus or gallbladder, or a blood vessel. Spasms are often accompanied by sharp pain.

spasmo- – Prefix designating spasm.

spasmodic – Pertaining to an area affected by spasm.

spasmolytic – An agent that relieves muscle spasm. For example, some anticholinergic drugs reduce spasms in the urinary tract.

spastic colon – *See irritable bowel syndrome.*

spasticity – Increased tone or force of muscle contraction leading to amplified reflexes.

spatula – A knife-like instrument with a flexible, flat blade used by pharmacists to compound drugs, particularly ointments and creams. Pharmacists often use spatulas to count tablets and capsules and to handle powders during weighing.

specialist – A physician who has received intensive training in a specific branch of medicine. Specialists must complete a residency and in some cases a fellowship in their chosen field. Medical specialties include cardiology, dermatology, thoracic surgery, neurology, and many others.

specimen – A small portion of a tissue or body fluid intended for testing. Specimens include biopsy material for pathologic study, and urine, stool, and blood samples intended for bacteriologic or chemical analysis.

spectrum – The range of microorganisms an antibiotic can be expected to inhibit.

sperm – The male germ cell. Each sperm carries half of the genetic code needed by an organism. Upon fertilization, an ovum provides the other half of the code. Thus the organism's genetic

S

code is comprised of equal parts of the mother's and father's genes.

sperma- – Prefix designating sperm or semen.

spermato- – Prefix designating sperm or semen.

spermatocide – An agent that kills sperm. Spermatocides are commonly used along with diaphragms and condoms to reduce the risk of conception following intercourse. *See also contraceptive foam, contraceptive jelly.*

spermatogenesis – The process of making sperm in the male reproductive system.

spermo- – Prefix designating sperm or semen.

SPF – *See sun protective factor.*

sphincter – A circular muscle whose contractions close access to an anatomic opening. For example, the anal sphincter closes the anus to prevent leakage of stool. The iris of the eye contracts and relaxes to reduce or increase, respectively, the amount of light that enters the eye.

sphygm- – Prefix designating pulse.

sphygmo- – Prefix designating pulse.

sphygmomanometer – An instrument used to measure blood pressure. A sphygmomanometer consists of an inflatable cuff and a gauge. The gauge may be either a dial or a mercury column.

spin- – Prefix designating the spine.

spinal – Pertaining to the spine.

spinal anesthesia – A route for administering a local anesthetic into the spinal column that causes deadening of sensations from the point of administration down to the feet. Spinal anesthesia is an alternative to general anesthesia for some types of surgery.

spinal cord – A column of nervous tissue approximately 18 inches long that runs through openings in the center of the spinal column. All nerves in the trunk and limbs connect to the spinal cords. The spinal cord is the communications link between peripheral nerves and the brain. Spinal cord injury can result in paralysis.

spine – The column of 33 small bones (vertebrae) that forms the support for the back, ribs, and head. The spine runs from the base of the skull to the pelvis.

spino- – Prefix designating the spine.

spirit – An alcohol-containing liquid that may be used pharmaceutically as a solvent, vehicle for medication, or a flavoring agent.

spirochete – A bacterium from the order Spirochaetales that has a spiral shape and long, flexible filaments. Spirochetes are capable of causing several diseases, including syphilis.

spirometer – An instrument that measures the amount of air inhaled and exhaled. Spirometers are often used to evaluate the need for asthma treatments.

spleen – An organ that lies in the upper left quadrant of the abdomen. The spleen stores blood within the body, filters bacteria and damaged cells out of the blood, and forms lymphocytes and monocytes.

splenomegaly – Enlargement of the spleen. Causes of splenomegaly include cirrhosis of the liver, hemolytic anemia, and leukemia.

spondyl- – Prefix designating the vertebrae.

spondylitis – An arthritic inflammation of one or more vertebrae. *Also see ankylosing spondylitis.*

spondylo- – Prefix designating the vertebrae.

spondylosis – A condition of osteoarthritis in the spinal column. As part of the degenerative process, two or more vertebrae may fuse with each other, causing an inflexible, painful joint.

spontaneous abortion – *See miscarriage.*

spore – Germ cell of fungi.

Also, a form some bacteria assume to increase their chances of surviving heat, dehydration, antiseptics, or antibiotics. Once the threat to their lives is removed, these bacteria resume their normal state and continue to live and reproduce.

S

sports medicine – The branch of medical practice that deals with the health of athletes and those pursuing athletic activities. Sports medicine includes diagnosis and treatment of sports-related injuries plus wellness activities that include diet and proper preparation for exercise.

spot – To discharge a small amount of blood from the vagina. Spotting may be a sign of hormonal imbalance and is common during the first few months of treatment with an oral contraceptive. During pregnancy, spotting may be a sign of potential miscarriage.

spotted fever – *See Rocky Mountain spotted fever.*

sprain – An injury to a joint in which a ligament is damaged by stretching the ligament beyond its normal capacities. Sprains are characterized by pain, swelling, and bruising.

sputum – Viscous fluid coughed up from the lungs. Sputum may consist of mucus, cellular debris, and bacteria. Discolored sputum may be a sign of infection or lung disease. Colloquially known as phlegm.

SQ – *See subcutaneous.*

sq – *See subcutaneous.*

squamous cell – A flat scale, usually the type of cell that covers tissues such as skin and mucous membranes.

squamous cell carcinoma – A flat skin cancer that most often forms in areas that have received long-term sun exposure. Squamous cell carcinoma seldom metastasizes to other organs; however, this type of cancer is highly invasive and can spread deep into tissues, causing disfiguration.

ss – Abbreviation often used on prescriptions for the Latin *semis,* meaning a half.

SSRI – *See selective serotonin reuptake inhibitor.*

stability – The degree to which or the length of time that a drug is resistant to change. For example, a dose of an injectable antibiotic may have a stability of 48 hours after it is prepared.

S

staff – A specific group of workers or employees. For example, a hospital medical staff is the group of physicians who are approved to practice in that hospital.

staff model HMO – A health maintenance organization that hires physicians as employees to service the medical needs of its members. Staff model physicians typically see patients in the HMO's buildings rather than private offices.

stain – A dye (e.g., Gram's stain) used to color cells and subcellular structures to facilitate microscopic examination.

standard treatment – A therapy that is typically used for a given condition. For example, diuretics are a standard treatment for hypertension.

staph – *See Staphylococcus.*

staphyloccocal – Pertaining to the bacterial genus *Staphylococcus*.

staphylococcemia – The presence of *Staphylococcus* bacteria in blood. Staphylococcemia may occur after minor trauma to the skin that allows bacteria to enter the bloodstream. Such cases are common and usually resolve without symptoms or treatment. In other cases, staphylococcemia may indicate serious infection that requires immediate and aggressive treatment.

staphylococci – Plural of staphylococcus.

***Staphylococcus* (staph)** – A genus of gram-positive bacteria commonly found in nature and in the normal flora of human skin. Most strains of staph are nonvirulent and cause no clinical problems. Other strains can be highly pathogenic and exhibit resistance to almost all known antibiotics.

Overgrowth of staph in improperly stored or inadequately cooked foods is the most common cause of food poisoning.

staphylodermatitis – Inflammation of the skin due to staphylococcal infection.

starch – A complex carbohydrate found in plants. As the body digests starch it converts it to simple sugars. These sugars may be used as energy, stored as glycogen, or stored as fat.

S

starvation – The physical state that results from inadequate intake or the inability to absorb and process essential nutrients. During starvation, the body loses weight, and burns stored glycogen, fats, and proteins for energy.

stasis – Slow down or stagnation of fluid in an area. For example, venous stasis is a condition where blood pools in blood vessels. Venous stasis may lead to thrombus formation.

stat – Abbreviation used on prescriptions and other medical orders for the Latin *statim*, meaning immediately.

state board of pharmacy – *See board of pharmacy.*

state insurance department – *See department of insurance.*

statin – A class of drugs that inhibits the activity of an enzyme that forms cholesterol in the body. These drugs are called statins because all of their generic names end with "statin" (e.g., lovastatin).

statistical significance – A mathematical test applied to research findings to determine the probability that chance occurrence may have altered the results of a study. In most cases, the probability of chance occurrence must be less than 5% in order for the findings to be accepted in the scientific community.

status – A state or condition. Normally combined with another term to describe a physical or medical condition. For example, status asthmaticus is an intense, prolonged asthma attack that is life-threatening due to impaired breathing and accompanying physical exhaustion. Status epilepticus is a series of convulsions that come so frequently that the patient does not recover consciousness between them.

STD – *See sexually transmitted disease.*

steal syndrome – A condition where blood is unintentionally diverted from one part of the body to another. For example, attempting to treat obstructed blood vessels in the legs with vasodilators causes blood to pool in the healthy vessels that respond to the treatment. These healthy vessels "steal" blood from all other areas of the body. Ironically, because of deterioration of vascular smooth muscle, the diseased vessels cannot respond to vasodilators

S

and actually have blood diverted away from them during vasodilator therapy.

steato- – Prefix designating fat.

steatorrhea – Elimination of large amounts of fat in the stool. Steatorrhea may be caused by malabsorption of nutrients or by liver or pancreatic disease.

stem cell – A type of cell in bone marrow that generates all other blood cells. Stem cells give rise to cells that eventually differentiate themselves into red and white blood cells and platelets.

stenosis – The narrowing of a passageway. For example, aortic stenosis is a narrowing of the valve that allows blood to flow from the heart to the aorta. Pyloric stenosis is a constriction of the passage from the stomach to the duodenum of the small intestine. Pyloric stenosis may be a birth defect or may be caused by a scar made by a peptic ulcer.

step therapy – A treatment protocol often used by managed care organizations that calls for a progression of treatments that begin with relatively inexpensive interventions and move up to more costly ones. The patient is maintained at the level of best response.

step-down unit – A specialized floor of a hospital where staff are trained to care for patients who are well enough to be discharged from an intensive care unit but still too ill to be cared for on a regular floor. Step-down units are usually equipped with more specialized technology than regular floors and are better staffed.

sterile – The state of being free of all living microorganisms.

Also, the inability to conceive a child.

sterilization – The process of removing or killing all microorganisms. Sterilization may be accomplished by using disinfectants, extreme heat, ultraviolet radiation, or by passing air or liquids through filters fine enough to remove microorganisms.

Also, a surgical process that causes a person to be unable to conceive. Examples include castration, vasectomy, and tubal ligation.

S

sternum – The breast bone. The bone that secures the first seven ribs on each side of the body and protects the heart from trauma.

steroid – A chemical that contains a cluster of three cyclohexane rings and one cyclopentane ring in its central structure. Naturally occurring steroids include estrogen, progesterone, testosterone, vitamin D, cortisol, bile acids, cholesterol, and others.

Steroids are often collectively named according to the part of the body they come from or for their physiologic function. For example, corticosteroids are produced in the cortex of the adrenal glands, androgenic steroids are male sex hormones, estrogenic steroids are female sex hormones.

Among health care professionals, the term "steroid" is normally used to refer to corticosteroids, the hormones that reduce inflammation and allergic reactions. Nonmedical people, however, normally think of "steroids" solely in the context of the testosterone-like hormones some athletes abuse.

steroidal – Pertaining to steroids, their characteristics, or their basic chemical structure.

stetho- – Prefix designating the chest.

stethoscope – An instrument originally designed to allow a physician to listen to heartbeats. Uses for stethoscopes now include listening to the sounds of the heart, blood flowing through blood vessels, air passing through the lungs, and food passing through the intestines.

stimulant – An agent that increases the activity of a cell, tissue, organ, or the whole organism. For example, a neurotransmitter such as epinephrine stimulates the heart to beat faster. Drugs such as amphetamine and caffeine stimulate the central nervous system to increase wakefulness.

stimulant laxative – A class of drugs that increase intestinal contractions in order to produce a bowel movement. Stimulant laxatives irritate the lining of the large intestine. In response, the intestine tries to eliminate the irritant by producing a bowel movement.

sting – The injection of venom by an insect such as a bee or wasp.

S

Also, a sharp sensation of pain of short duration such as that experienced by dabbing alcohol on a cut.

stom- – Prefix designating mouth.

stoma – An artificial opening in the wall of the abdomen such as that produced by a colostomy.

stomach – The digestive organ positioned between the esophagus and the small intestine. The stomach receives swallowed food from the mouth and esophagus and begins the process of diges- tion. When food enters, the stomach secretes hydrochloric acid and enzymes and churns those together with food to produce a substance called chyme. The acid and enzymes begin breaking proteins and other large molecules into simpler substances, preparing them for further digestion in the small intestine.

stomach flu – A colloquial term referring to a form of viral gastroen- teritis characterized by nausea, vomiting, and diarrhea.

stomat- – Prefix designating mouth.

stomatitis – Inflammation of the mucous membranes in the mouth. Stomatitis makes eating and drinking painful and may lead to ulcerations in the mouth. Stomatitis is a common complication of cancer chemotherapy.

stomato- – Prefix designating mouth.

-stomy – Suffix designating a surgical opening, e.g., colostomy.

stool – Solid waste from the intestinal tract. Defecation. Feces.

strain – A subgroup of a species of bacteria in which all members of the strain exhibit common characteristics, such as resistance or susceptibility to the same antibiotics or the ability to form the same endotoxins.

strength – The concentration or potency of a drug in a dosage form. For example, the strength of an ordinary aspirin tablet is 325 mil- ligrams.

strep – *See Streptococcus.*

streptococcal – Pertaining to the bacterial genus *Streptococcus*.

S

streptococcemia – The presence of *Streptococcus* bacteria in blood. Streptococcemia may occur following minor trauma to the skin or a dental procedure that allows bacteria to enter the bloodstream. Such cases are common and usually resolve without symptoms or treatment. In other cases, however, streptococcemia may indicate serious infection that requires immediate and aggressive treatment.

streptococci – Plural of streptococcus.

Streptococcus (strep) – A genus of gram-positive bacteria commonly found in nature and in the normal flora of human skin. Most strains of strep are nonvirulent and cause no clinical problems. Other strains can be highly pathogenic and exhibit resistance to almost all known antibiotics.

Streptococcus can cause infections as varied as endocarditis, pneumonia, impetigo, and pharyngitis. Some strains of *Streptococcus* can secrete toxins that cause rheumatic fever and kidney failure.

stress – The physical or psychological forces that may be placed on an organ, tissue, or person that may disrupt function.

Physical stresses include both harmful and therapeutic forces such as exercise, injury, surgery, and physical therapy.

Psychological stress is an adverse stimulus that causes emotional upset. Causes of psychological stress include financial problems, family discord, and job-related difficulties.

It is common to misinterpret the term stress. For example, stress formula vitamin products replace vitamins lost due to physical stress such as surgery. They have no effect on psychological stress or its consequences.

stress test – An evaluation of an organ or tissue in which the area of concern is exposed to controlled exertion. For example, a cardiac stress test usually requires that the patient walk briskly on a treadmill while heart function is monitored.

stria – A line or stripe of discoloration that appears on the skin. For example, the stretch marks of pregnancy or the stripes caused by prolonged use of corticosteroid drugs.

striae – Plural of stria.

S

stricture – The abnormal temporary or permanent narrowing of a passageway or hollow organ. Causes include inflammation, trauma, scarring, and spasm.

stridor – A high-pitched whistling sound during respiration caused by an airway obstruction. Causes include foreign bodies (e.g., a swallowed child's toy), inflammation (e.g., asthma), airway spasms, and tumors.

stroke – A neurologic problem caused by the sudden blockage of a blood vessel in the brain or sudden hemorrhage of a blood vessel with bleeding into the brain. Strokes lead to death of brain tissue with resulting problems that may range from mild to death. Complications of stroke may include paralysis, difficulty with speech, visual disturbances, and dementia.

structure – The pattern of attachment of atoms in a molecule.
Also the arrangement of the parts of an organism.

study – A detailed research investigation of a problem, physical function, or phenomenon. *Also see controlled study.*

stupor – An altered state of consciousness that causes an individual to be less aware of and less able to respond to physical or mental stimuli. Stupor often occurs following large doses of drugs that suppress the function of the central nervous system, including alcohol, tranquilizers, and narcotics.

styptic – An agent that stops bleeding upon physical contact with the site of hemorrhage.

sub- – Prefix designating below or less than.

subacute – Pertaining to a disease that has features of both acute and chronic manifestations.

subatomic – Pertaining to one or more parts of an atom. Subatomic particles include electrons, protons, and neutrons.

subclinical – Pertaining to an illness that does not yet produce detectable signs or symptoms. The subclinical stage of a disease often occurs in the early development of the disorder.

subcutaneous (sc, sq, subq) – Beneath the skin.

S

subcutaneous (sc, sq, subq) injection – The administration of medication by means of a needle and syringe into the layer of fat and blood vessels beneath the skin. Insulin and other self-administered injectable medications are frequently injected subcutaneously.

subject – The participating person or animal or object of a scientific experiment.

subjective – Not observable or perceptible by anyone other than the individual. For example, feelings, sensations, and emotions are subjective observances. Opposite of objective.

sublingual – Pertaining to the area under the tongue. For example, some drugs such as nitroglycerin are administered sublingually, causing them to have more complete absorption and more rapid onset of action.

submicroscopic – Pertaining to organisms (e.g., viruses) that are too small to be seen with a standard microscope.

subq – *See subcutaneous.*

subscriber – The individual who signs up for (subscribes to) insurance for himself and/or his family. The subscriber is responsible for the portion of premiums not paid by the employer and for any medical bills not covered by the insurance policy.

subscription – The part of a prescription that includes directions for compounding. Physicians seldom include this information anymore, leaving product preparation to the discretion of the pharmacist.

substance abuse – The overuse and, in some cases, dependence upon drugs that have stimulant, sedative, or hallucinogenic effects on the central nervous system. In many cases the abused substances are either illegal drugs or legal drugs that are illegally obtained. Alcohol is the most commonly abused substance.

substitution – *See generic substitution.*

substrate – A substance that is altered as part of a chemical reaction. For example, levodopa (substrate) is chemically altered in the brain to produce dopamine, a substance helpful in treating Parkinson's disease.

S

sucrose – Table sugar. Sucrose is a disaccharide, composed of one molecule of glucose and one molecule of fructose.

sudor- – Prefix designating sweat.

sudorific – An agent that causes sweating. For example, drugs that stimulate the cholinergic portion of the autonomic nervous system produce sweating as a side effect.

suffocation – The condition of being deprived of oxygen supply. Causes of suffocation include obstruction of the respiratory tract (e.g., asthma, chronic obstructive pulmonary disease), heart disease (e.g., heart failure), neurologic disease (e.g., stroke, Lou Gehrig's disease), and drowning.

sugar – A class of carbohydrates composed of one or two molecules that are soluble and taste sweet.

sulf- – Prefix designating sulfur.

sulfa drug – Colloquial term for a drug of the sulfonamide class.

sulfo- – Prefix designating sulfur.

sulfonamide – A class of drugs that interfere with bacterial growth and development by interfering with the enzymes susceptible bacteria need for normal metabolism, growth, and reproduction. Sulfonamides are commonly used to treat a wide variety of infections.

sulfonylurea – A class of orally administered medications that are used to treat type II diabetes mellitus. The sulfonylureas increase the amount of insulin the pancreas releases into the blood, consequently lowering blood sugar levels.

sun protective factor (SPF) – A numeric value given to sunscreen products that indicates the amount of protection against ultraviolet radiation. For example, a product with an SPF value of 15 in theory allows the user to stay in the sun 15 times longer than usual without burning. Even though a product may have a high SPF value, factors such as sweating, swimming, scratching, and friction against clothing, towels, etc. causes sunscreen to wear off prematurely, leaving the user at risk of burning.

S

sunblock – *See sunscreen.*

sunburn – Irritation to the skin caused by exposure to ultraviolet radiation. Repeated sunburn accelerates the skin aging process and increases the risk of developing skin cancer.

sunscreen – An agent that is applied to the skin for the purpose of absorbing ultraviolet radiation and reducing the risk of sunburn. *Also see sun protective factor.*

sunstroke – Heatstroke caused by excessive exposure to the sun. *See heatstroke.*

super- – Prefix designating excess or above.

superficial – Pertaining to an injury or illness that is not deep or dangerous. For example, a superficial infection is an infection that has not spread beneath the surface of the skin.

superinfection – An opportunistic infection that occurs during treatment of another infection. For example, antibiotic treatment of a bacterial infection may allow yeast to grow uncontrolled and infect the mouth or vagina.

superior – Pertaining to the upper surface of an organ. For example, the superior aspect of the liver refers to the top portion of the liver.

Also, when two anatomic structures are located one above the other, the superior structure is the higher of the two.

Opposite of inferior.

supernatant – The fluid that remains after solid particles have settled out of a suspension; for example, the clear fluid that collects above the pink sediment in a bottle of calamine lotion.

superscription – The area on a prescription form beneath the patient's name and address that begins the body of the prescription itself. The superscription is usually designated by the symbol Rx.

supine – The position of the body in repose with the face and front of the body upward.

supp – Abbreviation for suppository.

S

supportive treatment – Therapy intended to relieve symptoms without necessarily treating the cause of the problem. By contrast, definitive treatment is therapy administered to treat a specific disorder. For example, an antibiotic is a definitive treatment for an infection, but aspirin, which only reduces pain and fever, is a supportive treatment.

suppository – A bullet-shaped or cylindrical dosage form intended to be inserted into a body orifice. Suppositories contain medication usually intended for local effect at the site of insertion, although some are intended for absorption into the systemic circulation. Suppositories maintain their shape and consistency at room temperature but melt or dissolve when inserted. The most common sites of administration for suppositories are the rectum, vagina, and urethra.

suppressant – An agent that diminishes the normal activity of a cell, organ, or tissue. For example, sedative drugs are central nervous system suppressants.

suppuration – The production of pus.

supra- – Prefix designating a position above the root word.

supraventricular – Positioned above the ventricle of the heart.

supraventricular arrhythmia – An abnormal heart rhythm that originates in the atrium, the heart chamber located above the ventricle.

surfactant – A chemical agent that attracts both water and lipid molecules, allowing them to be combined in a mixture. Surfactants are used as detergents, emulsifiers, and cleansers.

surgeon – A physician who specializes in diagnosing and treating illness by means of surgery. Surgeons may be general surgeons (operating on almost any part of the body) or may specialize in particular types of surgery. Examples of surgical specialists include thoracic surgeons (chest and heart surgery), neurosurgeons (brain and nerve tissue), and vascular surgeons (blood vessels).

surgery – The specialty of medicine that deals with diagnosis and treatment of disease by means of operations. Surgery may be a

S

complicated procedure lasting for hours and requiring general anesthesia or may be as simple as removing or repairing a small lesion under local anesthesia.

surgical – Pertaining to surgery.

suspension – A pharmaceutical preparation in which an insoluble drug, when shaken, is held up in a fluid long enough for a dose to be prepared. Special additives called suspending agents disperse the drug evenly throughout the fluid and slow the settling process. Examples include calamine lotion and most oral liquid antibiotics.

swab – A piece of cotton, gauze, or other absorbent material attached to the end of a stick. Swabs are used to clean material from the skin or to apply a medication to a specific area.

swallow – The natural process of passing any material from the mouth to the stomach.

swelling – Enlargement of a tissue usually due to fluid accumulation. Swelling may be the result of inflammation, allergy, trauma, or disease process.

sympath- – Prefix designating the sympathetic nervous system.

sympathetic nervous system (SNS) – The part of the autonomic nervous system that increases heart rate and constricts blood vessels by secreting hormones, primarily epinephrine and norepinephrine, that increase the force and frequency of contraction of muscles in these organs. The SNS initiates the so-called "fight or flight" response, preparing the body to react to emergencies.

sympatheto- – Prefix designating the sympathetic nervous system.

sympathico- – Prefix designating the sympathetic nervous system.

sympatho- – Prefix designating the sympathetic nervous system.

sympatholytic – An agent that blocks or inhibits the effects of epinephrine or norepinephrine on the cells that normally react to them. Some drugs used to treat hypertension are sympatholytic agents.

S

sympathomimetic – An agent that acts on tissues in the same way as epinephrine or norepinephrine. These drugs may be used to treat shock, cardiac arrest, asthma, nasal congestion, and other conditions.

symptom – A subjective, nonobservable manifestation of a medical condition. Symptoms can only be felt and reported by the person experiencing them. Examples of symptoms include nausea, pain, hallucinations, etc. In some cases, a symptom may be accompanied by one or more objective signs. For example, vomiting (objective sign) and nausea (subjective symptom), itching (subjective symptom) with a skin rash or scratch marks (objective signs). *Also see sign.*

symptomatic – Pertaining to a symptom. Normally used in the context of a characteristic of a disease. For example, lack of energy is symptomatic of iron deficiency anemia.

symptomatic treatment – Therapy that treats a manifestation of disease rather than the cause of the disease. For example, use of a nighttime sleeping medicine only treats the symptoms of insomnia, not its cause.

symptomatology – The spectrum of signs and symptoms associated with a specific disease. For example, the symptomatology of diabetes mellitus includes increased urination, increased hunger, and increased thirst.

syn- – Prefix designating a joining together.

synapse – The juncture between a nerve cell and either the muscle or other cell it controls or another nerve cell. At their synapses, nerves pass chemicals to their receptors that either stimulate or inhibit the receptor cell from acting.

syncope – A sudden drop in blood pressure that leads to fainting or the sensation of fainting. Syncope can be a sign of cardiovascular disease or a side effect of drug therapy, particularly therapy for hypertension.

syndrome – A pattern of signs and symptoms that result from a common cause and but are usually not characteristic of a specific disease. For examples, see Sjögren's syndrome and Reye's syndrome.

S

synergism – A combined action of two or more agents that produce an effect greater than would have been expected from the two agents acting separately. Some drug interactions exhibit synergism, which depending upon the circumstances may be beneficial or harmful. For example, the combination of the antibacterial drugs trimethoprim and sulfamethoxazole is more effective for treating infections than either drug acting alone. However, the combination of aspirin and the anticoagulant warfarin can act synergistically to reduce blood clotting to the extent of spontaneous hemorrhage if doses are not carefully monitored.

synergistic – Pertaining to synergism.

synovia – The viscous fluid inside joints that lubricates their movements.

synovitis – An inflammation of the membrane that surrounds joints and contains the synovia. Synovitis is common in arthritis.

synthesis – The process of chemically uniting simpler chemicals into a larger molecule. When synthesis occurs in a living system it is sometimes called biosynthesis.

synthetic – Pertaining to a chemical formed in a laboratory or factory rather than in a living system. For example, synthetic drugs are medications developed in a research laboratory rather than from a natural source.

syphilis – A sexually transmitted disease cause by the spirochete *Treponema pallidum*. Untreated syphilis can lead to heart disease, birth defects in pregnant women, and mental illness.

syphilitic – Pertaining to syphilis or a person who has syphilis.

syringe – A hollow cylinder used along with a hollow needle to inject drugs or other materials into a tissue or to extract materials (e.g., blood) from the body. Syringes intended for injecting drugs are available in a variety of sizes ranging from less than 1 milliliter to over 50 milliliters. These syringes are sterile and the cylinder or barrel of the syringe is marked to assist in measuring doses accurately.

S

syrup – A pharmaceutical dosage form that consists of a high concentration of a sugar, usually sucrose, in water. A wide variety of medications are added to syrups to make them taste better, particularly for children.

system – A group of interrelated organs that perform similar and complimentary functions. For example, the digestive system includes the mouth, esophagus, stomach, liver, pancreas, small intestine, large intestine, rectum, and anus. All of these organs assist in the digestion of food, absorption of nutrients, and elimination of food wastes. Other systems include the central nervous system, endocrine system, reproductive system, and skeletal system.

systemic – Pertaining to the entire organism in contrast to a local effect. For example a systemic drug is one that is distributed to and has the potential to affect the entire body.

systole – The point in the cardiac cycle when the heart muscle contracts, forcing blood out of the heart and into a blood vessel.

systolic – Pertaining to the time when the heart contracts.

systolic blood pressure – The higher number of a blood pressure reading. For example, a blood pressure reading of 120/80 indicates a systolic pressure of 120 and a diastolic pressure of 80. The systolic pressure represents the highest pressure the blood reaches, while the diastolic pressure is the lowest.

T

tab – *See tablet.*

tablespoon – A kitchen measure that equals 1/2 fluid ounce or approximately 15 milliliters.

tablespoonful – A common measure for medication intended to deliver 15 milliliters of medicine. "Tablespoons" commonly used as flatware may measure significantly more or less than 15 milliliters. Consequently, they should not be used to give doses of medicine because they can result in significant overdoses or underdoses. Whenever a "tablespoonful" of medication is to be given, it should be carefully measured in either an accurate kitchen measuring spoon or in a specially made measure available in most pharmacies.

tablet – A pharmaceutical preparation made by compressing the powdered form of a drug and bulk filling material under high pressure. While most tablets are cylindrically shaped, they may take any form. Caplets, for example, are tablets that are stamped into a capsule shape. Tablets may or may not have special coatings or colorings.

Most tablets are intended to be swallowed whole for dissolution and absorption from the gastrointestinal tract. Some special forms, however, are intended to be dissolved in the mouth, dissolved in water, inserted as suppositories, etc.

Tablets are commonly mistakenly called pills. Pills are actually an entirely different type of pharmaceutical preparation.

Also see pill.

tachy- – Prefix designating fast or rapid.

tachyarrhythmia – An abnormal heart rhythm accompanied by a heart rate over 100 beats per minute.

tachycardia – A heart rate over 100 beats per minute. Tachycardia may or may not be accompanied by irregular heart rhythms or other forms of heart disease such as heart failure. Tachycardia also occurs naturally during vigorous exercise.

tachyphylaxis – The quick emergence of resistance of a disease to a drug treatment. For example, patients with insomnia may devel-

T

op resistance to sleeping medications after only a few nights' use.

tachypnea – Abnormally rapid breathing. Tachypnea often develops during fever and with respiratory disease.

tactile – Pertaining to the sense of touch or the ability to perceive touch.

tag – A radioactive atom that is chemically or otherwise attached to a molecule. Tags are used in research and diagnostic procedures to trace the path of drugs, hormones, or other substances through the body. For example, in bone scans radioactive technetium is tagged to a drug that deposits in rapidly growing bone tissue. When given intravenously to a patient with a hairline fracture, the technetium-drug complex accumulates at the site of the fracture and the radioactivity from the technetium can be detected and measured.

talc – A chalky, powdered form of magnesium silicate. Talc may be applied to the skin as a drying agent or may be used in pharmaceutical preparations to provide bulk.

talcum – See *talc*.

tamper-resistant packaging – Special seals or wrappers applied to medicine bottles at the manufacturing plant. Anyone who tried to gain access to the medication in one of these contains must damage the packaging to do so. The purpose of tamper-resistant packaging is to warn consumers that the integrity of the container has been compromised and the contents may have been adulterated before purchase.

tap – To puncture a body structure in order to withdraw fluid. For example, a spinal tap is a procedure where a needle is inserted into the spinal column in order to draw off spinal fluid for laboratory examination.

tar – A thick, dark fluid formed by the chemically-induced deterioration of carbon-containing materials such as petroleum, coal, shale, and wood. Coal tar is applied topically in ointments or shampoos to treat some dermatologic conditions such as psoriasis and seborrheic dermatitis.

T

tardive – Late or late-developing.

tardive dyskinesia – A movement disorder that may occur with long-term use of some antipsychotic medications. Tardive dyskinesia is characterized by writhing and jerking movements that intensify when a patient with the disorder tries to engage in physical activity. Tardive dyskinesia may affect any skeletal muscle group including the tongue, mouth, arms, legs, and trunk. Ironically, signs of tardive dyskinesia usually worsen when the causative medication is discontinued. It may take months to years for tardive dyskinesia to resolve.

tartar – Hardened material that accumulates on teeth at or below the gum line. Tartar accumulation is slowed with regular oral hygiene.

TB – *See tuberculosis.*

TCA – *See tricyclic antidepressant.*

tea – An extraction made by passing hot water over organic material, particularly whole or ground leaves. The water dissolves water-soluble chemicals in the organic material. The water is then filtered and drunk. Many herbal remedies are prepared in this fashion.

tear – The lubricating fluid in the eyes. The purpose of tears is to protect the eyes from damage to membranes that would be caused by drying.

teaspoon – A measure equivalent to 1/6 of a fluid ounce or approximately 5 milliliters.

teaspoonful – A common measure for medication intended to deliver 5 milliliters of medicine. "Teaspoons" commonly used as flatware may measure significantly more or less than 5 milliliters. Consequently, they should not be used to give doses of medicine because they can result in significant overdoses or underdoses. Whenever a "teaspoonful" of medication is to be given, it should be carefully measured in either an accurate kitchen measuring spoon or in a specially made measure available in most pharmacies.

T

teething – The emergence of a new tooth through the gum line. Teething normally begins at about six months of age and continues to about 2 1/2 years. Teething is a painful experience for a child and is usually accompanied by crying, drooling, and irritability. The affected gum area is usually inflamed and tender to touch.

telemetry – The process of transmitting information via radio signals from one location to another. In a hospital, sensors attached to a patient can transmit information to monitors in the nurses' station, allowing nurses at any time to observe medical data such as heart rate, blood pressure, and electrocardiogram patterns.

telemetry unit – A hospital floor that monitors patients by means of telemetry.

temperature – The measure of heat associated with metabolism. While it may vary slightly from one person to another, the normal body temperature is 98.6° Fahrenheit or 37° Celsius.

temporal – Pertaining to time. For example, temporal association is one factor in determining whether a drug produced a certain therapeutic or adverse effect. In order for the drug to have caused the effect, it must have been taken or administered at a time (before the event) when it would be possible for the drug to have produced the effect.

Also, pertaining to the temple of the skull.

tender – Pain or discomfort felt when a diseased or injured part of the body is touched or compressed. A tender spot or lesion is usually not painful unless it is touched.

tenderness – The state of being tender.

tendinitis – *See tendonitis.*

tendo- – Prefix pertaining to tendon.

tendon – A tough, fibrous band of tissue that attaches one end of a muscle to a bone or other structure.

tendonitis – Inflammation of a tendon. Tendonitis can be extremely painful and may last for weeks or months. Tendonitis is usually

T

treated with rest, analgesics and/or anti-inflammatory drugs, and sometimes with physical therapy or surgery.

tenesmus – Repetitive, painful spasms of the anus or urinary bladder accompanied by feeling the need to defecate or urinate, even if the bowel and bladder are empty. Tenesmus may also cause straining with little or no passage of stool or urine.

teno- – Prefix pertaining to tendon.

tenosynovitis – Inflammation of a tendon and the membrane that covers it. Causes of tenosynovitis include infection, physical strain, calcium deposits, and arthritis.

tension headache – A dull pain affecting primarily the front of the head. Tension headaches are so named because they are usually caused by physical or emotional stress (tension) that contracts the muscles of the face, neck, and scalp.

tera- – Prefix designating a malformed structure.

teratogen – A drug, chemical, or other substance (e.g., rubella virus) that causes damage to a developing fetus. Although there are many exceptions, drugs are most likely to cause teratogenic effects during the first trimester of pregnancy. This is the time when many of the fetus's organs are forming and they are most vulnerable to toxic effects.

teratogenic – Pertaining to a teratogen or its effects.

teratology – The study of birth defects, particularly their causes, risk factors for developing them, and their classification.

terminal – An end. For example, a terminal nerve is the last nerve of a nerve fiber. A terminal disease is a condition that is expected to progress to death in a short time.

termination – The end of insurance coverage. The most common causes for termination include filing fraudulent claims, switching to another insurance company, death of the member, and failure to pay premiums. The member or the new insurance company are responsible for payment for any services received after termination.

T

termination date – The day an insurance policy goes out of effect.

tertiary care – The most sophisticated medical care treatment available, usually obtainable only at a medical school-affiliated hospital that has specialists with extensive expertise in diagnosis and treatment of difficult conditions. Examples of tertiary care include burn centers, transplant units, and neonatal intensive care units.

test – A method of examination. Tests include physical (e.g., palpation, knee reflexes), chemical (e.g., cholesterol levels, liver enzymes), and microscopic (e.g., blood cell counts, identification of bacteria).

testes – Plural of testis.

testis – The primary male reproductive organ. The testes are located in the scrotum. Their functions include development of sperm, production of semen, and secretion of testosterone.

testosterone – The primary male hormone. In men, testosterone is produced mainly in the testes and is secreted into the blood. In women, a small amount of testosterone is produced in the ovaries. During menopause, the ovaries lose the ability to produce both testosterone and estrogen. Both men and women produce a small amount of testosterone in the adrenal glands.

In men, testosterone is responsible for the development of male characteristics, including sexual maturity, libido, body hair, deepening of the voice, and skeletal muscle development.

Testosterone is considered to be an androgenic steroid. Some athletes abuse testosterone and its chemical derivatives because of the hormone's abilities to increase muscle mass and endurance. The United States Drug Enforcement Agency (DEA) classifies all androgenic steroids as controlled substances.

tetanus – A sustained, strenuous, involuntary muscle contraction caused by a rapid succession of nerve impulses. The impulses come so rapidly that the muscle does not have time to relax between them.

Also, a potentially fatal infectious disease caused by *Clostridum tetani*, an organism that secretes a toxic that causes uncontolled

T

muscle contractions. Tetanus can be prevented with immunization.

tetany – Intermittent cramps or muscle contractions. Tetany may affect the hands, face, or trunk. Causes of tetany include calcium deficiency and electrolyte imbalance.

tetracycline – A class of antibiotics that are useful in treating a wide variety of conditions including acne, Rocky Mountain spotted fever, and some forms of pneumonia and urinary tract infection.

thalassemia – A hereditary disorder of hemoglobin that causes anemia and smaller than normal red blood cells. In its most serious form, patients may require frequent blood transfusions with the risk of developing iron toxicity due to the death of erythrocytes and deposition of iron in body tissues.

therapeutic – Pertaining to the treatment or the results of treatment of a medical condition.

therapeutic abortion – The termination of a pregnancy by a physician when the physician determines that the health of the mother may be at risk or that the baby, if born, is likely to have serious birth defects.

therapeutic class – A group of drugs that has in common the ability to treat the same type of conditions. Examples include antihypertensive drugs, antiarrhythmics, antivirals, and laxatives.

therapeutic equivalent – A drug that has the same actions as another drug and in most cases, can be expected to have the same effects on the majority of patients. Managed care organizations (MCOs) often encourage the use of therapeutic equivalents as a cost saving measure. In these cases, someone from the MCO or a contracted agency contacts prescribers to request a change to a less expensive drug in the same drug class.

therapeutic nihilism – A disbelief in the effectiveness of any treatment intervention.

therapeutics – The area of health care concerned with the treatment of disease, as opposed to diagnostics, the area concerned with diagnosis of disease.

T

-therapeutics – Suffix designating a type of treatment. For example, pharmacotherapeutics is treatment with drugs.

therapeutic substitution – The practice of dispensing one chemically different drug for another. Therapeutic substitution requires the prescriber's authorization before the substitution can be made. Managed care organizations frequently initiate therapeutic substitution programs as a cost saving measure.

therapy – The treatment of disease or an abnormal state. Types of therapy include drug therapy (pharmacotherapy), surgery, psychotherapy, electroconvulsive therapy, radiation therapy, physical therapy, occupational therapy, and many others.

therm- – Prefix designating heat.

thermo- – Prefix designating heat.

thermometer – A device used to measure temperature. Glass thermometers intended for measuring body temperature are typically designed to be used either in the mouth or rectum. Battery powered digital thermometers are designed for use in the mouth or the ear canal.

thermoregulation – Temperature control. The primary site for thermoregulation in the body is the hypothalamus in the brain. If the body is overheating, the hypothalamus may cause sweating and dilation of blood vessels in the skin. Evaporation of sweat reduces heat in the body and dilation of blood vessels increases heat dissipation.

Conversely, if body temperature is too low, the hypothalamus may constrict blood vessels in the skin and initiate shivering. Blood vessel constriction reduces heat loss and shivering increases heat production.

Drugs may also augment or inhibit the actions of the hypothalamus. For example, when given during fever, aspirin reduces shivering and dilates cutaneous blood vessels. Some antipsychotic drugs, however, override the influence of the hypothalamus and may cause the body temperature to shift in the direction of environmental temperature, similar to a cold blooded animal.

T

thinking – The intellectual process that includes cognition, reasoning, problem solving, and memory.

third party administrator (TPA) – An independent person or corporation (the third party) that administers insurance benefits and claims for a self-insured company or group. The TPA provides administrative services for the client company. Services may include collecting premiums, processing claims, and managing routine clerical functions. The TPA does not underwrite risk or otherwise act as an insurance company.

third party payer – An organization or corporation that pays medical claims on behalf of the recipient of service. In pharmacy, such claims are transmitted from the pharmacy directly to the payer (e.g., Medicaid, Blue Cross, an HMO) and the payer reimburses the pharmacy for service. The patient is only responsible for making any applicable copayments.

thirst – The uncomfortable feeling in the mouth and throat that accompanies the desire to drink fluids. Thirst is a mechanism to prevent dehydration.

thixotropy – The property of some gels to become less viscous when shaken or stirred and then to go back to their previous form when agitation ends. Some nasal medication vehicles exhibit this property. These products liquefy when shaken in the bottle and stay in liquid form until they are sprayed into the nose. Once they are left standing in the nose, they thicken again and cling to the nasal mucosa. This allows the medication to stay in contact with irritated tissue longer than a traditional nasal spray.

thorac- – Prefix designating the chest.

thoracentesis – Insertion of a needle through the chest wall and into the pleural space surrounding a lung. Thoracentesis is used to drain fluids secreted from the lungs as the result of cancer, infection, or other lung disease.

thoracic – Pertaining to the thorax.

thoracico- – Prefix designating the chest.

thoraco- – Prefix designating the chest.

T

thoracotomy – Surgical incision into the chest.

thorax – The chest. The upper part of the trunk of the body. The thorax begins at the base of the neck and extends down to the diaphragm. The ribs shape and protect the thorax.

threatened abortion – A condition during some pregnancies where the mother experiences uterine cramps and vaginal bleeding, indicating that a miscarriage may be imminent.

threshold dose – The minimum amount of medication that is needed to produce an effect.

thrill – A vibration of the chest wall caused by a heart murmur. When present, thrills can be felt by placing a hand over the heart.

thromb- – Prefix designating a blood clot.

thrombi – Plural of thrombus.

thrombin – An enzyme in blood that converts fibrinogen to fibrin. Thrombin is necessary for blood to clot normally.

thrombo- – Prefix designating a blood clot.

thromboangiitis – Inflammation of the inside wall of a blood vessel along with the formation of a blood clot at the site.

thrombocyte – *See platelet.*

thrombocytopenia – A deficiency of platelets in circulating blood. Severe thrombocytopenia can allow spontaneous hemorrhaging. The most common cause of thrombocytopenia is cancer chemotherapy.

thrombolysis – The process of dissolving a blood clot.

thrombolytic agent – A drug that dissolves blood clots. Several medications are effective for clot dissolution when given immediately following heart attacks or strokes. If given soon enough, they restore blood flow to the affected area and limit tissue damage from thrombosis or embolization.

thrombophlebitis – Inflammation inside a vein along with the formation of a blood clot at the site. Thrombophlebitis is a dangerous situation since the thrombus can break away and lodge in a vital

T

organ. Thrombophlebitis is treated with anticoagulants and anti-inflammatory drugs.

thrombosis – The formation of a blood clot, usually along the wall of a blood vessel. Thrombosis reduces blood flow to the area normally supplied by the blood vessel.

thrombotic – Pertaining to thrombosis.

thrombus – A blood clot that forms in the cardiovascular system. Thrombi may form in a blood vessel or in a chamber of the heart. A thrombus that breaks away from its site of formation and floats through the bloodstream is called an embolus.

thrush – Yeast infection in the mouth caused by *Candida albicans*. Thrush most commonly occurs after a course of antibiotic treatment.

thyr- – Prefix designating the thyroid gland.

thyro- – Prefix designating the thyroid gland.

thyroid – A gland located in the neck. The thyroid gland weighs about one ounce and produces thyroid hormone, a biochemical that stimulates the body's rate of metabolism, rate and force of heart contractions, and increases muscle tone. Hypersecretion of thyroid hormone causes all of these functions to be dangerously accelerated. Deficiency of thyroid hormone causes lack of energy, weight gain, and fluid accumulation. Severe deficiency of thyroid hormone can be life-threatening.

thyroidectomy – The surgical removal of all or part of the thyroid gland.

thyroiditis – Inflammation of the thyroid gland. Causes of thyroiditis include infection, autoimmune disease, radiation poisoning, and cancer.

thyrotoxicosis – The medical condition caused by excessive amounts of thyroid hormone. The excess may be naturally produced or the result of overdose of thyroid hormone supplements.

TIA – *See transient ischemic attack.*

T

tic – A repetitive, uncontrollable spasm of a muscle or group of muscles. Tics may be the result of habit or a neurologic problem.

t.i.d. – Abbreviation commonly used on prescriptions for the Latin *ter in die*, meaning three times a day.

tincture (tr) – An alcoholic solution of a drug. In some cases, the solution may also contain water.

tinea – A fungal infection of the skin or skin-related structures. The location of the infection is usually indicated in the Latin name of the disorder. Also known as ringworm. Tinea is most commonly treated with topical antifungal medications but in some cases oral therapy may be necessary.

tinea barbae – A fungal infection of the bearded area of the face.

tinea capitis – A fungal infection of the scalp.

tinea corporis – A fungal infection of the trunk or any other part of the body.

tinea cruris – A fungal infection of the groin. Jock itch.

tinea manus – A fungal infection of the hand, usually the palm.

tinea pedis – A fungal infection of the foot. Athlete's foot.

tinea unguium – A fungal infection of the fingernails or toenails.

tinea versicolor – A fungal infection of the skin that causes brownish discoloration of infected areas. In sunlight these patches fail to tan, appearing as light colored areas in contrast to tanned skin.

tingling – A sensation of stinging, tickling, or prickling. Tingling may be caused by damage, pressure, or trauma to a nerve, exposure to cold, or emotions.

tinnitus – Uncontrollable ringing, buzzing, or whistling sound in the ear. Causes of tinnitus include nerve damage to the ear and drug toxicity.

tissue – A group of cells of identical or similar composition that act together to perform a specific function. Examples of tissues include bone, blood, cartilage, muscle, and nerve.

T

tissue plasminogen activator (TPA) – A substance that occurs naturally in the walls of blood vessels that helps to dissolve the clots that form during a bleeding episode. Large amounts of TPA are produced through genetic engineering processes. The drug is administered to patients experiencing myocardial infarctions, strokes, and pulmonary emboli in order to dissolve the clots that are causing these problems. TPA and similar drugs must be given as soon as possible after development of the condition, usually within a few hours, to prevent permanent damage to the affected areas. When given quickly enough, TPA can be a lifesaving treatment.

titration – The slow, methodical addition of a chemical to a solution or other medium until a desired change is effected. In pharmacy, dose titration is the gradual, systematic increase of dose of a medication until the patient either exhibits a desirable response or experiences undue side effects.

toco- – Prefix designating childbirth.

tocolytic – A drug that slows or stops labor contractions and childbirth. Tocolytics are used to try to stop premature labor and premature birth.

tolerance – The development of resistance to the effects of a drug such that doses must be continually raised in order to elicit the desired response. Tolerance is often experienced in relation to drugs of abuse. Cross-tolerance occurs when a person develops a resistance to all the drugs in a class.

tone – The tension or degree of firmness exhibited by a muscle or group of muscles.

tonic – A medication, usually containing alcohol, that is supposed to restore vitality and function to the body as a whole or to one or more specific organs, such as the heart, liver, intestines, etc. In the past, many tonics were quack remedies.

tonsil – Lymphoid tissue located in the throat. The tonsils facilitate formation of white blood cells and protect the body from infection by trapping bacteria before they reach the lungs.

T

tonsillitis – Inflammation of a tonsil, usually due to infection. Signs and symptoms include fever, difficulty swallowing, sore throat, and enlarged lymph nodes in the neck. Tonsillitis may or may not be due to streptococcal (strep) infection.

toothache – Acute pain in a tooth or gum due to decay or infection that reaches the nerve in the pulp of the tooth.

tophi – Plural form of tophus.

tophus – A deposition of uric acid in a joint or other tissue. Tophi often accompany gout.

topical – Pertaining to a drug that is applied to the surface of the body. For instance, topical anesthesia is the application to the skin of a drug that temporarily deadens nerve sensations. Topical anesthetics are most commonly used in aerosol, cream, or lotion form and may be used for conditions that include burns, insect bites, and itching.

torpid – Inactive, sluggish, lethargic.

torticollis – A neuromuscular disorder characterized by muscle contractions in the neck that cause the head to twist to one side with the chin pointed in the opposite direction. Torticollis may occur as a side effect of some antipsychotic medications.

total parenteral nutrition (TPN) – An intravenous feeding that supplies all of the nutrients necessary for life. *Also see parenteral nutrition.*

tourniquet – A constricting band applied to one or more limbs to restrict blood flow. Tourniquets may be used to treat arterial bleeding or to temporarily reduce blood return to the heart in conditions such as pulmonary edema.

tox- – Prefix designating poison.

toxemia of pregnancy – *See preeclampsia.*

toxi- – Prefix designating poison.

toxic – Pertaining to a poison or symptoms of poisoning.

toxicity – The state of being noxious or the degree of noxiousness.

T

toxico- – Prefix designating poison.

toxicologist – A person with an advanced degree in toxicology. A toxicologist may or may not be a pharmacist or physician.

toxicology – The basic science that deals with poisoning, particularly the effects of drugs or other chemicals on the intracellular function of tissues and organs.

toxic shock syndrome (TSS) – A rare but potentially fatal illness caused by certain strains of *Staphylococcus aureus* that secrete a unique toxin. The condition most commonly affects women who wear highly absorbent tampons for long intervals during their menstrual periods but has also occurred in men and infants. Signs and symptoms include fever, rash, inflammation of mucous membranes, and headache. The condition may progress to kidney failure, liver impairment, unstable blood pressure, mental confusion, and death. Treatment consists of intravenous fluids and other measures to support blood pressure.

toxin – A poison. A toxin may be a synthetic chemical or a chemical naturally produced in a plant or microorganism.

toxo- – Prefix designating poison.

toxoid – A toxin, usually one produced in a microorganism, that is specially treated to destroy its toxic properties and yet retain its antigenic properties. Toxoids are used as vaccines to prevent some infectious diseases (e.g., tetanus toxoid).

TPA – See *third party administrator.*

TPA – See *tissue plasminogen activator.*

TPN – See *total parenteral nutrition.*

TPR – Abbreviation for temperature, pulse, and respiration. Abbreviation for total peripheral resistance. See *peripheral resistance.*

tr – See *tincture.*

trace element – A chemical element that is needed in minute quantities for nutrition. Many of these are needed for proper function

T

of proteins or enzyme systems. Trace elements include chromium, copper, cobalt, iodine, selenium, and zinc.

trachea – The tubular structure in the neck through which air passes. The trachea is located between the nose and mouth and the lungs. The windpipe. The trachea is formed by a cartilage that protects it from trauma and prevents it from collapsing as air passes within.

tracheal – Pertaining to the trachea.

tranquilizer – A drug that acts on the central nervous system to reduce anxiety or emotional stress, ideally without altering other mental functions or causing sedation. Tranquilizers are often used to treat anxiety disorders.

trans- – Prefix designating across or over.

transdermal – Pertaining to passage through the skin. For example, transdermal patches are dosage forms that release minute amounts of drug at a consistent rate. As the drug is released from the patch it is absorbed into the skin and carried off by the capillary blood supply. Examples of drugs administered transdermally include nitroglycerin, estrogen, testosterone, and nicotine.

transfusion – The intravenous injection of blood taken from one person (donor) into another (recipient). Transfusions may consist of whole blood or any component of blood such as packed red cells, platelets, plasma, etc. Transfusions may be administered as a treatment for acute blood loss or to treat a disease that causes a deficiency of a blood component.

transient – Temporary, of short duration, or quickly passing.

transient ischemic attack (TIA) – A brief episode of insufficient blood flow to part of the brain. The most common causes of TIA are a partial blockage of a cerebral artery or a small embolus. Signs and symptoms may include visual disturbances, lightheadedness, dizziness, weakness, falling, loss of feeling in one or more extremities, and loss of consciousness.

transmission – Transfer or passage from one person to another or from one part of the body to another. For example, an infectious

T

disease such as influenza may be transmitted from an infected person to an uninfected person. An impulse may be transmitted from a nerve cell to a muscle fiber.

transplantation – The surgical transfer of a living body part from one person to another or from one part of a person's body to another (e.g., skin graft). Tissues or organs that may be transplanted from one person to another include corneas, livers, lungs, hearts, kidneys, bone, cartilage, blood vessels, and bone marrow. Transplantation often requires the use of drugs that suppress the immune system in order to prevent rejection.

transport – The movement of biological fluids and/or the substances dissolved in them across cell membranes.

traum- – Prefix designating injury.

trauma – Any physical or emotional injury caused by physical contact or harrowing experience. Physical trauma may be caused by surgery, falls, motor vehicle accidents, gunshots, drowning, suicide attempts, etc. Emotional trauma may be caused by witnessing or experiencing violent events such as war, murder, financial ruin, divorce, physical or emotional abuse, etc.

traumat- – Prefix designating injury.

traumatic – Pertaining to trauma.

traumato- – Prefix designating injury.

treatment – An intervention or procedure intended to improve symptoms of disease or other medical condition. *Also see therapy.*

tremor – An uncontrollable rhythmic shaking or trembling. Tremors may affect either the limbs or the trunk. Tremors may be of short duration or chronic. They may be caused by neuromuscular disease (e.g., Parkinson's disease), psychological conditions (e.g., anxiety), or by drug toxicity (e.g., caffeine).

trending – An analytical technique of examining current and past costs in order to forecast future expenses. For example, an insurer uses pharmacy claims information to try to determine the impact of drug costs on the plan for the coming year. Insurers use this information to adjust premiums from one year to the next.

tricho- – Prefix designating hair.

trichomoniasis – Any infection by a species of *Trichomonas*. Various *Trichomonas* species may infect the intestines or the mouth, but trichomoniasis is most commonly used in reference to genitourinary infections. In women, vaginal trichomoniasis causes inflammation, itching, burning, and a foul-smelling, discolored, watery discharge. Men may carry the infection but seldom have symptoms. If untreated during pregnancy, the infection may be passed to the baby during delivery. In order to eradicate the infection, all sexual partners must be treated simultaneously.

trichosis – Any disease that affects the hair or abnormal growth patterns of hair.

tricyclic antidepressant (TCA) – A group of drugs that are effective for treating depression. Major disadvantages of the TCAs are that they usually take as long as two weeks of daily use to exert their therapeutic effect, and they may cause a wide spectrum of side effects.

triglyceride – A chemical compound composed of a molecule of glycerol with three fatty acids attached. Excessive levels of triglyceride in the blood increases the risk of cardiovascular disease.

trimester – A three-month period. Most commonly used in the context of pregnancy. The term of pregnancy is normally divided into three trimesters of three months each. Although some drugs used by a pregnant woman can be dangerous to a fetus at any point of pregnancy, as a general rule, drugs are most likely to cause birth defects during the first trimester. This is the time when many of the fetus's organs are forming and they are most vulnerable to toxic effects.

trismus – A spasm of the muscles that control the jaw. Lockjaw. Trismus can occur as a result of infections in or around the mouth or with tetanus.

trituration – The process of grinding crystals or other particles into fine powders, often by using a mortar and pestle.

Also, a pharmaceutical technique for combining two or more powders to assure that all ingredients are uniformly mixed.

T

troche – A lozenge. A hard or semisolid dosage form containing a medication intended for local application in the mouth or throat. Typically, a troche is placed on the tongue or between the cheek and gum and left in place until it dissolves. The medications most commonly administered by means of troches include cough suppressants and treatments for sore throat.

tropical medicine – The branch of medicine that specializes in the diagnosis and treatment of disease indigenous to the areas within approximately 30° north and south of the equator.

trough – Low point. A term commonly used in pharmacy to describe the lowest point a drug blood level reaches between doses. Depending upon the drug involved, a low trough may be desirable or undesirable. In the case of aminoglycoside antibiotics for serious infections, blood level troughs must fall below a certain value in order to reduce the risk of side effects. In other cases, allowing a blood level to fall too low may allow symptoms of the illness to return. For example, low troughs of anticonvulsant medications in an epileptic may increase the risk of seizures.

TSS – *See toxic shock syndrome.*

tubal ligation – A surgical sterilization procedure where a woman's fallopian tubes are obstructed in order to prevent sperm from uniting with the woman's ovum.

tubercle – The typical lesion caused by *Myobacterium tuberculosis*, the organism that causes tuberculosis. Tubercles represent the body's attempt to wall off invading organisms before they can cause disease. Tubercles may range in size from 0.5 up to 3 millimeters. Healthy persons exposed to tuberculosis may form tubercles that last for a lifetime. Typically the disease stays dormant unless the immune system is compromised, allowing the organisms to break out of the tubercles.

tubercul- – Prefix designating tuberculosis.

tuberculo- – Prefix designating tuberculosis.

tuberculosis – An infection caused by *Myobacterium tuberculosis*. While tuberculosis most commonly affects the lungs, it can also invade any part of the body, including bone, the gastrointestinal tract,

T

and the kidneys. Tuberculosis lesions are characterized by death of affected tissue with sloughing of tissue and formation of cavities. General signs and symptoms include weakness, lack of energy, profuse sweating at night, and pain at the site of infection. In the lungs, the most common site of infection, signs and symptoms include coughing, coughing blood, and difficulty breathing. Treatment consists of a combination of drugs that must be taken consistently for months.

tubule – A small canal. For example, the renal (kidney) tubules cause urine to concentrate and then convey the urine to a collection point.

tumor – An abnormal growth of new tissue that forms itself into a mass. Tumors may be benign or malignant, invasive or localized.

Also, a swelling or enlargement of tissue.

tumor antigen – A protein produced by a tumor that the body's immune system recognizes as foreign. Future cancer treatments will identify tumor antigens and allow for vaccinations that will allow the immune system to selectively attack malignant tumors without affecting normal tissue.

tunnel – A passageway that is open at both ends. For example, the carpal tunnel is a channel through the bones of the wrist that the median nerve and flexor tendons pass through.

turbidity – Cloudiness in a normally clear liquid caused by insoluble particles, sediment, or by microorganisms. For example, turbidity in urine is often a sign of urinary tract infection or some other urinary tract disease.

turgid – Swollen, usually because of accumulation of fluid as in inflammation or congestion.

turgor – The normal tension of a cell or structure. For example, skin turgor is a function of the body's state of hydration. Excessively tight skin may be a sign of fluid accumulation, as occurs in heart failure. Poor skin turgor may be a sign of dehydration.

twitch – An involuntary muscle spasm.

T

tympanic membrane – The covering that separates the outer ear from the middle ear. The eardrum. The tympanic membrane transmits sounds from the external ear to the auditory structures of the middle and inner ear.

U – *See unit.*

U&C – *See usual, customary, and reasonable.*

UCR – *See usual, customary, and reasonable.*

ulcer – An erosion in a surface membrane caused by loss or destruction of tissue. Sites where ulcers may occur include the skin (e.g., decubitus ulcer), gastrointestinal tract (e.g., peptic ulcer), and mucous membranes (e.g., apthous ulcer).

ulcerate – To form or produce an ulcer.

ulceration – An ulcer or the process of forming an ulcer.

ulcerative – Pertaining to an ulcer.

ulcerative colitis – A chronic inflammation of a portion of the large intestine and rectum. Inflammation is accompanied by erosion of patches of the mucous membrane lining the interior of the structures. Signs and symptoms of ulcerative colitis include abdominal pain, diarrhea, rectal bleeding, intestinal abscesses, fever, and weight loss. The condition may cause metabolic problems including anemia, loss of protein, and electrolyte imbalance.

ultra- – Prefix designating beyond or above.

ultrasonic – Pertaining to sound waves beyond the range that can be heard by humans.

ultrasonogram – The image produced by ultrasonography. Ultrasonograms, also called sonograms, may be recorded on photographic film or electronic media.

ultrasonography – The process of examining structures within the body by the use of high frequency sound waves. Advantages of ultrasonography are that it does not involve radiation and that images can be immediately viewed on a monitor. Ultrasonography is commonly used to monitor fetal health during pregnancy and to diagnose problems in deep organs or tissues such as the gallbladder, urinary bladder, heart, lungs, and tumors.

ultrasound – High energy sound waves that are used in ultrasonography. Ultrasound waves have a frequency greater than 30,000 hertz.

ultraviolet radiation – Energy waves that range from the highest portion of the visible spectrum (violet) up to x-rays. Ultraviolet radiation is useful in the treatment of some skin disorders (e.g., psoriasis) and for the conversion of vitamin D in the skin to its active form. However, most of the effects of ultraviolet radiation are harmful. These include skin burning, skin aging, skin discoloration, and skin cancer.

UM – *See utilization management.*

umbilical cord – The flexible strand of tissue that connects the fetal umbilicus with the mother's placenta during pregnancy. The umbilical cord allows passage for all of the fetus's metabolic and nutritional needs.

umbilicus – The indentation or protrusion in the abdomen where the mother's placental cord joined the fetal abdomen during pregnancy. Colloquially called the belly button or navel.

un- – Prefix designating reversal or not.

uncompensated care – Services provided by health care professionals or institutions (e.g., hospitals) for which payment is not received. Uncompensated care may include *pro bono* care for indigent or uninsured patients or may be the result of bad credit extended to the patient.

unconsciousness – A state of dulled mental alertness in which the person is unaware of the environment and demonstrates limited response to external stimuli. Levels of unconsciousness range from normal sleep to coma.

unction – The act of rubbing or applying an ointment or oil.

unctuous – Greasy or oily.

underinsured – Pertaining to people who do not have adequate insurance to pay their health care expenses.

ung – An abbreviation for the Latin *unguentum*, meaning ointment.

unguent – Ointment.

uninsured – Pertaining to people who have no health care insurance at all.

unit – A standard of measurement based on the biological activity of a drug rather than its mass or weight. While most drugs are measured in milligrams or similar designations, some drugs' potencies vary significantly from batch to batch. Drugs from natural sources may also vary according to the source of the drug. For example, the activity of the anticoagulant heparin depends upon whether it is extracted from lung or intestinal tissue. Assigning a unit of activity value to these drugs assures dose-to-dose consistency. Examples of drugs that are measured in units include insulin, heparin, vitamin A, vitamin D, and vitamin E.

United States Pharmacopoeia (USP) – A reference book that contains the official standards for drug preparation and manufacture. The first American pharmacopoeial convention of physicians and pharmacists was held on January 1, 1820 for the purpose of initiating an authoritative national literature on pharmacy and medicine. The first edition of the USP was released on December 15, 1820. The first edition contained one section for "articles of decided reputation or general use" and a second section for "those the claims of which are of a more uncertain kind."

Today, the USP provides the guidelines that manufacturers must follow to assure drug potency and purity. The USP has merged with the *National Formulary* and the combined publication contains all official standards. *Also see* National Formulary.

unofficial – The designation for a drug that is not listed in either the *United States Pharmacopoeia* or the *National Formulary*.

unsaturated – Pertaining to an organic chemical that has at least one double or triple bond between carbon atoms. In this sense, an unsaturated compound does not have all of its potential binding sites saturated with other atoms, particularly hydrogen.

Also, a solution that is capable of dissolving more solute.

unsaturated fatty acid – A fatty acid that has at least one double or triple bond in its carbon chain. Some studies indicate that diets

U

that substitute unsaturated fatty acids in place of saturated fatty acids promote cardiovascular health. *Also see fatty acid.*

upper respiratory infection (URI) – A bacterial or viral infection of any of the structures of the upper respiratory tract. URIs include the common cold, influenza, sinusitis, laryngitis, and tonsillitis.

upper respiratory tract – The anatomical structures lying above the lungs that are involved in breathing. The upper respiratory tract includes the nose, sinuses, larynx, and trachea.

UR – *See utilization review.*

ure- – Prefix designating urine or urea.

urea – The primary form of nitrogen waste produced by humans. Urea is formed in the liver from ammonia that is liberated during protein metabolism. Urea itself is not harmful, but elevated levels of urea in the blood usually indicate that the kidneys are not clearing waste products effectively. Low levels of urea may indicate an inadequate dietary intake of protein, or liver disease.

urea- – Prefix designating urine or urea.

uremia – The presence of high levels of urea and/or ammonia in the blood.

uremic – Pertaining to uremia.

ureo- – Prefix designating urine or urea.

ureter – The tubular structure that conveys urine from the kidneys to the urinary bladder.

ureteral – Pertaining to the ureter.

urethra – The tubular structure that conveys urine from the urinary bladder and allows it to be discharged from the body. In adult females the urethra is less than 1 1/2 inches long. In males, it is approximately eight inches long. Because of their shorter urethras, women experience more urinary tract infections than men.

urethral – Pertaining to the urethra.

Also, a route of administration for specially formulated suppositories.

U

urethritis – An inflammation of the urethra. Urethritis is painful, especially when passing urine, and is most commonly caused by infection.

urgent care center – A medical facility where ambulatory patients can be evaluated and treated for nonemergency problems without an appointment. Urgent care centers may be located in a hospital separate from the emergency room or they may be free-standing in the community.

urgi-center – *See urgent care center.*

URI – *See upper respiratory infection.*

uri- – Prefix designating uric acid.

uric- – Prefix designating uric acid.

uric acid – A waste product produced during the metabolism of proteins. Uric acid is only slightly soluble in water and is normally eliminated in the urine. Excessive production of uric acid causes it to crystallize in the joints, initially in the joints of the toes. Accumulation of uric acid leads to gout and sometimes kidney failure.

urico- – Prefix designating uric acid.

uricosuria – The presence of excessive amounts of uric acid in urine.

uricosuric – A class of drugs that promotes the elimination of uric acid in urine. These drugs are used to treat gout.

urin- – Prefix designating urine.

urinalysis – A chemical and/or microscopic examination of the urine intended to detect the presence of pathogenic bacteria, blood cells, crystals, protein, glucose, or any other abnormalities.

urinary – Pertaining to urine.

urinary tract – The structures involved in the production and elimination of urine. The urinary tract includes the kidneys, ureters, urinary bladder, and urethra.

urinary tract infection (UTI) – An infection of any part of the urinary tract. Most urinary tract infections are caused by gram-negative

U

bacteria. Signs and symptoms include fever, pain especially on urination, and frequent urination.

urinate – The process of passing urine.

urine – The fluid waste produced by the kidneys. Urine is composed of water and dissolved metabolic waste materials.

urino- – Prefix designating urine.

urography – A radiologic examination of the urinary tract. Typically, a radiopaque dye is injected intravenously into the patient. X-rays are taken as the dye is eliminated in the urine. These films show any strictures or other deviation from normal structure of the urinary organs.

urologic – Pertaining to urology or the urinary tract.

urological – Pertaining to urology or the urinary tract.

urologist – A physician who specializes in urology.

urology – The specialty of medicine that deals with the diagnosis and treatment of diseases of the urinary tract. Urology also deals with conditions of the male reproductive system. In contrast to nephrology, urology is primarily a surgical specialty while nephrology is an internal medicine specialty.

uropathy – A disease of any part of the urinary tract.

urticaria – A skin eruption characterized by small, itchy bumps. Hives. Urticaria is most commonly part of an allergic reaction.

urticarial – Pertaining to urticaria.

USP – See *United States Pharmacopoeia*.

usual and customary (U&C) – See *usual, customary, and reasonable*.

usual, customary, and reasonable (UCR) – The fee a managed care organization is willing to pay to a health care provider based on the normal fees for the same service in the same geographic area.

ut dict – Abbreviation sometimes used on prescriptions for the Latin *ut dictum*, meaning as directed.

uter- – Prefix designating uterus.

uterine – Pertaining to the uterus.

utero- – Prefix designating uterus.

uterus – The female reproductive organ that holds, protects, and nourishes the fetus throughout pregnancy. The womb.

UTI – *See urinary tract infection.*

utilization – The frequency with which a particular benefit or health care service is used.

utilization management (UM) – The process of administering resources in order to meet the greatest need for service at the lowest cost. Utilization management uses programs such as utilization review and case management to review the necessity for costly services such as hospitalizations, emergency room visits, and specialist referrals and to determine where savings can be made. Utilization management is typically most successful when it is done with the cooperation of patients, employers, providers, and payers.

utilization review (UR) – A clinical quality improvement program and cost containment system that includes a formal assessment of the medical necessity, efficiency, and appropriateness of the health care services provided. Utilization review may be prospective, concurrent, and/or retrospective.

uveitis – Inflammation of the iris of the eye and related structures. Causes of uveitis include infection, allergy, and diabetes mellitus.

vaccinate – To give a vaccine, usually by injection.

vaccination – The act of giving a vaccine, usually by injection.

vaccine – A preparation of material derived from microorganisms administered for the purpose of conferring immunity to one or more infectious diseases. While most vaccines are administered by injection, a few are given orally (e.g., poliovirus vaccine) or by other means. Vaccines may be prepared from bacteria, viruses, or rickettsiae.

Vaccines may be composed of live, attenuated microorganisms, killed microorganisms, toxins extracted from microorganisms, or proteins or other substances extracted from microorganisms.

vagin- – Prefix designating the vagina.

vagina – The passageway, approximately four inches long, between the uterus and the vulva. The vagina is lined with a mucous membrane and serves as the birth canal during childbirth.

vaginal – Pertaining to the vagina.

Also, a route of administration for creams, suppositories, and other locally acting medications.

vaginitis – An inflammation, usually due to infection, of the mucous membrane of the vagina. Common causes of vaginitis include bacterial and yeast infections.

vagino- – Prefix designating the vagina.

vaginopathy – Any disease of the vagina.

vago- – Prefix designating the vagus nerve.

vagolytic – An agent that suppresses the activity of the vagus nerve.

vagus nerve – A major nerve originating in the cranium. The vagus has a wider distribution through the body than any other nerve of its type. The vagus affects functions in the pharynx, larynx, lungs, heart, esophagus, stomach, and intestines. The vagus influences speech, swallowing, heart rate, and digestive secretions.

valence – In chemistry, the number assigned to an element or ion to indicate its ability to share electrons with other elements or ions. Hydrogen, with a valence of one, is the standard for comparison.

value-added service – Extra assistance offered, often by a pharmaceutical manufacturer, to help a managed care plan provide better service or control costs. For example, a pharmaceutical manufacturer may offer to send the male members of an HMO literature and a screening questionnaire for prostate disease.

valve – A flap-like structure that prevents backflow of fluid. For example, the valves of the heart open to allow blood to be pumped forward during a heart contraction, but close to prevent regurgitation back into the chamber once it is empty. Damaged or diseased heart valves cause the blood turbulence that is heard as a murmur.

vapor – The gaseous form of any substance that is normally found in the solid or liquid state.

Also, a medication intended to be administered by inhalation.

vaporizer – A device that causes liquids and any medications dissolved in them to be discharged into the air as a fine mist or vapor. Typically, vaporizers turn water into steam and expel the steam into the air. The vaporized water and medication are inhaled by the patient, usually to treat a respiratory condition.

varicella – An infection of the varicella-zoster virus commonly known as chickenpox. Varicella is highly contagious and causes fever with a rash that turns into blisters. Infected blisters may cause permanent scars.

varicose vein – A contorted, bulging vein with defective valves. Because the valves do not function properly, blood is allowed to stagnate and pool in the veins. Varicose veins can occur in various parts of the body but most commonly occur in the legs.

variola – A highly contagious, often fatal, viral illness commonly known as smallpox. Because of extensive worldwide immunization programs, smallpox appears to have been eradicated.

vas- – Prefix designating a blood vessel.

vascular – Pertaining to one or more blood vessels.

vascular surgeon – A physician who specializes in performing surgical operations on blood vessels.

vasculitis – Inflammation of a blood vessel.

vasculo- – Prefix designating a blood vessel.

vasectomy – A male surgical sterilization procedure where the vas deferens is severed, prohibiting the passage of sperm.

vaso- – Prefix designating a blood vessel.

vasoactive – Pertaining to an agent that causes either vasoconstriction or vasodilation.

vasoconstriction – A narrowing of blood vessels that reduces blood flow. Vasoconstriction may occur naturally (e.g., to reduce heat loss in cold weather) or may be induced by drugs that raise blood pressure (e.g., treatment of shock).

vasoconstrictor – An agent that causes blood vessels to narrow, restricting blood flow and raising blood pressure in the affected area.

vasodilation – An increase in the size of blood vessels. Vasodilation increases blood flow through the affected area and may occur naturally (e.g., to dissipate heat in hot weather) or may be induced by drugs (e.g., treatment of angina pectoris, hypertension).

vasodilator – An agent that causes blood vessels to expand, increasing blood flow and lowering blood pressure in the affected area.

vasopressor – A drug or naturally occurring substance that causes vasoconstriction and raises blood pressure.

vasospasm – A sudden and uncontrollable contraction of the smooth muscles in the walls of one or more blood vessels.

VD – See *venereal disease*.

vector – An organism that harbors microorganisms that cause disease in organisms of a different species. A carrier. Vectors are usually arthropods (e.g., ticks, mites) or insects (e.g., mosquitoes, flies) that allow disease-causing microorganisms to live within them.

V

Bites from these vectors inject some of these microorganisms into the victim. Examples of diseases transmitted in this fashion include malaria, Rocky Mountain spotted fever, plague, and Lyme disease.

vehicle – A pharmacologically inert substance that provides a medium for the administration of a medication. The medication is mixed in or dissolved in the medium and then given to a patient. Examples of vehicles include syrups, elixirs, ointment bases, lotions, etc.

vein – A blood vessel that carries blood back to the heart. All veins except the pulmonary vein carry dark, oxygen-depleted blood. Veins are different from arteries in that veins are more numerous and hold a greater volume of blood. Veins also contain valves that prevent blood from flowing backward.

venereal – Pertaining to or associated with sexual intercourse.

venereal disease (VD) – *See sexually transmitted disease.*

venereal wart – *See condylomata acuminata.*

veni- – Prefix designating vein.

venipuncture – The intentional piercing of a vein for any purpose. The most common reasons for venipuncture are withdrawal of blood for a laboratory test or blood donation and administration of an intravenous medication or fluid.

veno- – Prefix designating vein.

venom – A poison secreted by animals such as snakes, spiders, and insects. Venom is injected into the victim by means of a bite or sting. Some venoms are universally toxic (e.g., rattlesnake), while others cause only local reactions for most people but can cause fatal allergic reactions for others (e.g., honeybee).

venomous – Pertaining to an animal that has poison-producing glands. Examples include rattlesnakes and black widow spiders.

venous – Pertaining to a vein or group of veins.

venous return – The blood that comes back to the heart by means of the venous side of the circulatory system.

ventilation – The movement of air in and out of the lungs. Ventilation may be the result of normal breathing or may be mechanically assisted for patients with respiratory conditions.

ventricle – A hollow chamber in the heart or brain. The ventricles of the brain secrete and store cerebrospinal fluid. The ventricles of the heart are responsible for ejecting blood out of the heart. The right heart ventricle pumps blood into the blood vessels of the lungs, where it is oxygenated. The left ventricle pumps blood into the general circulation for distribution to remote organs and tissues of the body.

ventricular arrhythmia – Any of several types of irregular heartbeats that originate in or affect one or both of the ventricles of the heart.

ventricular fibrillation – A series of disorganized electrical firings in the heart that result in unproductive twitching of the heart muscle instead of normal, forceful contraction. During ventricular fibrillation the heart is not capable of pumping blood. The condition is fatal if not treated immediately.

ventricular premature contractions – A type of ventricular arrhythmia where, instead of synchronizing contractions with the atria, the ventricles contract in an irregular pattern. Patients may report that they feel that their heart skips beats.

ventricular tachycardia – A type of ventricular arrhythmia where the ventricles accelerate the heart rate to a dangerous velocity. Ventricular tachycardia may precede ventricular fibrillation.

ventriculo- – Prefix designating a ventricle.

venule – A small blood vessel on the venous side of the circulatory system. Venules are the small blood vessels that make the transition from the capillaries to the larger veins.

vertebra – One of the small bone segments that constitute the spinal column. The human body has 33 vertebrae. The vertebrae hold the body erect and protect the spinal cord.

vertebrae – Plural of vertebra.

vertebral – Pertaining to one or more vertebrae.

V

vertebro- – Prefix designating a vertebra.

vertigo – A feeling of dizziness in which victims feel that they or their surroundings are spinning around. Causes of vertigo include middle ear disease and drug toxicity.

very low-density lipoprotein (VLDL) – A protein in circulating blood that consists of triglyceride along with small amounts of cholesterol. VLDL transports triglycerides from the liver to peripheral blood vessels for metabolic use. Excessive levels of VLDL are thought to contribute to heart disease by depositing too much triglyceride in the vascular spaces.

vesicant – An agent that causes blisters to develop.

vesicle – A raised sac of skin filled with fluid. A blister.

veterinarian – An individual who holds a doctor of veterinary medicine (D.V.M.) degree. Veterinarians specialize in the diagnosis, prevention, and treatment of disease in animals.

veterinary – Pertaining to animal health.

viable – Living or capable of living. Often used in the context of a fetus that has reached a gestational age (usually 24 weeks) that would allow it to survive outside of the uterus.

vial – A small glass or plastic bottle intended to hold medicine. Pharmacists dispense tablets and capsules in clean, nonsterile vials. Some injectable drugs are aseptically placed in sterile vials at the manufacturing plant.

viral – Pertaining to a virus.

viral shedding – The spread of a virus by an infected host. Viruses may be shed in any body fluid or secretion (e.g., saliva, blood, semen, stool) by any means that causes emission of those fluids (e.g., coughing, sneezing, bleeding, sexual intercourse).

virilization – The development of secondary male sexual characteristics in a woman. Male effects may include skeletal muscle development, deepening voice, and growth of body hair. Virilization may occur due to hormonal imbalance or treatment with male hormones.

virologist – An individual who specializes in the study of viruses. A virologist may or may not be a physician.

virology – The branch of science that studies viruses and viral diseases.

virucidal – Pertaining to the ability to kill viruses.

virucide – An agent that kills viruses either in a living organism or on inanimate surfaces.

virulence – The degree to which a microorganism is capable of causing disease. A highly virulent organism would be expected to cause disease in a high percentage of persons exposed to it while an organism with low virulence causes infection in a low percentage of exposed persons.

virulent – Capable of causing disease, usually an infectious disease.

virus – A minute organism not visible with an ordinary microscope. Viruses do not exist as cells. Instead, they are composed only of a single strand of nucleic acid with an enveloping protein sheath. Viruses are not capable of growing or reproducing on their own; they must invade another cell for these functions. Viruses cause human diseases as varied as the common cold, influenza, sore throat, measles, AIDS, and smallpox. Over 200 viruses have been found to cause disease in humans.

viscera – Plural of viscus.

viscosity – Thickness or stickiness. The resistance of a fluid to flow. In a biologic fluid, viscosity is caused by the attraction of molecules or cells to each other.

viscous – Sticky, gummy.

viscus – Any internal organ contained within a cavity such as the chest and abdomen. Examples include the stomach, heart, liver, and gallbladder.

vision – The ability to see light and external forms and objects.

vision care – The portion of a health insurance policy that provides coverage for eye examinations and corrective lenses.

vital – Pertaining to life.

vital signs – The physical indications of life. Vital signs are usually considered to be body temperature, pulse rate, respiratory rate, and blood pressure.

vitamin – One of a group of organic substances that are essential for life but are not naturally produced in the body. Vitamins must be obtained from the diet or by means of supplements. Vitamins are normally considered to be either soluble in oil or soluble in water. The oil-soluble vitamins include vitamins A, D, E, and K. The water-soluble vitamins include the B vitamins and vitamin C.

vitamin supplement – A commercial product that provides vitamins intended to complement the diet. Vitamin supplements are typically available as tablets, capsules, and oral liquids. Vitamin supplements are particularly valuable for persons who are on weight loss diets and those who do not or cannot eat balanced meals.

vitiligo – A skin condition characterized by patches that lack pigmentation surrounded by normally pigmented skin. Vitiligo patches can be large and disfiguring, especially in those with dark skin tone.

vitreous humor – The semisolid fluid behind the iris of the eye. The vitreous humor gives the eye its firmness and shape.

VLDL – *See very low-density lipoprotein.*

vocal – Pertaining to the voice.

voice – The sound made as air passes through the larynx and vocal cords. The sounds pass through the mouth and include talking and singing.

volatile – Pertaining to a material that turns into vapor form easily (e.g., alcohol, acetone, gasoline).

voluntary – Pertaining to willful control. Not automatic.

voluntary muscle – Any muscle that can be controlled and moved by free choice. Skeletal muscles (e.g., muscles controlling movement of the arms and legs) are voluntary muscles.

V

vomit – To explosively expel stomach material through the mouth. Causes of vomiting include illness, emotional stress, and drug toxicity.

Also, the material expelled from the stomach.

vomitus – The material expelled from the stomach during vomiting.

vulgaris – The common type. Ordinary. For example, acne vulgaris is the typical form of acne.

vulva – The external female genitalia. The vulva includes the labia, clitoris, and vaginal opening.

vulvar – Pertaining to the vulva.

vulvitis – An inflammation of the vulva.

vulvo- – Prefix designating the vulva.

vulvovaginal – Pertaining to both the vulva and the vagina.

vulvovaginitis – An inflammation, usually due to infection, of the mucous membrane of the both the vulva and the vagina. Common causes of vulvovaginitis include bacterial and yeast infections.

v/v – Abbreviation for a volume to volume solution or mixture. The proportion of the volume of a solute per volume of the resulting solution. For example, a 10% v/v solution of alcohol in water indicates a proportion of 1 milliliter of alcohol for every 10 milliliters of the total solution.

v/w – Abbreviation for a volume to weight solution or mixture. The proportion of the volume of a substance per unit of mass of the total mixture. For example, a 10% v/w solution of alcohol in water indicates a proportion of 1 milliliter of alcohol for every 10 grams of the resulting solution.

WAC – *See wholesale acquisition cost.*

wafer – A pharmaceutical dosage form that uses a thin film of flour paste to envelop a powdered form of a drug. The purpose of the wafer is to allow the patient to swallow the drug without tasting it.

Also, a flat vaginal suppository.

waiting period – The time between starting employment and the beginning of health insurance benefits. Depending upon the company, there may be no waiting period (e.g., immediate eligibility) or the waiting period may be as long as several months.

wart – A defined elevation of skin with a rough surface caused by a local virus. Warts most commonly appear on the hands, face, neck, and knees. Genital warts are contagious.

wash – An irrigating solution (e.g., eyewash, mouthwash). Washes may or may not contain medications.

wasting – The loss of excessive body weight due to starvation or disease. Emaciation.

water – In pharmacy, a mixture of distilled water with an aromatic volatile oil. Waters may be used for medicinal purposes or as fragrances. Examples include peppermint water and rose water.

WBC – *See white blood cell.*

wean – To discontinue breastfeeding a baby. The weaning process requires the baby to adjust to new forms of nutrition and for the mother to stop secretion of milk. Medications are available that suppress milk production for those women who experience undue breast discomfort during this time.

wellness program – A plan that promotes healthy lifestyles among participants. Wellness programs typically seek to increase participants' awareness of health issues and assist them in changing unhealthy behaviors. Topics for wellness programs may include preventing osteoporosis, identifying prostate disease, increasing exercise, losing weight, or stopping smoking.

welt – *See wheal.*

W

wheal – An intensely itchy skin eruption larger than a hive. Wheals may be red, are rounded on top, and may expand or contract with time. Causes of wheals include allergic reactions and insect bites (e.g., mosquito).

wheeze – An abnormal whistling lung sound made during breathing, especially during expiration. Wheezing is commonly associated with asthma.

whey – The liquid portion of milk after it is separated from its casein (curd) component. Both casein and whey are sources of protein.

white blood cell (WBC) – A leukocyte. White blood cells are an important part of the body's defense against infection. Some WBCs phagocytize bacteria while others produce immune globulins. Five types of white blood cells circulate in human blood: neutrophils, basophils, eosinophils, lymphocytes, and monocytes.

Neutrophils, basophils, and eosinophils are called granulocytes because they all contain granules in their cytoplasm. The agranulocytes (no granules in the cytoplasm) are the lymphocytes and monocytes.

whitehead – *See comedo.*

wholesale acquisition cost (WAC) – The price a wholesale drug company charges a pharmacy for a drug. The WAC includes the price the manufacturer charges plus the wholesaler's handling fee.

windburn – Reddening of the face and other exposed areas due to irritation caused by wind exposure.

withdrawal syndrome – A pattern of physical changes that occur when a drug is abruptly discontinued or withheld from an addicted person. The various addicting drugs (e.g., narcotics, alcohol, cocaine) cause their own characteristic withdrawal syndromes.

withhold fund – The portion of the money owed to physicians that a managed care organization may hold back until the end of the year as an incentive to provide cost effective care. Physicians whose costs of care exceed local norms may lose their withhold fund.

womb – *See uterus.*

workers' compensation – A federally mandated system designed to pay medical expenses for work-related injuries. Under the system, employers pay into a pool that assumes the cost of medical treatment and wage losses arising from a worker's job-related injury or disease, regardless of who is at fault. In return, employees give up the right to sue their employers.

work-up – The process of establishing a diagnosis by performing a total evaluation of the patient. Components of the work-up may include physical examination, medical history, laboratory tests, and x-rays.

wound – Trauma to any part of the body. Wounds may be caused by accidental acts (e.g., motor vehicle accident), violence (e.g., gunshot), or may be intentional (e.g., surgical incision).

w/v – Abbreviation for a weight to volume mixture or solution. The proportion of the weight or mass of a substance per unit of volume of the total mixture. For example, a 10% w/v solution of sugar in water indicates a proportion of 1 gram of sugar for every 100 milliliters of the total solution.

w/w – Abbreviation for a weight to weight mixture or solution. The proportion of the weight or mass of a substance per weight or mass of the total mixture. For example, a 1% w/w mixture of hydrocortisone in a petrolatum ointment base indicates a proportion of 1 gram of hydrocortisone for every 100 grams of the total mixture.

xanth- – Prefix designating yellow.

xanthine derivative – A group of drugs chemically related to caffeine that dilate bronchioles in the lungs. Xanthines are most often used to treat asthma.

xantho- – Prefix designating yellow.

xanthoma – A flat, slightly elevated, yellowish patch of skin, usually on the eyelids. Xanthomas are often composed of cholesterol deposits.

xanthosis – A yellowish discoloration of the skin caused by destruction of tissue, often from cancer.

Also, a yellowish discoloration of the skin caused by excessive ingestion of foods with yellow pigments (e.g., carrots, squash). This form of xanthosis is usually harmless.

xenograft – The surgical transplantation of an organ tissue from one species to another. For example, skin from pigs is sometimes temporarily grafted to humans who have suffered extensive burns.

xero- – Prefix designating dry.

xeroderma – A dermatologic condition characterized by rough, dry skin.

xerosis – Excessive dryness of the skin, mucous membranes, or eyes.

xerostomia – Excessive dryness of the mouth. Causes of xerostomia include dehydration, radiation to the mouth, cancer chemotherapy, or side effects from other drugs.

x-ray – A high-energy form of radiation just above the ultraviolet range. X-rays are commonly used to diagnose and evaluate fractures and diseases of internal structures.

yeast – A general term for a type of single-celled fungus that reproduces by budding. Some yeasts ferment carbohydrates, forming alcohol. Others (e.g., *Candida albicans*) are capable of causing clinical infection, especially in the mouth, damp skin folds, and vagina.

Z

zone of inhibition – The clear area that appears around an antibiotic disc in an antibiotic sensitivity test. Once a specific bacterium has been determined to be the cause of a clinical infection, the laboratory usually tries to determine which antibiotics it is most likely to respond to. One of the techniques used is to grow the bacteria on a petri dish along with antibiotic impregnated discs. An area that is free of bacteria (zone of inhibition) surrounds the antibiotics that inhibit growth of the bacteria. The size of the zone of inhibition is a rough indication of the degree of sensitivity to the antibiotic.

zoonosis – An infectious disease that infected animals can transmit to humans under natural conditions (e.g., rabies).

zoster – *See herpes zoster.*

zygote – An ovum fertilized by a sperm.

Appendix A

Pharmaceutical Manufacturers

3M Pharmaceutical
3M Center
Building 275-3W-01
St. Paul, MN 55133
651-736-4930
800-328-0255

Abbott Laboratories
100 Abbott Park Rd.
Abbott Park, IL 60064-3500
800-633-9110
www.abbott.com

Adria Laboratories
See Pharmacia & Upjohn

A. H. Robins, Inc.
See Whitehall-Robins Healthcare

Akorn, Inc.
2500 Millbrook Dr.
Buffalo Grove, IL 60089
800-535-7155
www.akorn.com

Alcon Laboratories, Inc.
6201 S. Freeway
Ft. Worth, TX 76134
800-757-9195
www.alconlabs.com

Allen & Hanburys
See Glaxo Wellcome

Allergan, Inc.
2525 DuPont Dr.
P.O. Box 19534
Irvine, CA 92715-9534
714-246-4500
800-347-4500
www.allergan.com

Allermed Laboratories, Inc.
7203 Convoy Ct.
San Diego, CA 92111
858-292-1060
800-221-2748
www.allermed.com

Alpharma USPD, Inc.
7205 Windsor Blvd.
Baltimore, MD 21244
800-638-9096
www.alpharmauspd.com

Alpha Therapeutic Corp.
5555 Valley Blvd.
Los Angeles, CA 90032
323-225-2221
800-421-0008

Almay, Inc.
1501 Williamsboro St.
P.O. Box 6111
Oxford, NC 27565
800-473-8566

Alza Corp.
1900 Charleston Rd.
Mt. View, CA 94039
650-564-5000
800-634-8977
www.alza.com

American Dermal Corp.
See *Rhone-Poulenc Rorer*

American Home Products
See *Whitehall-Robins Healthcare*
www.ahp.com

American Red Cross
1616 N. Ft. Myers Dr.
Arlington, VA 22209
800-446-8883
www.redcross.org/plasma

Amgen Inc.
Amgen Center
Thousand Oaks, CA 91320
805-447-1000
800-772-6436
www.amgen.com

Apothecon, Inc.
Div. of Bristol-Myers Squibb
P.O. Box 4500
Princeton, NJ 08543-4500
609-897-2000
800-321-1335
www.apothecon.com

Applied Biotech, Inc.
10237 Flanders Ct.
San Diego, CA 92121
858-587-6771

Applied Genetics
205 Buffalo Ave.
Freeport, NY 11520
516-868-9026

Applied Medical Research
308 15th Ave. N.
Nashville, TN 37203
615-327-0676

Ascent Pediatrics, Inc.
187 Ballardvale St., Suite B125
Wilmington, MA 01887
978-658-2500
www.ascentpediatrics.com

AstraZeneca LP
50 Otis St.
Westborough, MA 01581
508-366-1100
800-237-8898
www.astrazeneca-us.com

AstraZeneca LP
725 Chesterbrook Blvd.
Wayne, PA 19087
610-695-1000
800-237-8898
www.astrazeneca-us.com

AstraZeneca Pharmaceuticals LP
1800 Concord Pike
P.O. Box 15437
Wilmington, DE 19850
302-886-3000
800-456-3669
www.astrazeneca-us.com

AutoImmune, Inc.
128 Spring St.
Lexington, MA 02173
781-860-0710
www.autoimmune.com

Aventis Behring
1020 First Ave.
King of Prussia, PA 19406
610-878-4000
800-504-5434
www.aventisbehring.com

Aventis Pasteur, Inc.
Discovery Dr.
Swiftwater, PA 18370-0187
570-839-7187
800-822-2463
www.aventispasteur.com/usa

Aventis Pharmaceuticals
399 Interpace Parkway
Parsippany, NJ 07054
973-394-6000
www.aventispharma-us.com

Baker Norton Pharmaceuticals
4400 Biscayne Blvd.
Miami, FL 33137
800-735-2315
www.ivax.com

Barr Laboratories, Inc.
2 Quaker Rd.
Pomona, NY 01970
914-362-1100
800-222-0190
www.barrlabs.com

Bausch & Lomb North American
Vision Care
1400 N. Goodman St.
P.O. Box 450
Rochester, NY 14692-0450
716-338-6000
800-553-5340
www.bausch.com

Bausch & Lomb
Pharmaceuticals
8500 Hidden River Pkwy.
Tampa, FL 33637
813-975-7770
800-323-0000
www.bausch.com

Baxa Corporation
13760 Arapahoe Rd.
Englewood, CO 80112
800-525-9567
www.baxa.com

Baxter Healthcare
One Baxter Parkway
Deerfield, IL 60015
847-948-4770
800-422-9837
www.baxter.com

Baxter Hyland Immuno
550 N. Brand Blvd.
Glendale, CA 91203
818-956-3200
800-423-2862
www.baxter.com

Bayer Allergy Products
See Bayer Pharmaceutical
Divison
www.bayerus.com

Bayer Consumer Care Division
36 Columbia Rd.
P.O. Box 1910
Morristown, NJ 07962-1910
973-254-5000
800-331-4536
www.bayerus.com/consumer/
index.html

Bayer Diagnostics
914-631-8000
www.bayerus.com/diagnostics/
index.html

Bayer Pharmaceutical Division
400 Morgan Lane
West Haven, CT 06516
203-812-2000
800-288-8371

B. Braun Medical
P.O. Box 19791
Irvine, CA 92713-9791
949-660-2000
800-227-2862
www.bbraunusa.com

Becton Dickinson & Co.
1 Becton Dr.
Franklin Lakes, NJ 07417
201-847-6800
888-237-2762
www.bd.com

Becton Dickinson Biosciences
2350 Qume Drive
San Jose, CA 95131
410-316-4000
800-638-8663
www.bdbiosciences.com

Beiersdorf, Inc.
360 Martin Luther King Dr.
S. Norwalk, CT 06856-5529
203-854-8000
800-233-2340
www.beiersdorf.com

Berlex Laboratories, Inc.
300 Fairfield Rd.
Wayne, NJ 07470
888-237-5394
www.berlex.com

Biogen
14 Cambridge Center
Cambridge, MA 02142
617-679-2000
800-262-4363
www.biogen.com

BioGenex Laboratories
4600 Norris Canyon Rd.
San Ramon, CA 94583
925-275-0550
800-421-4149
www.biogenex.com

Biomerica, Inc.
1533 Monrovia Ave.
Newport Beach, CA 92663
949-645-2111
800-854-3002
www.biomerica.com

Biomira USA, Inc.
1002 East Park Blvd.
Cranbury, NJ 08512
609-655-5300
www.biomira.com

Bio-Technology General Corp.
70 Wood Ave. S.
Iselin, NJ 08830
732-632-8800
www.btgc.com

Block Drug Co., Inc.
257 Cornelison Ave.
Jersey City, NJ 07302
201-434-3000
800-365-6500
www.blockdrug.com

Bock Pharmacal Co.
See Eli Lilly

Boehringer Ingelheim
Pharmaceuticals, Inc.
P.O. Box 368
900 Ridgebury Rd.
Ridgefield, CT 06877-0368
203-798-9988
800-542-6257
www.boehringer-ingelheim.com

Boehringer Mannheim
See Roche

Boots Pharmaceuticals, Inc.
See Knoll Laboratories

Braintree Laboratories, Inc.
P.O. Box 850929
Braintree, MA 02185-0929
781-843-2202
800-874-6756
www.braintreelabs.com

Bristol-Myers Squibb Company
Pharmaceuticals Group
Princeton House
905 Herrontown Rd.
Princeton, NJ 08540
800-321-1335
www.bms.com

Burroughs Wellcome Co.
See GlaxoWellcome

Cambridge NeuroScience
One Kendall Square
Building 700
Cambridge, MA 02139
617-225-0600

Carnrick Laboratories
65 Horse Hill Rd.
Cedar Knolls, NJ 07927
973-267-2670
www.elancorp.com

Carter-Wallace, Inc.
www.carterwallace.com

C. B. Fleet, Inc.
4615 Murray Place
Lynchburg, VA 24502
804-528-4000
800-999-9711

Celgene Corp.
P.O. Box 4914
7 Powder Horn Dr.
Warren, NJ 07059
732-271-1001
800-890-4619
www.celgene.com

Celltech Medeva
755 Jefferson Rd.
Rochester, NY 14623-0000
800-932-1950

Centeon
See Aventis Behring

Centers for Disease Control and
Prevention
1600 Clifton Rd. N.E.
Atlanta, GA 30333
404-639-7290
800-311-3435
www.cdc.gov

Centocor, Inc.
200 Great Valley Pkwy.
Malvern, PA 19355
610-651-6000
888-874-3083
www.centocor.com

Cephalon, Inc.
145 Brandywine Pkwy.
West Chester, PA 19380
610-344-0200
800-896-5855
www.cephalon.com

Cerenex Pharmaceuticals
See GlaxoWellcome

Chiron Corporation
4560 Horton St.
Emeryville, CA 94608
510-655-8730
800-244-7668

Ciba-Geigy Pharmaceuticals
See Novartis

Ciba Vision Corporation
11460 Johns Creek Pkwy.
Duluth, GA 30097
800-845-6585
www.cibavision.com

Clintec Nutrition
1 Baxter Pkwy.
Deerfield, IL 60015
847-948-2000
800-422-2751
www.baxter.com

CNS Inc.
4400 West 78th St.
Minneapolis, MN 55435
612-820-6696
800-441-0417
www.cns.com

CoCensys, Inc.
213 Technology Dr.
Irvine, CA 92618
949-753-6100
www.cocensys.com

Collagen Aesthetics
1850 Embarcadero Rd.
Palo Alto, CA 94303
800-722-2007
www.collagen.com

CollaGenex Pharmaceuticals,
Inc.
41 University Dr., Suite 200
Newtown, PA 18940
215-579-7388
888-339-5678
www.collagenex.com

Connaught Labs
See Pasteur-Mérieux-Connaught

ConvaTec
Div. of Bristol-Myers Squibb
P.O. Box 5254
Princeton, NJ 08543-5254
800-422-8811
www.convatec.com

CooperVision
200 Willowbrook Office Park
Fairport, NY 14450
949-597-8130
800-538-7850
www.coopervision.com

COR Therapeutics, Inc.
256 E. Grand Ave.
S. San Francisco, CA 94080
650-244-6800
888-267-4633
www.corr.com

Corixa
1124 Columbia St., Suite 200
Seattle, WA 98104
206-754-5711
www.corixa.com

C. R. Bard
8195 Industrial Blvd.
Covington, GA 30014
770-784-6100
800-526-4455
www.crbard.com

Cutter Biologicals
See Bayer Corp. (Biological and Pharmaceutical Div.)

Cynacon/OCuSOFT
5311 Ave. N
P.O. Box 429
Richmond, TX 77406-0429
281-342-3350
800-233-5469
www.ocusoft.com

Cytel Corp.
5820 Nancy Ridge Dr.
San Diego, CA 92121
858-860-2500
www.cytelcorp.com

Cytogen Corporation
600 College Rd. East
Princeton, NJ 08540
609-987-8200
800-833-3533
www.cytogen.com

Cytosol Laboratories
55 Messina Dr.
Braintree, MA 02184
800-288-3858

Derma Science
1065 Highway 315, Suite 403
Wilkes Barre, PA 18702
570-824-3605
800-825-4325
www.dermasciences.com

Dermik Laboratories, Inc.
See Arcola

Dista Products Co.
See Eli Lilly

DuPont Pharmaceuticals Co.
P.O. Box 80705
Wilmington, DE 19807
302-992-5000
800-474-2762
www.dupontpharma.com

E. Fougera Co.
60 Baylis Rd.
Melville, NY 11747
516-454-6996
800-645-9833

Elan Pharmaceuticals
800 Gateway Blvd.
S. San Francisco, CA 94080
650-877-0900
800-537-8899
www.elanpharma.com

Elan Research Co.
1300 Gould Dr.
Gainsville, GA 30504
770-538-6360

Eli Lilly and Co.
Lilly Corp. Center
Indianapolis, IN 46285
317-276-2000
800-545-5979
www.elililly.com

Elkins-Sinn, Inc.
See Wyeth-Ayerst

Endo Pharmaceuticals, Inc.
223 Wilmington Westchester
Pike
Chadds Ford, PA 19317
800-462-3636
www.endo.com

Enzon, Inc.
20 Kingsbridge Rd.
Piscataway, NJ 08854-3998
732-980-4500
www.enzon.com

E. R. Squibb & Sons, Inc.
See Bristol-Myers Squibb

ESI Lederle Generics
P.O. Box 8299
Philadelphia, PA 19101-8299
610-688-4400
www.ahp.com

Fisons Corp.
See Celltech Medeva Pharmaceuticals

Forest Pharmaceuticals, Inc.
13600 Shoreline Dr.
St. Louis, MO 63045
314-493-7000
800-678-1605
www.forestpharm.com

Freeda Vitamins, Inc.
36 E. 41st St.
New York, NY 10017-6203
212-685-4980
800-777-3737

Fujisawa USA, Inc.
3 Parkway N. Center
Deerfield, IL 60015-2548
847-317-8800
800-888-7704
800-727-7003
www.fujisawa.com

Galderma Laboratories, Inc.
P.O. Box 331329
Ft. Worth, TX 76163
817-263-2600
800-582-8225

Geigy Pharmaceuticals
See Novartis

Genentech, Inc.
1 DNA Way
S. San Francisco, CA 94080
650-225-1000
800-626-3553
www.gene.com

Genetic Therapy, Inc.
938 Clopper Rd.
Gaithersburg, MD 20878
301-590-2626

Genetics Institute
35 Cambridge Park Dr.
Cambridge, MA 02140
617-503-7332

Geneva Pharmaceuticals, Inc.
2599 W. Midway Blvd.
P.O. Box 469
Broomfield, CO 80038-0469
800-525-8747
800-622-9191
www.genevarx.com

Genzyme Corp.
One Kendall Square, Building 1400
Cambridge, MA 02139
617-252-7500
800-326-7002
www.genzyme.com

Glaxo Wellcome, Inc.
5 Moore Dr.
Research Triangle Park, NC 27709
919-248-2100
800-437-0992
www.glaxowellcome.co.uk

Greenstone
Div. of Pharmacia & Upjohn
Moors Bridge Rd.
Portage, MI 49002
800-447-3360

Hemotec Medical Products, Inc.
P.O. Box 19255
Johnston, RI 02919
401-934-2571

Henry Schein, Inc.
135 Duryea Rd.
Mail Route 150
Melville, NY 11747
516-843-5500
800-472-4346

Herald Pharmacal Inc.
See Allergan, Inc.

Herbert Laboratories
See Allergan, Inc.

Hoechst-Marion Roussel
Div. of Aventis
10236 Marion Park Dr.
P.O. Box 9627
Kansas City, MO 64134-0627
816-966-5000
800-362-7466
www.hmri.com

Hollister-Stier
See Bayer Corp. (Allergy Div.)

Hyland Immuno
Div. of Baxter
550 N. Brand Blvd.
Glendale, CA 91203
818-956-3200
800-423-2090
http://baxdb1.baxter.com

Hyland Therapeutics
See Baxter Hyland

ICI Pharmaceuticals
See Zeneca Pharmaceuticals

ICN Pharmaceuticals, Inc.
3300 Hyland Ave.
Costa Mesa, CA 92626
714-545-0100
800-556-1937
www.icnpharm.com

Immunex Corp.
51 University St.
Seattle, WA 98101
206-587-0430
800-IMMUNEX
www.immunex.com

Immuno Therapeutics
2135 N. Lakeshore Dr.
Moorhead, MN 27514
701-239-3775

Immuno U.S., Inc.
Div. of Baxter
1200 Parkdale Rd.
Rochester, MI 48307-1744
248-652-4760
www.baxter.com

Immunobiology Research Inst.
Route 22 East
P.O. Box 999
Annandale, NJ 08801-0999
908-730-1700

ImmunoGen
148 Sidney St.
Cambridge, MA 02139
617-497-1113

Immunomedics
300 American Rd.
Morris Plains, NJ 07950
973-605-8200
www.immunomedics.com

Interferon Sciences
783 Jersey Ave.
New Brunswick, NJ 08901
732-249-3250
888-728-4372
www.interferonsciences.com

Interneuron Pharmaceuticals,
Inc.
1 Ledgemont Center
99 Hayden Ave.
Lexington, MA 02421
781-861-8444
www.interneuron.com

IVAX Corporation
4400 Biscayne Blvd.
Miami, FL 33137
305-575-6000
www.ivax.com

Janssen Pharmaceutical, Inc.
P.O. Box 200
Titusville, NJ 08560-0200
609-730-2000
800-526-7736
www.us.janssen.com

Johnson & Johnson Medical
P.O. Box 90130
Arlington, TX 76004-0130
800-423-5850
www.jnjmedical.com

Jones Pharma, Inc.
P.O. Box 46903
St. Louis, MO 63146-6903
314-576-6100
800-525-8466
www.jmedpharma.com

KabiVitrum, Inc.
See Pharmacia & Upjohn

Kendall Health Care Products
15 Hampshire St.
Mansfield, MA 02048
800-962-9888
www.kendallhq.com

Kendall-McGaw Labs, Inc.
See B. Braun Medical

Key Pharmaceuticals
See Schering-Plough

Knoll Pharmaceuticals
3000 Continental Dr. N.
Mt. Olive, NJ 07828-1234
973-426-2600
800-526-0221
www.basf.com

Kremers Urban
9428 Baymeadows Rd., Suite
250
Jacksonville, FL 32256
800-625-5710

K.V. Pharmaceutical Co.
2503 S. Hanley Rd.
St. Louis, MO 63144
314-645-6600

Lederle Professional Medical
Services
Div. of Wyeth-Ayerst
401 N. Middletown Rd.
Pearl River, NY 10965-1299
914-732-5000
800-999-9384

Leeming
See Pfizer US Pharmaceutical Group

Lilly and Co.
(Eli Lilly and Co.)
Lilly Corp. Center
Indianapolis, IN 46285
317-276-2000
800-545-5979
www.elililly.com

Liposome Co.
One Research Way
Princeton, NJ 08540
609-452-7060
www.liposome.com

Mallinckrodt-Baker
222 Red School Lane
Phillipsburg, NJ 08865
908-859-2151
www.mallinckrodt.com

Mallinckrodt Chemical
16305 Swingley Ridge Dr.
Chesterfield, MO 63017
314-654-2000
800-325-8888
www.mallinckrodt.com

Mallinckrodt Medical, Inc.
675 McDonnell Blvd.
P.O. Box 5840
St. Louis, MO 63134
314-654-2000
888-744-1414
www.mallinckrodt.com

McGaw, Inc.
See B. Braun Medical
www.bbraunusa.com

Mead Johnson Laboratories
See Bristol-Myers Squibb

Mead Johnson Nutritionals
Div. of Bristol-Myers Squibb
2400 W. Lloyd Expressway
Evansville, IN 47721
812-429-5000
www.meadjohnson.com

Mead Johnson Oncology
See Bristol-Myers Oncology

Medeva Pharmaceuticals
See Celltech Medeva

MedImmune, Inc.
35 W. Watkins Mill Rd.
Gaithersburg, MD 20878
301-417-0770
800-934-7426
www.medimmune.com

Merck & Co.
P.O. Box 4
West Point, PA 19486
800-672-6372
www.merck.com

Merieux Institute, Inc.
See Pasteur-Mérieux-Connaught

Miles, Inc.
See Bayer Corp.

MSD
See Merck & Co.

Nephron Pharmaceuticals Corp.
4121 34th St.
Orlando, FL 32811
407-246-1389
800-443-4313
www.nephronpharm.com

NeuroGenesis, Inc.
2045 Space Park Dr., Suite 132
Houston, TX 77058
281-333-2153
800-862-5033
www.neurogenesis.com

Neutrogena Corp.
5760 W. 96th St.
Los Angeles, CA 90045-5595
800-421-6857
www.neutrogena.com

Neutron Technology Corp.
877 Main Street, Suite 402
Boise, ID 83702
208-345-3460
www.neutrontechnology.com

Norcliff Thayer
See SmithKline Beecham Consumer Healthcare

Novartis Consumer Health
560 Morris Ave., Bldg. F
Summit, NJ 07901
908-598-7600
800-452-0051
www.us.novartis.com

Novartis Nutrition
5100 Gamble Dr.
St. Louis Park, MN 55416
612-925-2100
800-999-9978
www.us.novartis.com

Novartis Pharmaceuticals Corp.
59 Route 10
East Hanover, NJ 07936
973-781-8300
888-669-6682
www.us.novartis.com

Novo Nordisk Pharmaceuticals, Inc.
100 Overlook Center
Princeton, NJ 08540
800-727-6500
www.novo-nordisk.com

Novopharm USA, Inc.
165 E. Commerce Dr.
Schaumburg, IL 60173-5326
847-882-4200
800-426-0769
www.novopharmusa.com

Nycomed Amersham
101 Carnegie Center
Princeton, NJ 08540-6231
609-514-6000
www.nycomed-amersham.com

Organon, Inc.
375 Mt. Pleasant Ave.
West Orange, NJ 07052
973-325-4500
800-241-8812
www.organoninc.com

Ortho Biotech, Inc.
Route 202 S.
P.O. Box 670
Raritan, NJ 08869-0670
800-325-7504
www.procrit.com

Ortho-McNeil Pharmaceutical
Route 202
P.O. Box 600
Raritan, NJ 08869-0600
908-218-6000
800-682-6532
www.ortho-mcneil.com

Parke-Davis
See Pfizer US Pharmaceutical Group

Pasteur-Mérieux-Connaught Labs
See Aventis Pasteur, Inc.
www.aventispasteur.com/usa

Pfipharmecs
See Pfizer US Pharmaceutical Group

Pfizer Consumer Health
235 E. 42nd St.
New York, NY 10017
212-573-5656
800-332-1240
www.pfizer.com

Pfizer US Pharmaceutical Group
235 E. 42nd St.
New York, NY 10017-5755
800-438-1985

Pharmacia & Upjohn
100 Route 206 N.
Peapack, NJ 07977
908-901-8000
888-768-5501
www.pnu.com

Plough, Inc.
See Schering-Plough Health Care
Products

Princeton Pharmaceutical
Products
See Bristol-Myers Squibb

Procter & Gamble Co.
1 Procter & Gamble Plaza
Cincinnati, OH 45202
513-983-1100
800-543-7270
www.pg.com

Procter & Gamble
Pharmaceutical
P.O. Box 231
Norwich, NY 13815-0191
607-335-3321
800-448-4878
www.pg.com

Purdue Pharma
100 Connecticut Ave.
Norwalk, CT 06856
203-853-0123
800-877-5666
www.pharma.com

Rhone-Poulenc Rorer
Consumer, Inc.
See Aventis

Rhone-Poulenc Rorer
Pharmaceuticals, Inc.
See Aventis

Richardson-Vicks, Inc.
See Procter & Gamble Co.

R.I.D., Inc.
609 N. Mednik Ave.
Los Angeles, CA 90022-1320
323-268-0635

A.H. Robins, Inc.
See Wyeth-Ayerst

Roche Pharmaceuticals
340 Kingsland St.
Nutley, NJ 07110-1199
973-235-5000
800-526-6367
www.rocheusa.com

Roerig
See Pfizer US Pharmaceutical Group

Ross Laboratories
Div. of Abbott Laboratories
23480 Aurora Rd.
Bedford, OH 44146
440-232-7676
www.abbott.com

Roxane Laboratories, Inc.
P.O. Box 16532
Columbus, OH 43216-6532
614-276-4000
800-848-0120
www.roxane.com

Sandoz Consumer
See Novartis

Sandoz Nutrition Corp.
See Novartis

Sandoz Pharmaceuticals
See Novartis

Schering-Plough Corp.
2000 Galloping Hill Rd.
Kenilworth, NJ 07033-0530
908-298-4000
800-526-4099
www.sch-plough.com

Schering-Plough Health Care
Products
110 Allen Rd.
Liberty Corner, NJ 07938
908-604-1995
800-842-4090
www.sphcp.com

Schiapparelli Searle
See SCS Pharmaceuticals

Schwarz Pharma
6140 W. Executive Dr.
Mequon, WI 53092
800-558-5114
www.schwarzusa.com

SCS Pharmaceuticals
P.O. Box 5110
Chicago, IL 60680
800-323-1603
www.monsanto.com

Searle
Box 5110
Chicago, IL 60680-5110
847-982-7000
www.searlehealthnet.com

Serono Laboratories, Inc.
100 Longwater Circle
Norwell, MA 02061
781-982-9000
800-283-8088

Sherwood Medical
See Kendall Health Care

SmithKline Beecham
Pharmaceuticals
1 Franklin Plaza
P.O. Box 7929
Philadelphia, PA 19101
215-751-4000
800-366-8900
www.sb.com

Solvay Pharmaceuticals
901 Sawyer Rd.
Marietta, GA 30062-2224
770-578-9000
800-354-0026
www.solvay.com

Stuart Pharmaceuticals
See Zeneca Pharmaceuticals

Synergen, Inc.
See Amgen

Syntex Laboratories
See Roche

Tap Pharmaceuticals
2355 Waukegan Rd.
Deerfield, IL 60015
800-621-1020
800-348-2779
www.tapholdings.com

Teva Pharmaceuticals USA
151 Donorah Dr.
Montgomeryville, PA 18936
888-838-2872
www.tevapharmusa.com

Thompson Medical Co.
777 S. Flagler
West Palm Beach, FL 33401
561-820-9900

Upjohn Co.
See Pharmacia & Upjohn

Upsher-Smith Labs, Inc.
14905 23rd Ave. N.
Minneapolis, MN 55447-4709
800-328-3344
www.upsher-smith.com

Wallace Laboratories
Div. of Carter Wallace
Half Acre Rd.
Cranbury, NJ 08512
609-655-6000
www.astelin.com

Wampole Laboratories
Half Acre Rd.
P.O. Box 1001
Cranbury, NJ 08512-0181
800-257-9525
www.wampolelabs.com

Warner Chilcott Laboratories
100 Enterprise Dr., Suite 280
Rockaway, NJ 07866
800-521-8813

Warner Lambert
See Pfizer US Pharmaceutical Group

Westwood Squibb
Pharmaceuticals
Div. of Bristol-Myer Squibb
100 Forest Ave.
Buffalo, NY 14213
800-333-0950

Whitehall-Robins Healthcare
Division of American Home
Products
5 Giralda Farms
Madison, NJ 07940-0871
800-322-3129
www.whitehallrobins.com

Wyeth-Ayerst
P.O. Box 8299
Philadelphia, PA 19101
610-688-4400
800-934-5556
www.ahp.com/wyeth

Zeneca Pharmaceuticals
See AstraZenecaPharmaceuticals LP
www.astrazeneca.com

Zenith Goldline
Pharmaceuticals
4400 Biscayne Blvd.
Miami, FL 33137
800-327-4114
www.zenithgoldline.com

Appendix B

Pharmacy-Related Web Sites

Neither the author nor the publisher guarantees the accuracy of health information on any Internet site. Nor do they endorse one site in preference to another.

Pharmacy Associations

www.aacp.org
American Association of Colleges of Pharmacy (AACP)

www.accp.com
American College of Clinical Pharmacy (ACCP)

www.amcp.org
Academy of Managed Care Pharmacy (AMCP)

www.aphanet.org
American Pharmaceutical Association (APhA)

www.ascp.com
American Society of Consultant Pharmacists (ASCP)

www.ashp.org
American Society of Health-System Pharmacists (ASHP)

www.iacprx.org/
International Academy of Compounding Pharmacists (IACP)

www.lowwwe.com/tippsa/index.html
Technical Industrial Pharmacists and Pharmaceutical Scientists Association

www.members.aol.com/naep/naep.htm
National Association of Employee Pharmacists (NAEP)

www.nabp.net
National Association of Boards of Pharmacy (NABP)

www.nabp.net/vipps/intro.aps
Verified Internet Pharmacy Practice Sites (VIPPS)

www.nacds.org National Association of Chain Drug Stores (NACDS)

www.ncpanet.org
National Community
Pharmacists Association
(NCPA/NARD)

www.nwda.org
National Wholesale Druggists'
Association

www.pcmanet.org
Pharmaceutical Care
Management Association
(PCMA)

www.pharmacoepi.org/
International Society for
Pharmacoepidemiology (ISPE)

www.phrma.org
Pharmaceutical Research and
Manufacturers of America
(PhRMA)

www.sidp.org
Society for Infectious Diseases
Pharmacists (SIDP)

www.ualberta.ca/~csps/
Canadian Society for
Pharmaceutical Sciences (CSPS)

Government—U.S.

www.ahcpr.gov
Agency for Healthcare Research
and Quality (AHRQ)

www.cdc.gov
Centers for Disease Control
(CDC)

www.dhhs.gov
Department of Health and
Human Services (DHHS)

www.fda.gov
Food and Drug Administration
(FDA)

www.fda.gov/medwatch/
index.html
MedWatch medical product
defect reporting program

www.nih.gov
National Institutes of Health
(NIH)

www.nlm.nih.gov
National Library of Medicine

Health Information for Consumers
Most of these sites include drug
information for consumers.

http://accenthealth.com
Accenthealth

http://clinicaltrials.gov
Current information about clinical research studies

http://cpmcnet.columbia.edu/
texts/guide/
Complete Home Medical Guide

http://drkoop.com/
Dr. Koop

http://health.msn.com
MSN Health

http://medlineplus.gov/
National Library of Medicine

http://yourhealthdaily.com/
Your Health Daily

www.cancerpage.com
Specific information on cancer

www.healthanswers.com
HealthAnswers

www.healthscout.com
HealthScout

www.healthtouch.com
Healthtouch Online

www.intelihealth.com
From Harvard Medical School

www.mayohealth.org
Mayo Clinic Health Oasis

www.medicinenet.com
MedicineNet.com

www.msnbc.com/news/HEALTH
_Front.asp
MSNBC health page

www.onhealth.com
Onhealth

www.thriveonline.com
ThriveOnline

www.vh.org
Virtual Hospital

www.webmd.com
WebMD

www.wellweb.com
WellnessWeb

www.yourhealth.com
YourHealth.com

www3.healthgate.com
HealthGate

**Health Information for
Professionals**

http://hazard.com/msds MSDS
Index

http://odp.od.nih.gov/ods/
databases/ibids.html
International Bibliographic
Information on Dietary
Supplements (IBIDS)

http://resistanceweb.mfhs.edu/
cit/Index.asp
Analysis of antibiotic resistance
patterns

http://sun2.lib.uci.edu/HSG/
Pharmacy.html
Martindale's Health Science
Guide

http://text.nlm.nih.gov
Links to AHCPR Guidelines

http://views.vcu.edu/dimlist
Links to primary care resources

http://wonder.cdc.gov
CDC Wonder

www.citeline.com/C1SE/search
Data search

www.drugdiscoveryonline.com
Internet community for professionals

www.drugfacts.com
Drug information portal

www.freemedicaljournals.com
Full text medical journals

www.geocities.com/WallStreet/
6589/index.html
Pharmaceutical representatives
home page

www.incadinc.com
FDA and European Union
Regulatory Information

www.medmatrix.org
Hundreds of physician-reviewed
links

www.medscape.com/
Medical news and literature
searching

www.merck.com/pubs/mmanual
Merck Manual full text

www.pharmaceuticalonline.com
Community for pharmaceutical
manufacturing professionals

www.pharmulary.com
Pharmacy professionals site

www.pharmweb.net
Collection of pharmacy-related
links

www.pslgroup.com
iMD

www.rphlink.com/rphlink3.html
Links for pharmacists

www.usp.org
United States Pharmacopoeia

Internet Pharmacies
Prescriptions filled and shipped
via the Internet

www.cvs.com
CVSPharmacy

www.drugemporium.com
DrugEmporium.com

www.drugstore.com
Drugstore.com

www.healthcentralrx.com
HealthCentral.com

www.orderdrug.com
OrderDrug.com

www.planetrx.com
PlanetRx.com

www.riteaid.com
Rite Aid Corporation

www.rx.com
Rx.com

Natural Product Information and Sources

www.botanical.com
Botanical.com

www.dietsite.com
Dietsite.com

www.enutrition.com
Enutrition

www.gnc.com
GNC.com

www.healthshop.com
Healthshop.com

www.herbnet.com
Everything Herbal

www.mothernature.com
MotherNature.com

www.vitamins.com
Vitamins.com

www.vitaminshoppe.com
VitaminShoppe.com

www.vitaminsplus.com
Vitaminsplus.com

Health Fakes and Frauds

www.ftc.gov/bcp/conline/pubs/
health/frdheal.htm
Fraudulent health claims

www.hcrc.org
Healthcare Reality Check

www.ncrhi.org
National Council for Reliable
Health Information

www.phys.com/b_nutrition/
02solutions/10tufts/may98/
herbs.html
Herbal Myths

www.quackwatch.com
Guide to health frauds

Pharmaceutical/Managed Care Consulting Services

http://home.att.net/~Sonya.
MCPS
Managed Care Pharmacy
Solutions

www.adpharmconcepts.com
Advanced Pharmacy Concepts

www.cpspharm.com
Comprehensive Pharmacy
Services

www.grogancommunications.
com
Patient education material
development

www.ipcinc.org
Independent Pharmaceutical
Consultants

www.msi21.com
Management Solutions Institute

www.pharmacyinnovations.com
Pharmacy Innovations